Families:
Intergenerational
and Generational Connections

The *Marriage & Family Review* series:

Families: Intergenerational and Generational Connections

Susan K. Pfeifer
Marvin B. Sussman
Editors

The Haworth Press
New York • London

1991

Families: Intergenerational and Generational Connections has also been published as *Marriage & Family Review*, Volume 16, Numbers 1/2/3/4 1991.

The Haworth Press, Inc. 10 Alice Street, Binghamton, NY 13904-1580
EUROSPAN/Haworth, 3 Henrietta Street, London WC2E 8LU England

Library of Congress Cataloging-in-Publication Data

Families : intergenerational and generational connections / Susan K. Pfeifer, Marvin B. Sussman, editors.
    p. cm.
    Published as Marriage & family review, v. 16, no. 1/2/3/4 1991.
    ISBN 0-86656-864-6 (alk. paper)
    1. Family—United States. 2. Intergenerational relations—United States. I. Pfeifer, Susan K. II. Sussman, Marvin B.
HQ536.F3338   1991
306.87—dc20
                    91-6838
                    CIP

Families: Intergenerational and Generational Connections

CONTENTS

GENERATIONAL AND INTERGENERATIONAL CONNECTIONS WITHIN THE FAMILY AND THE COMMUNITY

ABOUT THE EDITORS

Susan K. Pfeifer, PhD, is Program Development/Planning Specialist with the State of Delaware in the Department of Health and Social Services, Division of Alcoholism, Drug Abuse and Mental Health. She is a member of the Gerontological Society of America, the National Council of Family Relations, and Omicron Nu. She also serves on the Board of Associate Editors for *Marriage & Family Review*. Dr. Pfeifer's area of specialization is intergenerational relations.

Marvin B. Sussman, PhD, is UNIDEL Professor of Human Behavior Emeritus at the College of Human Resources, University of Delaware. A member of many professional organizations, he was awarded the 1980 Ernest W. Burgess Award of the National Council on Family Relations. In 1983, he was elected to the prestigious academy of Groves for scholarly contributions to the field, as well as awarded a life-long membership for services to the Groves Conference on Marriage and the Family in 1984. Dr. Sussman received the Distinguished Family Scholar Award of the Society for the Study of Social Problems in 1985.

THEORETICAL
AND CONCEPTUAL
PERSPECTIVES

Reflections on Intergenerational and Kin Connections

Marvin B. Sussman

Intergenerational connections and interpersonal relationships, especially in the later years of life and the life cycle, is a "hot" issue for study by social scientists. It is so much in the forefront as an area for research that in the last few years innumerable conferences have been held on this theme, e.g., the Gerontological Society of America, November, 1990. Also U.S. Government agencies such as the Administration on Aging and the National Institute on Aging have issued calls for proposals on intergenerational phenomena with the promise of adequate funding for the winning applications.

Why, one may ask, is this largely unheralded issue gaining increasing attention not only from researchers but from governmental legislators, administrators, and policy makers? To begin the explanation I will take a step back into history. In part, it is my own history.

Intergenerational relations can best be understood within the context of social structures and modernization theories in vogue since the beginning of the twentieth century. The essential idea was that the family had to and did change from a multi-generational unit to a nuclear form. A large- became a small-sized unit, best suited to meet the normative demands of an emergent complex, occupationally differentiated, urban society. The economy based on the technology of the interchangeable part viewed labor as a commodity to be fitted into the industrial process. Hence, labor, vis-à-vis, small-size families were most suited for movement from one place of work to another. Thus, "the long arm of the job," as noted by Robert Lynd, going to the place where work could be found, characterized this new industrial age. The ease for small- compared to large-size families to move and the higher cost of housing and other amenities in urban contrasted to rural societies was believed to favor the nuclear family of procreation. This family consisted of husband and wife, usually the latter being the homemaker, and former, the breadwinner, living with their issue in a dwelling unit apart from either set of parents.

The ideology of twentieth century political, social, and economic systems embraced achievement and opportunity. Advancement in any of society's social systems would be based on merit. Large family and kin units with their endemic filial responsibilities were viewed as too demanding and cumbersome in the struggle for upward social and economic status. Individuation over group, smallness over largeness, became manifest in belief and practice. The large-size family, multi-generational and with bilateral kin or extended kin groups as units of being and analysis, were relegated to the museum of ancient history.

Another notion exacerbating the philosophy of the modernization of the family was the increasing dependence of the family on institutions and organizations usually large in size and bureaucratic in structure. W.F. Ogburn's classic analysis of the changing functions of the family, how other institutions, e.g., schools and factories, took over traditional family functions added to this dependency notion. Portrayed was the helplessness of the family, living in isolation and bereft of relationships and exchanges of help, and care with kin family members.

In review, the social and political theorists of the first half of this century postulated that the family was shorn of its functions or at best shared them with large scale systems, e.g., socialization of children with the schools. This was a consequence of industrialization, occupational specialization, and urbanization. Dependency upon the economic system determined where individuals would work and live, a readiness and expectation to move became part of the cultural baggage of the "new" family. The consequences, it was believed, resulted in a weak, isolated, fractured, and dependent family system.

An opportunity arose to challenge this mind set of family diminution in size and importance in modern, complex societies. The result was a doctoral dissertation I completed at Yale University in 1951, entitled, "Intergenerational Continuity: A Study of Factors

which Affect Relations between Families at Generational Levels."
Serendipity played a role in selecting this topic for research. A proposal to study group formation and interaction of ethnic adolescents
in New Haven, Connecticut was rejected for being too psychological in theory and substance. A paragraph in Reuben Hall's and Wil-
lard Waller's family text indicated that family connections, generational ties and supports remained largely unstudied. I took up the
challenge in the 1950-1951 study. Intensive interviews were conducted with parents of 97 middle-class, white, protestant families
whose children had married and left home. One hundred ninety-five
parent-child relationships comprised the final sample. The findings
indicated

> . . . the continuity of intergenerational family relationships
> tends to increase when marriage partners share similarity of
> background, observe the traditional conventions regarding
> courtship and the marriage ceremony, have been raised to be
> family-minded and self reliant, continue in moderation a pat-
> tern of economic help and service with their parents, and live
> in the same or nearby community as the elders. (Sussman,
> 1951)

Subsequent studies and reviews of intergenerational relationships
established their viability as units of activity and family continuity
(Sussman, 1953; Sussman & Burchinal, 1963; Litwak & Szelenyi,
1969; Farber, 1973; Schneider, 1980; Sweetser, 1963; Troll et al.,
1979). Throughout the decades of the 60s and 70s, a plethora of
research sustained the view that family members did not sever connections with their children, parents, or kin in their new urban environments. While there was a reduction in the number of generations
living within a household, the structural properties of kinships were
evident. Most individuals, culturally imprinted with the values and
ideologies of service, respect, and honor to members of their families and kin, continued in this kin network mode, even though they
could opt out of this commitment. Engaging family and kin members is voluntary and not legally binding.

The plethora of studies examining the notion of kin structure and
intergenerational functioning in the urban environment led to an

outcry that sufficient work had been done to now probe more deeply into this phenomena (Sussman, 1965). Investigations were now needed on the meaning and significance of activities and relationships of intergenerational and kin connections. How did such connections and activities fit in or collide with families of orientation and procreation? What were their relationships with larger groups such as organizations and institutions whose normative demands were expected to be met? Studies on inheritance, caregiving, support of nuclear families in need of help, family businesses, single parents, divorced families, economic maintenance, and linkages with bureaucratic organizations are examples of in-depth investigations on the relevance, importance, and meaning of these networks in the everyday lives of individuals.

For the most part, these studies were completed by social scientists who identified themselves as family or marriage experts. A few individuals from mainstream sociological theory and organizational analysis whose curiosity was piqued, if they did not research the topic, at least examined the evidence and did commentary. The point is that the myth of institutional domination over smaller units like families and kin networks in complex societies was so encrusted in the ideologies and phenomenologies of social science that this myth was accorded reality. Evidence to the contrary; that which is believed, is the truth.

During the 1980s, there is increased interest in studying kin networks, particularly the intergenerational connection. This concern of social scientists is not an outcome of their conceptual transformation, discarding an old for a new myth and concomitant realities. It is due largely to events and situations occurring in complex societies which place the intergenerational nexus on center stage.

The first of these is the curtailment of federal and state expenditures for health care of the general population, and services for the elderly. With few exceptions most leaders of highly industrialized societies, especially the United States, believe that they have reached the absorptive capacity in regard to state expenditures and continued investments in institutions for the care of its citizens. They are looking to families to provide substantial caretaking activities and, in some instances, the major burden of long-term care. Since 1980, and during the Reagan Presidency, the "return to the family" and its reinvigoration became a national goal helped along by a reduction in financial support of health and welfare programs. This diminution of third party transfers on a national scale led to increased interest in generational transfers within families. The concern is with the potential supports and transfer of resources from parents to children and children to parents over different periods of the life course. Also, the role of sibs and bilateral kin such as uncles, aunts, and cousins are being viewed as potential players in support networks of family members.

Reduction in the amount of funds for human services is juxtaposed with a radically altered demographic profile. This portraiture suggests that during this decade and well into the 21st century, there will be a tremendous increase in the prevalence of surviving older adults over retirement age, with a dramatic increase in the number of persons over age 85. Decreasing morbidity because of technical advances in medicine, improved nutrition, and increased concern to improve or maintain mental and physical well-being has resulted in these improved survival rates.

The increasing incidence and prevalence of older adults has the potential of increasing the current burdens of families whose members usually associated with caretaking are in competitive jobs or careers in the work force. There is also an increasing number of four and five generation families and it is becoming not unusual for the generation of middle-aged parents to care for their parents and young children. Sixty-year-olds caring for an 85-year-old parent, their divorced daughter, and two very young grandchildren is becoming a normal scenario.

The lowered fertility rate of the baby boom generation may provide a critical situation for individuals reaching their golden years in the 2010-2020 period. Many may be in search of a relative. The potential paucity of blood or marriage relatives may result in family formations varied from existing structures but still providing family-like responses (Marciano, 1988; Sussman & Pfeifer, 1987).

Older adults are forming morally armed constituencies; formidable lobbies who also engage in varied service activities for its members. The American Association for Retired Persons, with over 25 million members, is one such example. Generational conflict or harmonious relationships and activities between the generations is dependent on how these elder organizations use their newly acquired power.

Attention is now being directed by researchers to internal family distributions, inter vivos transfers, and bequests through inheritance (Cates & Sussman, 1982; IRS, 1990). These family transfers are becoming increasingly important in determining generational continuity, its symbolic and mythic components, and its potential for negotiating caretaking arrangements for older members. A hypothesis is that there will be more openness regarding the contests of wills and their intended economic transfers as older adults arrange with children or grandchildren for their care when they are no longer independent. Under the aegis of distributive justice one expects that the designated caretaker will receive a larger share of the inheritance and in most situations such distributions will be approved by other heirs and legatees who stand to benefit under conditions of testacy or intestacy.

The consequences of birthquaking research on generational and kin family relationships remains problematic. Policy makers, governmental administrators, practitioners, and researchers share a common interest in such undertakings. However, each group has an approach in consonance with their special interest, ideology, and mandate.

Various perceptions of reality remain and an integrated holistic view and solution may never be in the offing. Movement to closure, to a policy and practice, cost effective, and beneficial to all individuals and interest groups, is to initially determine what each group does best. Once this is decided cooperation may result around a superordinate goal. This is an objective which cannot be achieved without all groups participating and cooperating. The move is toward shared visions and reduction of intolerance.

Researchers are best doing research, family members are best in physical and caretaking domains; federal governments can supplement the economic contributions made by families and the vested pensions of the care receivers. Practitioners are the leaders and operate best when supplied with adequate resources and reduce the tunnel vision which is endemic to their professionalization. Policy makers can best function as thinkers and philosophers with proposals for partnering families, federal administrators, and caretakers in complementary activities of benefit to these groups. Such division of appropriate functions is a paradigm worth exploring. It has the potential of affecting a deeper understanding of each other's domain and a moral commitment to harmonize and cooperate in a common endeavor to serve others.

REFERENCES

Adams, B. (1968). *Kinship in an urban setting*. Chicago: Markham.

Cates, J. & Sussman, M. (1982). *Family systems and inheritance patterns*. New York: Haworth Press.

Farber, B. (1973). *Family and kinship in modern society*. Glenview: Scott, Foresman & Co.

Litwak, E. & Szelenyi, I. (1969). Primary group structures and their functions. *American Sociological Review, 34*, 465-481.

Internal Revenue Service (1990). Intergenerational wealth study. Washington, DC: Statistics of Income Division, IRS.

Schneider, D.M. (1980). *American kinship: A cultural account*. Chicago: The University of Chicago Press.

Sussman, M.B. (1951). *Family continuity: A study of factors which affect relationships between families at generational levels*. Doctoral dissertation, Yale University, New Haven, CT.

Sussman, M.B. (1953). The help pattern in the middle-class family. *American Sociological Review, 18*, 22-28.

Sussman, M.B. & Burchinal, L. (1962). Kin family network: Unheralded structure in current conceptualization of family functioning. *Marriage and Family Living, 24*, 320-332.

Sussman, M.B. & Pfeifer, S. (1987). *Youth connecting with older adults: Implications for improved life experiences and learning*. AARP Andrus Foundation.

Sweetser, O.M. (1962). Asymmetry in intergenerational relationships. *Social Forces, 41*, 346-352.

Troll, L., Miller, S.J., & Atchly, R.C. (1979). *Families in later life*. Belmont: Wadsworth Publishing Co.

Intergenerational Solidarity in Families: Untangling the Ties That Bind

Robert E. L. Roberts
Leslie N. Richards
Vern L. Bengtson

INTRODUCTION

One of the fundamental sociological insights is that human groups manifest properties which are not completely reducible to the characteristics of their individual members. Group properties such as cohesiveness, membership exclusiveness, and demand extensiveness generalize across groups whose individual members may differ greatly. It has long been argued, in fact, that the study of these emergent group properties represents the distinctive domain of sociological inquiry (e.g., Comte, 1875; Durkheim, 1938).

Another fundamental insight in sociology is the notion that the continued existence of human groups depends on some level of cohesion or solidarity being engendered among group members. Since its earliest sociological formulations (e.g., Comte, 1875; Durkheim,

Robert E.L. Roberts is Research Associate, Gerontology Research Institute, University of Southern California, Los Angeles, CA 90089-0191; Leslie N. Richards is Assistant Professor, Human Development and Family Sciences, Oregon State University, Corvallis, OR 97331-5102; and Vern L. Bengtson is AARP/ University Professor of Gerontology and Professor of Sociology, University of Southern California, Los Angeles, CA 90089-0191.

This research was supported by the National Institute on Aging (grant #R37-AG07977).

The authors wish to acknowledge the contributions of Margaret Gatz, co-PI of this research project on the conceptualization and design of the research, and Linda Hall for her expert technical assistance in preparing the manuscript.

[1893] 1933; Tönnies, [1887] 1957), the term *solidarity* has been used to describe the "glue" which overcomes the centripetal tendencies of human self-interest (e.g., Hobbes' ([1651] 1950) "war of all against all"), thus accounting for social order. While the view that solidarity forms the basis for social order has not gone unchallenged (e.g., Dahrendorf, 1959; Marx, 1920; Simmell, 1966), the construct has continued to occupy a central place in both the sociological mainstream (e.g., Parsons, 1951; Hechter, 1987) and in many of its various sub-specialties, including research on community (Sampson, 1988), work (Lincoln & Kalleberg, 1985), and social movements (Hechter, 1987).

The imagery of group cohesiveness has been central in the development of research on the intergenerational family as well. Family researchers have long recognized that families, as special instances of human groups, can be distinguished from one another on the basis of differences in levels of solidarity, cohesion, or integration (Angell, 1965; Hill, 1949; Jansen, 1952; Nye & Rushing, 1969; Thomas & Znaniecki, 1927). Most often solidarity in families, like solidarity in society, has been treated as the engine driving the pursuit of the common good within families. From this perspective, variation in family solidarity, both between families and within families over time, has been seen as reflecting and affecting the social, economic, and psychological well-being of the individuals entwined in intergenerational family relationships.

The purpose of this paper is to assess the state of research and theory devoted to understanding intergenerational cohesion, integration, or solidarity in families. For the sake of clarity, we employ "solidarity" in the remainder of this paper as a meta-construct subsuming characteristics of intergenerational bonds in families. The paper is organized around four distinct issues confronting researchers interested in explicating the bases, determinants, and consequences of family solidarity. In the first section, we assess the historical development of theoretical taxonomy of the essential behavioral and attitudinal elements of solidarity, both as evident in human groups generally and in families specifically. The second section provides an overview of efforts made to specify just how the unique elements of solidarity are related to one another. In the third section, we present a summary of empirical examinations of the individual and family characteristics found to predict higher or lower levels of intergenerational family solidarity. The final section is an examination of what is known about the consequences of intergenerational solidarity for individual and family well-being.

THE ELEMENTS OF SOLIDARITY

Classical Sociological Formulations

Understanding the nature of the ties which bind individuals into coherent collectivities has been a longstanding concern of social theorists (see reviews by Hechter, 1987; McChesney & Bengtson, 1988; and Turner, 1988). Owing to the complexity of the phenomenon under study, early research was by no means unifocal. A number of distinct theories of human bonding emerged, some diverging on the basis of disciplinary or ideological differences, others varying due to differences in scope. However, these early efforts were and continue to be important in their explicit or implicit identification of the particular group characteristics related to solidarity. Here, we focus briefly on the contribution of two of these early theorists, Emile Durkheim and Ferdinand Tönnies.

Among the classical treatments of the issue, Durkheim's (1933) distinction between mechanical and organic solidarity is probably the most well-known. His distinction between the two types of solidarity was driven by his concern over the impact of the industrial revolution on European society. He reasoned that before industrialization, individual ties to the collectivity were conditioned by internalization and endorsement of traditional norms and customs. This "mechanical" form of group solidarity encouraged relatively strong bonds between individuals based upon the power of collective standards of conduct—power derived from historical tradition and collective assession. Durkheim held that the strength of tradition as a cohesive social force was weakened by the progression of industrialization and the subsequent allocation of laborers into increasingly distinct yet interdependent functions. Solidarity between individuals in industrial society would, he suggested, increasingly derive from their mutual dependence upon one another as imposed by their relations in the division of labor. Durkheim labeled this latter form of solidarity "organic," and implied that it would produce weaker bonds than those in societies characterized by mechanical solidarity. In focussing on differences between traditional and modern industrial societies, Durkheim thus identified two bases of solidarity — normative prescriptions toward cohesion and functional interdependency of group members.

Ferdinand Tönnies (1957) also observed the potential for differing basis of solidarity in human relations. His primary distinction centered on the extensivity of normative obligations between persons engaged in social relationships. Tönnies noted that stronger bonds were likely to develop between individuals who had extensive, normatively prescribed obligations to one another (e.g., family members). Such highly cohesive social relations (*Gemeinschaft*), were contrasted with less cohesive relationships between individuals involved in voluntary exchanges (*Gesellschaft*). Solidarity between persons involved in *Gesellschaft* relations was not based on extensive mutual obligation but on consensus over the "rules" of reciprocity. The mutual obligations in this case are restricted to those agreed upon by the individuals in their implicit or explicit contract of exchange. According to Tönnies, *Gesellschaft* relations are characterized by weaker bonds due to the restrictedness of obligations and the tenuousness of contractual consensus. Thus Tönnies, like Durkheim, identified normative commitment and obligation as a powerful base for group solidarity. Alternately, however, Tönnies noted that consensus over rules of exchange could also form the basis for solidarity, albeit weaker than in *Gemeinschaft* relations.

Later theorists (e.g., Weber, [1922] 1968; Parsons, 1973) recognized weaknesses in the inherent dualisms implied by the mechanical/organic and *Gemeinschaft/Gesellschaft* distinctions. The central criticism was that neither dualism contrasted mutually exclusive forms of solidarity. The critiques cited examples of social relations which evidenced elements of *Gemeinschaft* and *Gesellschaft* relations, or mechanical and organic solidarity simultaneously. The importance of these critiques for later work was in the implicit observation that various bases of solidarity might be operating at the same time in any given set of social relations. The central contribution of the classical theorists to later work on solidarity in social psychology and in family sociology was thus in the description of the relevant bases of group solidarity, including: normative prescriptions internalized by group members (mechanical/*Gemeinschaft*), functional interdependencies among group members (organic), and consensus between members over rules of exchange (*Gesellschaft*).

The Contribution of Social Psychology

A great deal of empirical and theoretical work done by social psychologists in the 1950's and 1960's was devoted to understanding group dynamics (Back, 1951; Collins & Raven, 1969; Deutsch, 1968; Deutsch & Krauss, 1965; Festinger, Schachter, & Back, 1950; Turner, 1957). Much of the work focussed on identifying characteristics of interaction related to group cohesion and, in many ways, derived from and extended the classical formulations of solidarity. One of the more cogent theoretical taxonomies of the elements of group solidarity was developed by Homans (1950) and later amplified and extended by Fritz Heider (1958) (McChesney and Bengtson, 1988).

Homans emphasized the importance of four characteristics of human interaction in determining group solidarity. The first component, "interaction," referred to the degree of interconnectedness between the actions of one group member and another member. Homans' use of "interaction" was consistent with the notion of functional interdependence in Durkheim's organic solidarity. A second related component of group solidarity was the extensivity of "activity" involving group members. This construct subsumed the breadth of activities in which group members mutually engaged. Homan's third component—"sentiment"—referred to the degree of mutual affection obtaining between members of the group. The fourth dimension in Homans' scheme was indexed by group members' "norms" toward group membership and interaction. More cohesive groups were those in which members interacted often, liked each other, and shared similar normative commitments to group activities.

Heider's (1959) balance theoretical approach was similar to Homans' in that he emphasized the importance of interaction ("contact") and sentiment ("liking"). Heider also posited that similarity between actors would lead to cohesion between group members.

Heider's larger contribution was in suggesting that particular configurations of interaction, similarity, and sentiment may be more stable than others. In Heider's formulation, if both "contact" and similarity were present, then sentiment — and cohesion in general — would be stronger than if only contact or similarity was present alone. For example, a group of frequently interacting individuals with highly similar interests will exhibit greater solidarity than a group whose members interact as often but share few interests.

A number of other researchers focussed on the ways in which levels of similarity, affection, and interaction among group members contributed to cohesion or solidarity. Wilkening (1954), Cartwright and Zander (1960), and Smith (1969) all focussed on the importance of similar goals and interests among group members in promoting solidarity. Fiedler and Neuwese (1965) and Thibaut and Kelley (1959) examined the importance of mutual attraction among group members. Deutsch (1968), Lott and Lott (1961), and Kipnis (1957), among many others, examined the role of interaction dynamics in fostering group cohesion.

The general contribution of the social psychological laboratories, especially as codified in the theoretical work of Homans (1950) and Heider (1958), was to supplement the classical formulations of solidarity, which emphasized normative integration and functional interdependencies, with additional bases of cohesion. In the social psychological formulations, levels of both mutual affection and interaction were recognized as further elements of manifest solidarity among group members. In addition, the social psychologists expanded the classical version of consensus over rules of exchange to incorporate the notion of similarity among group members in general. Thus, five elements of solidarity can be identified by combining the classical and social psychological formulations: normative integration, functional interdependence, similarity or consensus, mutual affection, and interaction.

Family Sociology Approaches

Family researchers traditionally have been concerned with issues of cohesion, integration, and solidarity in families. Some of the earliest research in the field attempted to distinguish the characteristics of families which were more resilient in the face of external strains (Angell, 1936; Hill, 1949; Koos, 1946). Although the family is a markedly different type of group than the macro-social collectivities of concern to the classical theorists or the small experimental groups studied in the social psychology laboratory, the conceptual development of a theory of intergenerational solidarity has been highly influenced by the classical and social psychological approaches. Much of the early research in family studies has conceptualized solidarity in terms of "family integration," which was variously defined in terms of "common interests," "affection," and "interdependence" (McChesney & Bengtson, 1988).

The most significant gains made by family researchers in understanding intergenerational solidarity resulted from an attempt in the 1960's to improve the state of conceptualization and measurement in the field (see Christiansen, 1964). A number of investigators wished to parallel the advances made by psychologists and social psychologists in measuring individual-level phenomena by developing more sophisticated measures of family-level phenomena (e.g., Hill & Hansen, 1960; Rogers & Sebald, 1962; Strauss, 1964). The first benefit of this push for greater methodological precision was in encouraging greater conceptual precision in specifying the relevant elements of solidarity to be measured. For example, Nye and Rushing (1969) attempted to provide a single conceptual framework under which both previous research findings and future efforts to improve family measurement could be organized. The framework they adopted was built around the notion of family integration and incorporated many of the elements of solidarity identified in the sociological and social psychological traditions. They proposed that the best measures of family life would be those which assessed each of several bases of family integration. Building upon the work of Landecker (1951) and Jansen (1952), Nye and Rushing (1969) enumerated six dimensions of family integration for which, they argued, precise measures should be developed. These dimensions included: associational integration; affectual integration; consensual integration; functional integration; normative integration; and goal integration.

A number of investigators have generally followed the Nye and Rushing (1969) prescription, and have offered both refinements to the list of solidarity components (Bengtson & Schrader, 1982) and/or have developed measures of some or all of the components (e.g.,

Mangen et al., 1988; Markides & Krause, 1985; Rossi & Rossi, 1990).

Bengtson and Schrader (1982) attempted to refine the Nye and Rushing (1969) list by substituting "intergenerational family structure" for "goal integration." By "structure" Bengtson and Schrader were referring to patterns of kinship ties as influenced by such factors as propinquity, fecundity, morbidity, and mortality. Their elimination of "goal integration" may or may not have been necessary, depending upon whether one sees goal integration as subsumed variously under "consensual," "functional," and/or "normative" integration. The full list of solidarity elements are listed below with their nominal definitions (adapted from McChesney & Bengtson, 1988):

1. associational solidarity—the frequency and patterns of interaction in various types of activities in which family members engage;
2. affectual solidarity—the type and degree of positive sentiments held about family members, and the degree of reciprocity of these sentiments;
3. consensual solidarity—the degree of agreement on values, attitudes, and beliefs among family members;
4. functional solidarity or exchange—the degree to which family members exchange services or assistance;
5. normative solidarity—the perception and enactment of norms of family solidarity;
6. intergenerational family structure—the number, type, and geographic proximity of family members.

A parallel development in family sociology with regard to the specification of elements of cohesion derives from the clinical tradition and the identification of problematic and optimal forms of family functioning. While the roots of this development can be traced to the 1950s (e.g., Hess & Handel, 1959), the most recent and comprehensive treatment of elements of cohesion in families have been offered by the various "systems" models, including the Circumplex Model (Olsen et al., 1983) and the Beavers Systems Model

(Beavers & Voeller, 1983). The Circumplex Model (Olsen et al., 1983), for example, specifies eight distinct elements of family cohesion, including: emotional bonding, boundaries, coalitions, time, space, friends, decision-making, and interests and recreation.

Though on the surface it may appear that the elements of family cohesion identified in the circumplex formulation are quite distinct from the solidarity elements identified by Nye and Rushing (1969) and Bengtson and Schrader (1982), there is a fair amount of overlap. Clearly, emotional bonding and affectual solidarity are related as are interests/recreation and associational solidarity. The other dimensions of cohesion identified in the circumplex model alternately appeared to be empirical indicators of several of the other solidarity dimensions. In fact, the differences in terminology between the circumplex and solidarity formulations may be due to differences in levels of abstraction at which the elements are identified. The solidarity elements are stated at a more formal conceptual level of abstraction than the cohesion indicators in the systems model. The derivation of the elements of cohesion in the systems model has been significantly influenced by empirical results in family assessment which may account for their greater specificity.

While the Bengtson and Schrader (1982) taxonomy may not be exhaustive, the six dimensions of family solidarity identified have been useful in both stimulating new research and organizing existing findings. For example, indicators of some or all of the six elements have been employed by a number of researchers interested in family solidarity in varying ethnic (Markides & Krause, 1985), life course (Rossi & Rossi, 1990), and national (Knipscheer, 1989; Morioka et al., 1985; Rosenthal, 1987) contexts. The taxonomy also provides a template for linking under a single conceptual rubric previous intergenerational research related to kinship structure (Adams, 1968; Burton, 1985; Sussman & Burchinal, 1962), association (Bengtson & Black, 1973; Hill et al., 1970), exchange (Hill et al., 1970; Kahn & Antonucci, 1980; Lopata, 1973; Shanas, 1982; Sussman, 1965), consensus (Bengtson, 1970), affection (Adams, 1968), and normative integration (Havighurst & Albrect, 1953). In the remainder of the paper, we will focus on these six elements in assessing work on determining the structure, predictors, and consequences of family solidarity.

THE STRUCTURE OF SOLIDARITY

Along with identifying the relevant elements of intergenerational solidarity, a thorough understanding of the phenomenon requires knowledge of the specific interrelationships obtaining between the elements. Are the elements of solidarity highly interdependent, such that finding high levels of one element necessarily means that one will find high levels of any of the others? Is there an independence between the elements of solidarity? Are some elements more closely related than others? If the elements are not independent, is the relationship between them linear? In this section we will assess the degree to which research in the field has provided answers to these questions and discuss what lies ahead for future investigation.

Early Formulations

Classical treatments suggested that some elements of solidarity may be antagonistic. For example, Durkheim's (1933) distinction between mechanical and organic solidarity implies that levels of normative solidarity in groups may be inversely related to functional interdependencies. Such a distinction is probably not useful in understanding the family since the functional roles reflected in the behaviors of different family members tend to be normatively prescribed. In addition, while the family exhibits a division of labor among members, the structure imposed by this division is not the vehicle through which members gain knowledge of each other and interact (as in Durkheim's usage) but is an example of one of those instances where neither ideal type is a sufficient model.

The social psychological literature offers some suggestions as to the structure of relations between some of the solidarity components. Both Homans and Heider implied that levels of affection, association, and consensus should be interrelated. Heider (1958) reasoned syllogistically that both similarity (consensus) and contact (association) would induce one person to like another (affection). Thus, in Heider's scheme, the higher levels of consensus or association found between two or more individuals, the higher one would expect the strength of their affection for one another to be.

Among family sociologists, the specification of the structure of solidarity has received relatively little attention. As stated above, most of the work in this area has been in specifying the relevant elements of family cohesion and developing adequate measures of each (Mangen et al., 1988, but cf. chapter 10). Similarly, systems approaches such as the circumplex model described above have implicitly assumed a unidimensional structure among the distinct elements they have identified.

An Initial Formal Model

Bengtson, Olander, and Haddad (1976), in developing a theoretical model of solidarity among parents and children in old age, specified a hypothetical structure between three of the six eventual Bengtson and Schrader (1982) solidarity components—affection, association, and consensus. These investigators thus focussed on Heider's (1958) three essential components of group cohesion (liking, contact, and similarity). They extended Heider's reasoning that the constructs were mutually related through the joint influence of consensus and association on affection to posit that the constructs were so highly interdependent as to be mutually reinforcing. According to the formulation, higher levels of any of the three subconstructs would lead to higher levels of the other two constructs— and solidarity as a whole. Thus, solidarity was ultimately conceived of as a unidimensional meta-construct indicated by levels of affection, association, and consensus.

Two subsequent empirical tests of the Bengtson et al. model, however, failed to support the central proposition that levels of affection, association, and consensus among elder parents and children were mutually reinforcing elements of a higher-order solidarity construct (Atkinson, Kivett, & Campbell, 1986; Roberts & Bengtson, 1990). In the first test (Atkinson et al., 1986), intercorrelations between indicators of affection, association, and consensus were too low to allow the variables to be combined into a scale (Cronbach's alpha = .30). A replication of the Atkinson et al. test which applied alternate measures and statistical methods to data gathered from a different sample (Roberts & Bengtson, 1990), produced similar results. However, an in-depth analysis of the measurement structure of solidarity revealed a moderate correlation between factors accounting for variability in measures of affection and association. No significant correlation was found between a consensus factor and either of the other factors. Taken together, the two tests indicated that viewing solidarity as a unidimensional meta-construct manifest in the mutual reinforcement of affection, association, and consensus is inappropriate, at least among elder parents and children. However, the second test offered some insight for a more accurate depiction of the underlying structure — one in which affection and association are seen as somewhat interdependent yet independent of levels of consensus.

In the closing analytic chapter of a monograph devoted to assessing measures of intergenerational relations, Mangen and McChesney (1988) tested the extent of unidimensionality among measures of four elements of solidarity (structural solidarity: indicated by propinquity; associational solidarity: indicated by interaction frequency and context; affectual solidarity: indicated by expressed closeness; and functional solidarity: indicated by patterns of assistance exchanged). These investigators found high correlations (i.e., .60 to .80) between measures of associational, functional, and structural solidarity. Correlations between these three solidarity elements and affectual solidarity were much lower; the correlations between affection, proximity, and assistance were near zero. Despite the fairly high correlations they did find, the researchers concluded that a non-linear, typological approach to understanding the structure of solidarity was probably most warranted. Mangen and McChesney (1988) interpreted their findings to "suggest that families develop unique patterns of solidarity within the intergenerational system."

A Second-Stage Theoretical Model

While there have been a few attempts to untangle the hidden structures linking the solidarity elements, most have been limited to a subset of the elements. Two recent efforts, however, have attempted to formulate and empirically test models specifying relationships between each of solidarity components identified by Bengtson and Schrader (1982). The first effort represents our own research team's further attempts to adequately specify the structure of intergenerational solidarity among elder parents and their middle-aged children (Bengtson & Roberts, under review; Roberts & Bengtson, 1990). The second statement and empirical test was provided by Rossi and Rossi (1990) in their recent monograph on the subject of intergenerational bonds over the life course.

Our attempt to accurately specify the structure of solidarity began with a reappraisal of past findings and a reexamination of the historical development of solidarity as a construct in social theory. On the basis of this reassessment, we developed a revised theoretical model of intergenerational family solidarity in old age (Roberts & Bengtson, 1990). Figure 1 provides a simplified schematic of the proposed relations among the solidarity components, stated here at a dyadic level of abstraction in order to facilitate comparison with the Rossi and Rossi (1990) model we discuss below.

The model in Figure 1 represents a refocus on the *Gemeinschaft* nature of families. Thus, there is an implicit expectation of normative primacy in fixing levels of intergenerational affection, association, and exchange. Higher levels of normative solidarity are anticipated to lead to higher levels of intergenerational affection, association, and exchange. Or, put slightly differently: the more parents and children believe they should love, visit, and help one another, the more they will actually do so.

The model also specifies that levels of objective intergenerational consensus, especially along attitudinal lines, will be independent of levels of the other solidarity elements. This, in part, reflects our focus on parent-child relations near the end of the life course and earlier empirical findings (Atkinson et al., 1986; Roberts & Bengtson, 1990). The model predicts that, given higher levels of normative solidarity, parents and children will develop strategies for overcoming patterns of attitude or value dissensus over their adult lifetimes, in order to facilitate affection, association, and exchange. The model also suggests, given the focus on older parents and children, that the exchange of resources will be a major reason for interaction, especially if elder parents become increasingly dependent on assistance from their children. Thus, incremental increases in exchange are expected to be an explanation for increasing association.

The broken arrow from exchange to affection reflects the expectation that affection will be enhanced when exchanges are charac-

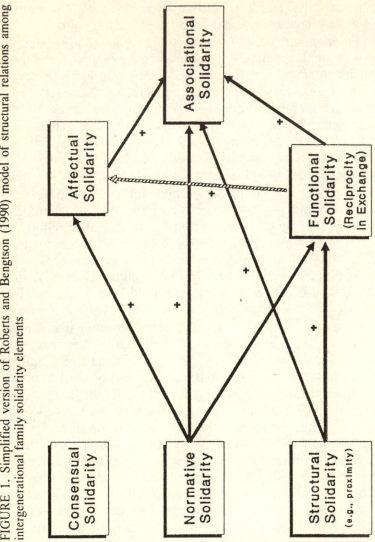

FIGURE 1. Simplified version of Roberts and Bengtson (1990) model of structural relations among intergenerational family solidarity elements

24

terized by reciprocity and diminished when a parent or child feels his or her contributions to the good of the other are not reciprocated. The model also specifies that greater levels of affection will lead to higher levels of association (following Schulman, 1975) and that particular structural configurations will constrain or enable levels of association and exchange (following Litwak, 1985; Morgan, 1982; Sussman, 1965).

The level of abstraction at which the model in Figure 1 is stated conceals the additional specification that levels of each element may exhibit some independence between parents and children. For example, while levels of normative commitment among parents and children may be associated in the aggregate, in any particular family, parent and child may differ markedly. Thus, their differing levels of normative commitment lead parent and child to differentially impact the dynamics through which solidarity is engendered.

Our first, partial test of the model (Bengtson & Roberts, under review) provides support for the notion of normative primacy in fixing levels of affection and association. Both the parent's and child's level of normative commitment to the intergenerational family predicted levels of affection between parent and child. Levels of affection, in turn, were found to lead to higher levels of association. In addition, measures of structural constraints (residential distance and poor parental health) were found to be negatively related to association. Unfortunately, adequate indicators of exchange given and received were not available for the subjects forming the basis for the initial test; thus the parts of the model involving exchange relationships were not tested.

An Alternative Model

As part of an examination of intergenerational bonds over the life course, Rossi and Rossi (1990) have developed and tested a model of solidarity similar to the model described in Figure 1 (see Figure 2). Though the Rossi and Rossi model is stated in longitudinal terms and is meant to encompass parent-child relations over the entire life course, there are few major differences between the structure of solidarity it implies and the structure implied by our model shown in Figure 1.

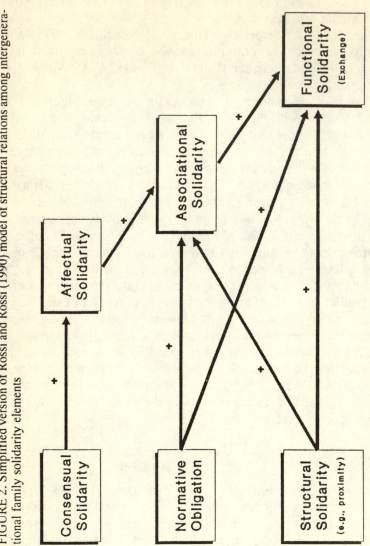

FIGURE 2. Simplified version of Rossi and Rossi (1990) model of structural relations among intergenerational family solidarity elements

26

The first difference is that consensus is not seen as independent of the other solidarity elements in the Rossi and Rossi model. Value consensus between parent and child is expected to lead to greater levels of affection. The second difference is that in the Rossi and Rossi formulation, while normative primacy is assumed with respect to fixing levels of association and exchange (as in Figure 1), normative obligations are not expected to lead to higher levels of affection. The last major difference between the models lies in the specification of the connections between exchange, association, and affection. Rossi and Rossi reverse the direction of the arrow between exchange and association and eliminate any direct connection between exchange and affection. Thus, exchange becomes the only completely endogenous construct in the Rossi and Rossi model, where association is the endogenous construct in ours. All other structural connections depicted in Figure 1 are consistent across the two models.

Rossi and Rossi provide a detailed empirical examination of variation in each of the solidarity constructs as well as the complex interrelations among constructs. Their data supported the connections implied by the model shown in Figure 2. All points of overlap between their model and the model in Figure 1 (i.e., the influence of norms, affection, and structural constraints on association and exchange) were supported. Rossi and Rossi also found subjective ratings of value consensus to be positively related to parent and child ratings of affection for one another. The greater the intergenerational consistency in values perceived by an individual, the more likely he or she was to express high levels of intergenerational affection. In addition, though not explicitly stated in their model, affection was found to exert a direct influence on the exchange of assistance among older parents and children in their sample.

Contrasts Between the Two Models

The convergent results of our efforts and those of Rossi and Rossi suggest that the reconsideration of the *Gesellschaft* nature of family relations, which assumes the primacy of normative solidarity, relative to other solidarity elements, is fruitful. In both examinations, the normative orientations of family members toward family roles were related to higher levels of association and exchanges of assistance. In addition, we have found endorsement of familistic norms to be associated with higher levels of intergenerational affection as well. Rossi and Rossi did not test this relationship.

The two points of greatest departure between the models of solidarity presented here — the independence or non-independence of consensus and the causal ordering of exchange and affection — may not be irreconcilable. First, the discrepancy between our finding consensus to be independent of the elements of solidarity (Roberts & Bengtson, 1990) and Rossi and Rossi (1990) finding value consensus and intergenerational affection to be related, may be due to differences in measurement. While we employed an objective measure of consensus, i.e., comparing independently measured attitude scales across parent-child dyads, Rossi and Rossi employed a subjective measure, i.e., the amount of consensus perceived by the respondent. In several preliminary analyses we found items which tapped the degree of subjective similarity between parent and child to load highly on a factor accounting for much of the variance in items forming a scale of intergenerational affection. It may be that subjective ratings of consensus and similarity are confounded in the phenomenological construction of affection between parents and children. It may be equally likely, however, that objective measures of consensus do not capture true consensus due to measurement imprecision. What is clear is that attention needs to be addressed to the different roles objective and subjective levels of consensus may play in engendering feelings of affection, as well as influencing levels of other elements of solidarity.

The second point of departure between the models is in their specification of the causal ordering of exchange and association. To some extent, any ordering is doomed to be flawed. Association and exchange are nearly completely dependent upon one another. In most respects exchange *is* association, and vice versa. However, one can think of exchange outcomes which might lead to greater or lesser association in the future. Exchanges which continually leave one of the parties feeling as if he or she has given more than received, might lead him or her to avoid association with the other party in the future. Similarly, a mutually rewarding exchange might lead to continued association in the future. We have suggested (Roberts & Bengtson, 1990) that some degree of the balance in exchange needs to be taken into account when attempting to specify the ordering of exchange and association. In this case we suggest that exchanges which are mutually rewarding to parent and child will lead to greater levels of association in the future.

Other Directions

In any event, this discussion shows that while some progress has been made in understanding the structure of intergenerational solidarity in families, a substantial amount of work lies ahead. Further empirical tests on the structure of solidarity need to be conducted, especially ones which include measures of all constructs. Longitudinal assessments of the relationships among solidarity elements are also required, in order to capture variability within families over time as well as to untangle the causal ordering among such variables as association and exchange. More accurate models need to be developed and evaluated as new information emerges from the empirical work.

Our one suggestion for future research is that the methodological focus should remain broad. More qualitative research is needed. At this early stage of understanding intergenerational solidarity, it is important that researchers remain flexible to new ways of putting together the pieces of the puzzle. As the foregoing discussion has demonstrated, the evolution of the solidarity constructs and models linking the constructs has proceeded largely deductively. Qualitative assessment of the subtleties of intergenerational relations affords the opportunity to augment this predominantly deductive focus with a more inductive approach. In addition, we feel future quantitative research should not be limited to applications of the linear model, but should also be attentive to non-linear approaches such as those suggested by Mangen and McChesney (1988).

PREDICTORS OF SOLIDARITY

This section presents a brief overview of research on the individual, familial, and cultural determinants of intergenerational solidarity. Given the current state of knowledge of the structure of solidarity, we have chosen to discuss the predictors of each of the six Bengtson and Schrader (1982) solidarity dimensions separately.

One could then employ either of the two models of the structure of solidarity to infer possible indirect connections between predictors of each solidarity element and the system of structural relations among the elements.

Normative Solidarity

The preceding discussion of the structure of solidarity in families points to the importance of normative commitments across generations in contributing to other dimensions of solidarity. However, there is a paucity of empirical research which attempts to assess predictors of normative obligations in the family. This lack of research may be due to a general decline in interest in social norms research among sociologists, due to difficulties in operationalization and measurement as noted by Mangen et al. (1988) and Rossi and Rossi (1990). In part, the problem stems from the fact that norms, by definition, tend to be collectively shared; yet the traditional behavioral scientific approach to measurement has been to capture maximal inter-individual variation (Rossi & Rossi, 1990).

A few studies have overcome the methodological difficulties posed by norms research and focussed on predicting normative commitments among family members. Differences in the strength of intergenerational normative solidarity have been found to be related to family ethnicity, characteristics of parents, and early family experiences of children. Bengtson, Manuel, & Burton (1981) found members of families of Mexican American heritage to exhibit higher levels of normative solidarity than members of Black and Anglo families. Rossi and Rossi (in press) found lower levels of normative commitment to primary kin among members of ethnically Black families than among members of families of other ethnic heritage. Among parental characteristics examined, widowhood, poor health, and low income have been found to predict higher levels of normative intergenerational obligation in families (Adams, 1968; Lopata, 1973, 1979).

Rossi and Rossi (1990) demonstrated that a number of early familial experiences impact on later levels of normative obligations among primary kin. Having been raised in a broken home was found to be negatively related to levels of normative obligation. In contrast, experiencing high levels of family cohesion and experiencing family adversities as a child were associated with greater levels of normative commitment in adulthood.

Affectual Solidarity

Ages of parents and children are fairly consistent predictors of the strength of intergenerational affection in families. Intergenerational affection has been found to be higher during the child's preadolescent years, to diminish during the child's adolescent years, and to rebound and remain higher during the child's adult years (Rossi & Rossi, 1990). Generational position in the family is an additional, related predictor of affectual solidarity, with members of older generations expressing more positive feelings about intergenerational relationships than do young family members (Bengtson, 1986). Bengtson and Kuypers (1971) labeled this phenomenon the "generational stake," referring to the greater investment that older family members may have in perceiving positive intergenerational relationships. This pattern of older generations perceiving greater affection in the family has been shown to be consistent over time (Richards, Bengtson, & Miller, 1989), although there is some evidence that the phenomenon may be culturally-specific (Morioka et al., 1985).

Attainment of adult status and establishment of separate households may also lead to more positive levels of affectual solidarity between parents and children (Baruch & Barnett, 1983; Bengtson & Black, 1973; Fischer, 1981). Along these lines, Rossi and Rossi (1990) have found that a child's becoming a parent increases levels of parental affection. Finally, there is some indication that gender may influence levels of affection, with higher levels of intergenerational affection being found between mothers and daughters (Rossi & Rossi, 1990).

Associational Solidarity

As one would expect, characteristics of the family structure greatly impinge on the amount of contact between generations in the family. Intergenerational interaction is enabled or constrained by such factors as kin proximity, number of kin, and competing occupational and filial demands. In fact, residential proximity of kin to one another is the strongest predictor of intergenerational association (Adams, 1968; Shanas et al., 1968). Residential proximity has been found to account for as much as 30 to 60 percent of the variance in measures of parent-child contact (e.g., Atkinson et al., 1986; Crimmins & Ingegneri, 1990; Roberts & Bengtson, 1990; Rossi & Rossi, 1990).

Proximity alone, however, does not account for all of the variance in intergenerational contact. As discussed above, higher levels of intergenerational affection and normative solidarity have been found to lead to greater association. Other research indicates that interaction patterns in the family vary by gender, with women more likely to associate more frequently than men (Aldous & Hill, 1965; Atkinson et al., 1986), perhaps reflecting the "kin keeping" role commonly taken by women.

Marital status, educational level, and urban residence are among characteristics of parents that have been found to influence intergenerational association. A parent who is divorced or separated, is more highly educated, and lives in an urban setting is likely to experience lower levels of contact with his or her children (Crimmins & Ingegneri, 1990). Widowhood, on the other hand, is associated with increased intergenerational contact (Anderson, 1984).

Age and health of older parents indirectly influence the amount of intergenerational contact taking place in the family. Both older and more physically debilitated parents are more likely to report living with a child and thus report higher levels of intergenerational association (Crimmins & Ingegneri, 1990).

Functional Solidarity (Exchange)

A large number of studies have attempted to assess the conditions under which assistance flows both up and down generational lines in the family (e.g., see Cheal, 1983; Cicirelli, 1983; Dean et al., 1989; Litwak, 1985; Matthews, 1987; Morgan, 1982). Aldous (1987) has observed that patterns of intergenerational support tend to reflect the giving of a resource which one generation has in excess, e.g., money, physical ability, to a generation which lacks that resource. Thus, those family members who have higher income and education, have been found to be more likely to provide financial assistance to a parent or child in need (Hoyert, 1989). Similarly, children are more likely to provide physical assistance to aging parents with poor health and physical disabilities (Mutran & Reitzes, 1984; Rossi & Rossi, 1990).

Marital status has been shown to be associated with intergenerational exchange patterns (Mutran & Reitzes, 1984). Married parents are more likely to provide greater support to children than either widowed or divorced parents who, in turn, are more likely to receive assistance from their children (Rossi & Rossi, 1990). In contrast, unmarried children, especially daughters, have been found to give more financial support to parents than married children, possibly reflecting the competing fiscal demands of one's own spouse and children (Hoyert, 1989).

Family size has also been found to influence patterns of intergenerational assistance. Rossi and Rossi (1990) report that parents with large numbers of children give less in the way of material and emotional intergenerational support but receive somewhat more support than parents with fewer children. In essence, having more children may provide a larger support resource base while not increasing intergenerational resource demands.

Consensual Solidarity

The most common explanation for intergenerational attitude and value continuity in the family is that shared socialization experiences produce shared orientations (Glass, Bengtson, & Dunham, 1986). Two types of socialization experiences are often implicated in producing similarities between parents and children. First, convergence is thought to result from direct transmission of attitudinal orientations from parent to child as part of early family socialization experiences. A number of studies have demonstrated that parental attitudes do predict child attitudes in adulthood (Acock & Bengtson, 1978; Jennings & Niemi, 1981; Smith, 1983). However, the predictive power of early parental attitudes for later child attitudes is fairly limited.

A second source of attitude and value consensus is in the sharing of experiences common to members of a particular social stratum or class. The central idea is that one's placement in the structure of society influences the nature and kind of activities, e.g., work and recreation, in which one engages. Individuals who share structural positions within society should be more likely to endorse similar attitudes, values, and beliefs (on the basis of common experience). In addition to transmitting attitudes directly, parents also transmit, to some extent, the location in society which their children will occupy. A number of studies provide evidence that intergenerational similarities in financial status, education, and religious affiliation are associated with greater intergenerational consensus on attitudes and values (Glass et al., 1986; Bengtson & Roberts, 1988; Rossi & Rossi, 1990).

Structural Solidarity

The number, availability, distance, marital status, and ages of the members of intergenerational families is influenced by the macro- and micro-social phenomena (Treas & Bengtson, 1982). Changes in birth and mortality rates, divorce rates, the gender composition and mobility of the labor force all impact on family structure. Decreased mortality among the oldest members of society, coupled with diminishing birth rates (Fowles, 1984; Rice & Feldman, 1983) has led to what Bengtson and Dennefer (1987) described as the "beanpole" family structure — characterized by families with living members in three or more generations but with few members in any particular generation. High divorce rates among younger generations also contribute to the vertical streamlining of family structure (Masnick & Bane, 1980; Smyer & Hofland, 1982; Uhlenberg & Myers, 1981). The increased participation of middle aged women in the labor force (Kamerman & Hayes, 1982; Stoller, 1983) also potentially impacts the availability of the traditional primary caregiver for dependent elders.

Many micro-level events and/or characteristics of family members influence family structure. Often, sources of change tend to be idiosyncratic, e.g., reflecting aspirations for family size or expectations of marital happiness, or unexpected, e.g., death of a child. However, a few studies have examined a number of micro-level influences on the family structure which generalize across families. For example, urban residence and poor parental health are associated with greater parent-child residential proximity in adulthood

(Crimmins & Ingegneri, 1990). On the other hand, residential proximity as well as number of children are negatively associated with higher levels of education (Crimmons & Ingegneri, 1990).

CONSEQUENCES OF SOLIDARITY

In this final section, we turn to the question of what is good or bad about intergenerational solidarity in families. Do members of families with higher levels of intergenerational solidarity fare better in life? Despite the fact that researchers have been interested in family solidarity for many years, these questions remain unanswered. Intuitively one might expect that high levels of solidarity would be uniformly good for individuals, but this relationship has not been clearly demonstrated empirically.

Research has established that early positive experiences of family solidarity contribute to health development during infancy, yet the links between family solidarity and psychological well-being in later life are still underdeveloped. This is in part due to the difficulties in untangling influences on development beyond the early childhood period. By the time individuals reach adulthood, their lives have been influenced by many events and many individuals, reaching far beyond the confines of the nuclear family. Nevertheless, there is some evidence that high levels of parent-child solidarity over the life course may buffer the negative impact of disruptive normative and non-normative life events.

Indications of the importance of early family solidarity come in part from the literature on attachment and bonding. Work by Bowlby (1969, 1973), Ainsworth (1973), Blehar (1974), Maccoby and Masters (1970) and others, points to the importance of the mother-infant attachment bond and the implications of such attachment for growth and development in early childhood. Parental warmth and positive regard (presumably indications of affectual solidarity) have also been shown to be related to higher levels of self-esteem in older children (Bachman, 1982).

The importance of continued social support and attachment across the life span has only recently begun to receive attention (Cohler, 1983; Kahn & Antonucci, 1980; Lerner & Ryff, 1978; Roberts & Bengtson, 1988; Rossi & Rossi, 1990) although it is not yet clear the extent to which high levels of family solidarity are more advantageous than support from friends. While there are numerous studies indicating that social network support is beneficial during times of crisis such as illness, divorce, or death, non-kin social support may be just as beneficial as support from kin. Additionally, the mechanisms through which high family solidarity translates to better psycho-social functioning need to be identified.

A number of early studies in family sociology examined the relationship between "family integration" and resiliency to life strains, typically in response to some sort of crisis (Angell, 1936; Hill, 1949; Koos, 1946). Greater family integration was found to lead to better adjustment by family members to the crisis. More recent studies have focussed on the effects of intergenerational functional support, or the enactment of functional solidarity, on psychological well-being. Much of this research suggests that intergenerational support does not tend to increase the psychological well-being of elder members of the family (Lee, 1980; Mutran & Reitzes, 1984; Wood & Robertson, 1976) and in some instances may lower it (Roberts & Bengtson, 1988).

Finally, there are some indications that under some circumstances, high family solidarity contributes to *poor* mental health. Families under severe economic stresses, for example, may find that high family solidarity leads to oppressive demands on time and resources (Belle, 1986). In other families, too much closeness can lead to enmeshment, with family members having no sense of individuality (Beavers, 1982; Epstein, Bishop, & Baldwin, 1982; Minuchin, 1974).

SUMMARY AND CONCLUSION

In this paper we have attempted to provide the reader with a brief but comprehensive perspective on research and theory development pertaining to intergenerational solidarity in families. In so doing, we identified four major directions in which work in this area is proceeding.

First, we reviewed efforts made to identify the concrete aspects of intergenerational relations thought to contribute to solidarity in the family. The intellectual roots of a list of six dimensions of solidarity were traced from classical macro-social theory, social psychology, and family sociology. The six bases of solidarity we identified included associational, affectual, consensual, functional (exchange), normative, and structural aspects of intergenerational relations.

Next, we summarized work which has attempted to specify the structure of interrelations among the solidarity elements. Two independent attempts to empirically assess that structure were reviewed, the first by our research team (Bengtson & Roberts, under review; Roberts & Bengtson, 1990) and the second by Rossi and Rossi (1990). Results from both attempts provided support for the view that higher levels of normative solidarity in the family are likely to lead to higher levels of intergenerational association, exchange, and affection. Affectual solidarity was found to lead to greater association in both analyses and to greater exchange in one (Rossi & Rossi, 1990). In both analyses, structural constraints imposed by residential distance were found to depress levels of association.

Third, we presented a number of empirical findings regarding exogenous predictors of each of the solidarity dimensions. Among the strongest predictors of normative solidarity were low income, poor parental health, parental widowhood, early experience of family cohesion, and an intact family of procreation. Predictors of affectual solidarity included child's age and child's attainment of adult status. Beyond that which can be accounted for by residential proximity, higher levels of associational solidarity are predicted by female-female gender linkages and parental widowhood. Lower levels of associational solidarity are predicted by higher levels of education, parental divorce, and urban residence. Functional solidarity tends to follow the rule that resources which are not scarce in one generation flow toward scarcity in another generation. While being a married parent leads to providing more intergenerational support, the greater the number of children one has, the less support one is likely to give and the more support one is likely to receive. Finally, structural solidarity varies with macro-social phenomena such as birth and death rates, divorce rates and changes in occupational structures. Among the micro-level predictors of residential proximity were urban residence, poor parental health and education.

In the last section, we outlined some potential implications of intergenerational solidarity for individual outcomes such as self-esteem, psychological well-being, and the provision and receipt of support. It appeared to us that the most important beneficial aspects of intergenerational solidarity pertained to the cultivation of high self-esteem among children and adolescents and as a force mobilizing family members to provide emotional and material support for one another over the adult life course.

We wish to conclude by noting that while the notion of solidarity has been a useful heuristic in family research and much has been learned already, a thorough understanding of solidarity in families requires a substantial amount of additional work. First, investigators should assess the degree to which the diverse bases of solidarity have been captured in the six dimensions listed above. One potentially fruitful direction to take in this respect would be to more closely examine the similarities and differences between elements of solidarity specified by Bengtson and Schrader (1982) and those identified by the system-oriented researchers (e.g., Beavers & Voeller, 1983; Olsen et al., 1983).

A second need is to gain a better understanding of the structure of solidarity. While the work which has been completed to date has been successful in demonstrating the importance of normative solidarity in predicting levels of some of the other solidarity elements (i.e., affection, exchange, and association), more needs to be known about the ways in which consensus and exchange fit into the puzzle. We suggest that an openness to alternative theoretical perspectives (e.g., critical and/or rational choice approaches) and the application of qualitative methodologies should be central to efforts in grappling with these issues.

A third requirement for future work is to incorporate predictive models of each element of solidarity with a model of the structure of solidarity. While knowledge of the structure of solidarity is useful, such a model remains acontextual until combined with a specification of other family and individual characteristics which lead to higher or lower levels of the separate solidarity elements. In addition, when such models are combined, one can determine the possible indirect influences of predictors of one solidarity element on the other elements.

Fourth, a complete theory of solidarity needs to draw explicit linkages between aspects of intergenerational solidarity and individual well-being. More needs to be known, both about the positive and negative psycho-social outcomes of family solidarity as well as the importance of family solidarity over the life course relative to solidarity in other human associations, e.g., among friends, in the work place, etc.

In closing, we suggest that movement toward a better understanding of solidarity will come only through closely connected theory development and empirical verification. Continual reference to the empirical world facilitates explicit model building through verifying or refuting expectations as well as providing serendipitous insights into unexpected relationships (Turner, 1986). The groundwork for an explicit model of intergenerational solidarity is in place; future work should build upon that foundation in iterations between theoretical codification and empirical verification.

REFERENCES

Acock, A. C. & Bengtson, V. L. (1978). On the relative influence of mothers and fathers: A covariance analysis of political and religious socialization. *Journal of Marriage and the Family, 40*, 519-530.

Adams, B. N. (1968). *Kinship in an urban setting*. Chicago: Markham Publishing Company.

Aldous, J. (1985). Parent-adult child relations as affected by the grandparent status. In V. L. Bengtson & J. F. Robertson (Eds.), *Grandparenthood* (pp. 117-132). Beverly Hills: Sage Publications.

Aldous, J. (1987). Family life of the elderly and near-elderly (NCFR presidential address). *Journal of Marriage and the Family, 49*, 227-234.

Aldous, J. & Hill, R. (1965). Social cohesion, lineage type and intergenerational transmission. *Social Forces, 43*, 471-482.

Ainsworth, M. D. S. (1973). The development of infant-mother attachment. In B. N. Caldwell & H. N. Ricciuti (Eds.), *Review of child development research*, Vol. 3. Chicago: University of Chicago Press.

Anderson, T. B. (1984). Widowhood as a life transition: Its impact on kinship ties. *Journal of Marriage and the Family, 46*, 105-114.

Angell, R. C. (1965). *The family encounters the depression*. Gloucester, Massachusetts: Peter Smith (Original work published 1936).

Atkinson, M. P., Kivett, V. R., & Campbell, R. T. (1986). Intergenerational solidarity: An examination of a theoretical model. *Journal of Gerontology, 41*, 408-416.

Bachman, J. G. (1982). Family relationships and self-esteem. In M. Rosenberg & H. B. Kaplan (Eds.), *Social psychology of the self-concept* (pp. 356-364). Arlington Heights, Illinois: Harlan Davidson, Inc.

Back, K. W. (1951). Influence through social communication. *The Journal of Abnormal and Social Psychology, 46,* 9-23.

Baruch, G. & Barnett, R. C. (1983). Adult daughters' relationships with their mothers. *Journal of Marriage and the Family, 45,* 601-606.

Beavers, W. R. (1982). Healthy, midrange, and severely dysfunctional families. In F. Walsh (Ed.), *Normal family processes.* New York: Guilford Press.

Beavers, W. R. & Voeller, M. N. (1983). Family models: Comparing and contrasting the Olson Circumplex Model with the Beavers Systems Model. *Family Process, 22,* 85-98.

Belle, D. E. (1986). The impact of poverty on social networks. In L. Lein & M. B. Sussman (Eds.), *The ties that bind: Mens' and womens' social networks.* New York: Haworth Press.

Bengtson, V. L. (1970). The 'generation gap': A review and typology of social-psychological perspectives. *Youth and Society, 2,* 7-32.

Bengtson, V. L. (1986). Sociological perspectives on aging, families, and the future. In M. Bergener (Ed.), *Perspectives on aging: The 1986 Sandoz Lectures in Gerontology,* (pp. 237-263). New York & London: Academic Press.

Bengtson, V. L. & Black, K. D. (1973). Intergenerational relations and continuity in socialization. In P. B. Baltes & K. W. Schaie (Eds.), *Life-span developmental psychology and socialization* (pp. 207-234). New York: Academic Press.

Bengtson, V. L. & Dannefer, D. (1987). Families, work and aging: Implications of disordered cohort flow for the 21st century. In R. A. Ward & S. S. Tobin (Eds.), *Health in aging: Sociological issues and policy directions,* (pp. 256-289). New York: Springer.

Bengtson, V. L. & Kuypers, J. A. (1971). Generational difference and the "developmental stake." *Aging and Human Development, 2,* 249-260.

Bengtson, V. L., Manuel, R. C., & Burton, L. M. (1981). Competence and loss: Perspectives on the sociology of aging. In R. H. Davis (Ed.), *Aging: Prospects and issues,* (pp. 22-39). Los Angeles: University of Southern California Press.

Bengtson, V. L., Olander, E. B., & Haddad, A. A. (1976). The 'generation gap' and aging family members: Toward a conceptual model. In J. E. Gubrium (Ed.), *Time, roles and self in old age* (pp. 237-263). New York: Human Sciences Press.

Bengtson, V. L. & Roberts, R. E. L. (1988). Stability and change in value orientations over time: Some implications of an aging society for the family. A paper presented at the Annual Meetings of the American Sociological Association, Atlanta, Georgia, August 1988.

Bengtson, V. L. & Roberts, R. E. L. (under review). Parent-child solidarity in aging families: An example of empirically-driven theory construction.

Bengtson, V. L. & Schrader, S. (1982). Parent-child relations. In D. Mangen &

W. A. Peterson (Eds.), *Research instruments in social gerontology*, (Volume 2) (pp. 115-186). Minneapolis: University of Minnesota Press.

Blehar, M. C. (1974). Anxious attachment and defensive reactions associated with day care. *Child Development*, *45*, 683-692.

Bowlby, J. (1969). *Attachment and loss, Volume I: Attachment*. New York: Basic Books.

Bowlby, J. (1973). *Attachment and loss, Volume II: Separation anxiety and anger*. New York: Basic Books.

Burton, L. M. (1985). *Early and on-time grandmotherhood in multigeneration black families*. Unpublished doctoral dissertation. University of Southern California.

Cartwright, D. & Zander, A. (1960). *Group dynamics: Research in marriage*. New York: Harper & Row.

Cheal, D. J. (1983). Intergenerational family transfers. *Journal of Marriage and the Family*, *45*, 805-813.

Christiansen, H. T. (1964). Development of the family field of study. In H. Christiansen (Ed.), *Handbook of marriage and the family*. Chicago: Rand-McNally.

Cicirelli, V. G. (1983). Adult children's attachment and helping behavior to elderly parents: A path model. *Journal of Marriage and the Family*, *45*, 815-823.

Cohler, B. (1983). Autonomy and interdependence in the family of adulthood: A psychological perspective. *The Gerontologist*, *23*, 33-40.

Collins, B. E. & Raven, B. H. (1969). Group structure: Attraction, coalitions, communication, and power. In G. Lindzey & E. Aronson (Eds.), *The handbook of social psychology*, Vol. 4, (pp. 102-204). Reading, MA: Addison-Wesley.

Comte, A. (1875). *System of positive polity of treatise on sociology*. London: Burt Franklin.

Crimmins, E. M. & Ingegneri, D. G. (1990). Interaction between older parents and their children: Past trends, present determinants, future implications. *Research on Aging*.

Dahrendorf, R. (1959). *Class and class conflict in industrial society*. Stanford, CA: Stanford University Press.

Dean, A., Kolody, B., Wood, P., & Ensel, W. M. (1989). Measuring the communication of social support from adult children. *Journal of Gerontology*, *44*, 71-79.

Deutsch, M. (1968). Field theory in social psychology. In G. Lindzey & E. Aronson (Eds.), *The handbook of social psychology*, Vol. 1 (pp. 412-487). Reading, MA: Addison-Wesley Publishing Co.

Deutsch, M. & Krauss, R. M. (1955). *Theories in social psychology*. New York: Basic Books.

Durkheim, E. (1933). In G. Simpson (Translator), *The division of labor in society*. New York: Free Press.

Durkheim, E. (1938). *The rules of sociological method*. Glencoe, Illinois: Free Press.

Epstein, N. B., Bishop, D. S., & Baldwin, L. M. (1982). McMaster model of family functioning: A view of the normal family. In F. Walsh (Ed.), *Normal family processes*. New York: Guilford Press.

Festinger, L., Schachter, S., & Back, K. (1965). The Operation of Group Standards. In H. Proshansky, & B. Seidenberg (Eds.), *Basic studies in social psychology* (pp. 471-485). New York: Holt, Rinehart & Winston.

Fiedler, F. W. & Nuewese, W. (1965). Leaders contribution to task performance in cohesive and uncohesive groups. In I. Steiner & M. Fishbein (Eds.), *Current Studies in Social Psychology*.

Fischer, L. R. (1981). Transitions in the mother-daughter relationship. *Journal of Marriage and the Family, 43*, 613-622.

Fowles, D. (1984). The numbers game: A look at the future. *Aging*, 46-47.

Glass, J., Bengtson, V. L., & Dunham, C. C. (1986). Attitude similarity in three-generation families: Socialization, status inheritance, or reciprocal influence? *American Sociological Review, 51*, 685-698.

Havighurst, R. & Albrect, R. (1953). *Older people*. New York: Longmans Green.

Hechter, M. (1987). *Principles of group solidarity*. Berkeley: University of California Press.

Heider, F. (1958). *The psychology of interpersonal relations*. New York: John Wiley.

Hess, R. & Handel, G. (1959). *Family worlds: A psychological approach to family life*. Chicago: University of Chicago Press.

Hill, R. (1949). *Families under stress*. New York: Harper.

Hill, R., Foote, N., Aldous, J., Carlson, R., & MacDonald, R. (1970). *Family development in three generations*. Cambridge, Mass: Schenkman.

Hill, R. & Hansen, D. A. (1960). The identification of conceptual frameworks utilized in family study. *Marriage and Family Living, 12*, 299-311.

Hobbes, T. ([1651] 1950). *Leviathan*. New York: Dutton.

Homans, G. F. (1950). *The human group*. New York: Harcourt, Brace and World.

Hoyert, D. L. (1989). The elder parent's report of intergenerational exchange. A paper presented at the 1989 Annual Meeting of the American Sociological Association, San Francisco, CA, 1989.

Jansen, L. T. (1952). Measuring family solidarity. *American Sociological Review, 17*, 727-733.

Jennings, M. K. & Niemi, R. G. (1981). *Generations and politics: A panel study of young adults and their parents*. Princeton, New Jersey: Princeton University Press.

Kahn, R. L. & Antonucci, T. C. (1980). Convoys over the life course: Attachment, roles and social support. In P. B. Baltes & O. G. Brim, Jr. (Eds.), *Lifespan development and behavior*, Vol. 3, (pp. 253-286). New York: Academic Press.

Kipnis, D. M. (1957). Interaction between members of bomber crews as a detriment of sociometric choice. *Human Relations, 10*, 263-270.

Knipscheer, C. P. M. (1988). Temporal embeddedness and aging within the multigenerational family: The case of grandparenting. In J. E. Birren & V. L. Bengtson (Eds.), *Emergent theories of aging* (pp. 426-446). New York: Springer.

Koos, E. L. (1973). *Families in trouble*. New York: Russell and Russell. (Original work published in 1946).

Landecker, W. S. (1951). Types of integration and their measurement. *American Journal of Sociology*, *56*, 332-340.

Lee, G. R. (1980). Kinship in the seventies: A decade review of research and theory. *Journal of Marriage and the Family*, *42*, 923-934.

Lee, G. R. & Ellithorpe, E. (1982). Intergenerational exchange and subjective well-being among the elderly. *Journal of Marriage and the Family*, *44*, 217-224.

Lerner, L. M. & Ryff, C. D. (1978). Implementation of the life-span view of human development: The sample case of attachment. In P. B. Baltes (Ed.), *Life-span development and behavior*, Vol. 1, (pp. 1-44). New York: Academic Press.

Lincoln, J. R. & Kalleberg, A. L. (1985). Work organization and commitment. *American Sociological Review*, *50*, 738-760.

Litwak, E. (1985). *Helping the Elderly*. New York: Guilford Press.

Lopata, H. Z. (1973). *Widowhood in an American city*. Cambridge: Sheckman Publishing Company.

Lopata, H. Z. (1979). *Women as widows: Support systems*. New York: Elsevier Horth-Holland.

Lott, A. J. & Lott, B. E. (1961). Group cohesiveness, communications level, and conformity. *Journal of Abnormal and Social Psychology*, *62*, 408-412.

Maccoby, E. E. & Masters, J. C. (1970). Attachment and dependency. In P. H. Mussen (Ed.), *Carmichael's manual of child psychology*, Vol. 2. New York: Wiley.

Mangen, D. J. & McChesney, K. Y. (1988). Intergenerational cohesion: A comparison of linear and nonlinear analytical approaches. *Research on Aging*, *1*, 121-136.

Mangen, D. J., Bengtson, V. L., & Landry, P. H. (1988). *Measurement of intergenerational relations*. Beverly Hills: Sage Publications.

Markides, K. S. & Krause, N. (1985). Intergenerational solidarity and psychological well-being among old Mexican Americans: A three-generation study. *Journal of Gerontology*, *40*, 506-511.

Marx, K. (1920). *The poverty of philosophy*. Translated by H. Quelch. Chicago, IL.

Masnick, G. & Bane, M. J. (1980). *The nation's families: 1960-1990*. Cambridge, MA: Joint Center for Urban Studies.

Matthews, S. H. (1987). Perceptions of fairness in the division of responsibility for old parents. *Social Justice Research*, *1*, 425-437.

McChesney, K. Y. & Bengtson, V. L. (1988). Solidarity, integration, and cohesion in families: Concepts and theories. In D. Mangen, V. Bengtson, & P.

Landry, Jr. (Eds.), *Measurement of intergenerational relations* (pp. 15-30). Newbury Park, CA: Sage Publications.

Minuchin, S. (1974). *Families and family therapy*. Cambridge, MA: Harvard University Press.

Morgan, J. N. (1982). The redistribution of income by families and institutions and emergency help patterns. In G. J. Duncan & J. N. Morgan (Eds.), *Five thousand American families—patterns of economic progress*, Vol. X, (pp. 1-45). Ann Arbor: Institute for Social Research.

Morioka, K., Sugaya, Y., Okuma, M., Nagayama, A., & Funjii, H. (1985). Intergenerational relations: Generational differences and changes. In K. Morioka (Ed.), *Family and life course of middle-aged men*. The Family and Life Course Study Group.

Mutran, E. & Reitzes, D. C. (1984). Intergenerational support activities and well-being among the elderly: A convergence of exchange and symbolic interaction perspectives. *American Sociological Review*, *49*, 117-130.

Nye, F. I. & Rushing, W. (1969). Toward family measurement research. In J. Hadden & E. Borgatta (Eds.), *Marriage and family*. Illinois: Peacock.

Olsen, D. H., Russell, C. S., & Sprenkle, D. H. (1983). Circumplex model of marital and family systems: VI Theoretical update. *Family process*, *22*, 69-83.

Parsons, T. (1951). *The social system*. New York: Free Press.

Parsons, T. (1973). Some afterthoughts on *Gemeinschaft* and *Gesellschaft*. In W. J. Cahnman (Ed.), *Ferdinand Tönnies: A New Evaluation* (pp. 140-150). Leiden: Brill.

Rice, D. P. & Feldman, J. J. (1983). Living longer in the United States: Demographic changes and health needs of the elderly. *Milbank Memorial Fund Quarterly*, *61*, 362-396.

Richards, L. N., Bengtson, V. L., & Miller, R. B. (1989). The 'generation in the middle': Perceptions of adults' intergenerational relationships. In K. Kreppner & R. M. Lerner (Eds.), *Family systems and life-span development* (pp. 341-366). Hillsdale, New Jersey: Erlbaum.

Roberts, R. E. L. & Bengtson, V. L. (1988). Intergenerational cohesion and psychic well-being: Implications over the adult life course. Paper presented at the annual meeting of the American Sociological Association, San Francisco, CA, August.

Roberts, R. E. L. & Bengtson, V. L. (1990). Is intergenerational solidarity a unidimensional construct?: A second test of a formal model. *The Journal of Gerontology*, *45*, S12-20.

Rogers, E. M. & Sebald, H. (1962). Familism, family integration, and kinship orientation. *Marriage and Family Living*, *24*, 27.

Rosenthal, C. J. (1987). Aging and intergenerational relations in Canada. In Victor W. Marshall (Ed.), *Aging in Canada: Social perspectives*, 2nd edition (pp. 311-342). Toronto: Fitzhenry & Whiteside.

Rossi, A. S. (1986). Sex and gender in an aging society. *Daedalus*, *115*, 141-169.

Rossi, A. S. & Rossi, P. H. (1990). *Of human bonding: Parent-child relationships across the life course*. New York: Alydine De Gruyter.

Sampson, R. J. (1988). Local friendship ties and community attachment in mass society. *American Sociological Review, 53*, 766-752.

Schulman, N. (1975). Life-cycle variations in patterns of close relationships. *Journal of Marriage and the Family, 37*, 813-821.

Shanas, E. (1980). Older people and their families: The new pioneers. *Journal of Marriage and the Family, 42*, 9-15.

Shanas, E. (1982). *National Survey of the Aged*. (Prepared for the Administration on Aging, U.S. Dept. of Health and Human Services, Washington, D.C. (Dec) DHHS Pub. No. (OHDS) 83-20425.

Shanas, E., Townsend, P., Wedderburn, D., Friis, H., Milhoj, P., & Stehouwer, J. (1968). *Old people in three industrial societies*. New York: Atherton.

Simmel, G. (1966). *Conflict*. Translated by Kurt H. Wolff. Glencoe, IL: Free Press.

Smith, M. B. (1969). *Social psychology and human values*. Chicago: Aldine.

Smith, T. E. (1983). Parental influence: A review of the evidence of influence and theoretical model of the parental influence process. In A. Kerkhoff (Ed.), *Research in Sociology of Educational Socialization*, Vol. 4, pp. 13-45.

Smyer, M. A. & Hofland, B. F. (1982). Divorce and family support in later life. *Journal of Family Issues, 3*, 61-77.

Soldo, B. J. (1981). The living arrangements of the elderly. In S. B. Kiesler, J. N. Morgan, & V. K. Oppenheimer (Eds.), *Aging: Social change*. New York: Academic Press.

Stoller, E. P. (1983). Parental caregiving by adult children. *Journal of Marriage and the Family, 45*, 851-858.

Strauss, M. (1964). Measuring Families. In H. T. Christiansen (Ed.), *Handbook of marriage and the family* (pp. 335-400). Chicago: Rand McNally.

Sussman, M. B. (1965). Relationships of adult children with their parents in the United States. In E. Shanas & G. F. Streib (Eds.), *Social structure and the family: Generational relations*. Englewood Cliffs: Prentice-Hall, Inc.

Sussman, M. B. & Burchinal, L. (1962). Kin family network: Unheralded structure in current conceptualizations of family functioning. *Marriage and Family Living, 24*, 231-240.

Thibaut, J. W. & Kelley, H. H. (1959). *The social psychology of groups*. New York: Wiley.

Thomas, W. I. & Znaniecki, F. (1927). *The Polish peasant in Europe and America* (2 vols). New York: Dover Publications.

Tönnies, F. ([1887] 1957). *Community and society*. Translated and edited by Charles P. Loomis. East Lansing: Michigan State University Press. (Originally published in 1887).

Treas, J. & Bengtson, V. L. (1982). The demography of the mid- and late-life transitions. In F. M. Berardo (Ed.), *The Annals of the AAPSS, 464*:11-21 (November). Chicago, IL: University of Chicago Press.

Treas, J. & Bengtson, V. L. (1987). The family in later years. In M. B. Sussman & S. K. Steinmetz (Eds.), *Handbook of marriage and the family* (pp. 625-648). New York: Plenum Press.

Turner, A. N. (1957). Foreman, job and company. *Human Relations*, *10*, 99-112.

Turner, J. H. (1986). *The structure of sociological theory*. Chicago: The Downey Press.

Turner, J. H. (1988). Toward a synthetic model of motivation. *A theory of social interaction* (pp. 55-69). Palo Alto, California: Stanford University Press.

Uhlenberg, P. & Myers, M. A. P. (1981). Divorce and the elderly. *The Gerontologist*, *21*, 276-282.

Weber, M. (1968). *Economy and society*. Edited by Guenther Roth and Claus Wittich. New York: Bedminster Press. [Originally published 1922].

Wilkening, E. A. (1954). Change in farm technology as related to familism, family decision making, and family integration. *American Sociological Review*, *19*, 29-37.

Wood, V. & Robertson, J. F. (1976). The significance of grandparenthood. In Jaber B. Gubrium, (Ed.), *Time roles and self in old age*, (278-304). New York: Human Sciences Press.

Families:
Intergenerational and Generational Connections — Conceptual Approaches to Kinship and Culture

John Mogey

The thesis of this essay is that intergenerational rules are now changing. As a result, theories to interpret these changes need to be examined. Up to about 1960, a generation ago, self-regulating mechanisms in the private sector worked well enough to transfer resources between different generations. Since then, public bureaucracies have been more and more involved. This has happened because more citizens live longer, more households are daily empty of persons who could give services to others, and more communities lose the obligation to provide group quarters for those who cannot fully meet the normal activities of daily living. We view these changes as readjustments in the institutional framework of industrial societies as markets and government bureaucratic agencies assume obligations formerly left entirely to informal and self-regulating personal relations. We will discuss some concepts that may relate social theory to the on-going debate between the generations in modern societies.

John Mogey is Adjunct Professor of Sociology, Arizona State University, Tempe, AZ 85287.

This paper benefitted from critical readings by Dr. Bernard Farber, Arizona State University, Dr. Edward Sabin, Towson State University, and Dr. Barry Wellman, University of Toronto. The editors and librarians at the University of Delaware and Anne Arundel Community College helped with the references. The author wishes to thank them all.

Some ten years ago, a review of research concluded with two theory statements: (1) parent-child solidarity or attachment represents an interpersonal norm found in all strata of contemporary American culture; and (2) the strength, the closeness or the intensity of the parent-child bond cannot definitely be linked neither to similarity of attitudes nor behavior of individuals in the two generations (Troll & Bengston, 1979).

Generation as a concept creates a class of individuals. Intergenerational connections, then, refer to interactions between generations. Data about the social behavior of groups or classes uses averages or summary measures of what is observable about individual members of those groups or classes. In other words, theory statements about intergenerational connections depend on to what social units membership in the class is assigned, and on the ways in which the generation as a class behaves in some social setting. Behavior in a class rests on indicators that are common to each unit within it.

To be members of a generation, individuals must be similar on three independent measures: by birth, by age, and by time, or period. Using birth and time independently gives us two different possibilities for the concept 'generation.' First, all human beings born into a society during a specified period of time are a generation, or as demographers would say, a 'cohort.' The time period could be a year, or a decade, or the average interval between the birth of a child and the birth of a child of that person, usually taken to be 25 or 30 years. Since many time periods are marked by special events, like World War I or II, or the Great Depression, or sudden changes in fertility as in the years of the 'baby boom' generation, cohort combines birth with the special social experiences shared during the lifecourse of its members (Eisenstadt, 1956; Fortes in Kertzer & Keith, 1984; Mannheim, 1952; Riley et al., 1972).

Second, a generation may refer to all who share a common parent. In this sense of the concept, members of a generation share both birth and a place in a time sequence made up of ancestors and descendants. This is the network that connects persons who choose to accept those obligations associated with kinship. We can underline the distinction by saying that individuals make up the membership of a cohort and that persons make up the kinship network (Dumont, 1980). Cohorts are aggregates of individuals in which criteria for entry to the aggregate are decided by a theorist. The theorist often assumes that each individual actor in such collectivities will be found to share, as a minimum, some other cultural attribute. They may have in common an attitude, an expectation, or a value. Members of generations as networks share both birth, a purely biological event, and kinship, a social bond. Their members are persons because they can and do identify with their parents and their other relatives and are aware as part of their self identity of that filiation. Although no one directly chooses their parents, the parents make a free choice of each other, if and when they marry. Choices among available relatives are relatively free, whatever kinship pattern of counting distance between relatives is involved (Farber, 1981). These attachments connect each person to a network of kin. Each self bases its expectations on a unique position in a network of generations that moves through the lifecourse stages of that society (Litwak & Kulis, 1987; Parsons, 1971; Wellman, 1979).

Whether generation is conceived as cohort or as network, its meaning derives from the cultural values sanctioned by members of a societal community. I use this term in the sense of 'a complex network of interpenetrating collectivities and collective loyalties' (Parsons, 1971, p. 13). It directs our attention more to the normative aspects of belonging to a social group than to the mere fact of being a member. It allows us to keep in mind that beyond any single loyalty norm there exists a hierarchy of expectations or beliefs from which any self can choose. This richness of choices is found in all human societies. Both the number and the variety of choices increased enormously in modern times. Nonetheless, it is important to remember that freedom to choose from a wide variety of behaviors has always been part of the human condition.

So defined, cohort, network, kinship, and self, allow us to approach the discussion of intergenerational connections between family members as examples of loyalties or attachments between members of human societies. This structural approach gives a view of human behavior different from, though perhaps parallel to, the developmental one. The stages of growth or decline of the human body, whether studied by biologists, or as mental development by psychologists, or as performance by gerontologists, have not yet been connected in any formal theoretical sense to the structural concept of generations used in this paper (Palmore, 1981; Riley et al., 1972; Shock et al., 1984).

The basic biological fact that human babies are born knowing nothing about social structures has, however, been anticipated by all societies. Everywhere there exist cultural norms that delineate obligations towards the newborn during the years of learning not only to speak a language but also the art of using that language as a means of self regulation through internal feedback. Language users have to learn both to respond to commands to start an activity and also to develop the skill to respond to an internal conversation that stops an action before it can be seen by others. This inhibitory function of language has to be general enough to be useable in a wide variety of social structures.

These structural norms underlie kinship and kinship sets the rules that govern marriage, parenthood, and preferences for contacts between relatives in general (Farber, 1975; 1977; 1981; Hoyt & Babchuk, 1983). These rules channel a flow of resources to those persons of a network generation who follow marriage rules, obey parental obligations, and work within the system of their society.

For our present purposes, the modern world is distinct from previous centuries because parents have little control over the marriage choices of their children. The law may set an age for marriage, and forbid incestuous unions, and parents may appeal to shared normative rules such as race, ethnicity, or social class to persuade their children of their opinion about their future spouse. They cannot compel, for to be legal, those intending to marry should freely choose each other (Fortes, 1969; Goode, 1963; MacFarlane, 1985). In other words, modern marriage differs from birth in that persons have to do something for themselves in order to reach that status; this act symbolizes achievement, not ascription. Having given that sign in a public ritual, other persons in networks that connect with the new marital pair find themselves in the ascribed roles of in-laws and generational relatives, without their consent being necessary or sought. So a marriage bargain creates personal obligations for others than the principals. These are not entered into by contract or bargaining; these intergenerational expectations operate as custom or tradition, through peer pressures. Only when they falter do they become of immediate interest to the political institutions of the societal community.

The structural divide that liberates persons to make a free choice at marriage separates the societal community into two sections; (1) an informal, private, self-regulating one consisting of marriages, households, interaction networks that link persons to kin, friends and associates, and (2) a formal, public one in which legal authority gives commands, guarantees the freedom of bargaining in markets and in which legal coercion supplements the persuasions of peers.

The sign that this degree of cultural complexity has been reached is the use of absolute age in place of relative age to decide on membership in a generation. Birth registration using a calendar date, whether by the church or by the state, marks the commencement of the use of an absolute age scale. The life of the newborn begins with a public record of the birthdate to symbolize that the event interests the community as well as the ancestors and the kin. Thereafter, lifestyles begin at zero age, the birthdate. The zero point is the key to the formation of cohorts as generational units, composed of individual citizens grouped together with peers of equivalent ages. Citizens placed in groups that have ranks form social class strata. Only in modern nation states are the inhabitants citizens in this sense (Cutler & Bengston, 1974; Eisenstadt, 1956; Marshall, 1950).

Unlike absolute age, relative age is a universal feature of all societal communities. Every human being moves irreversibly through a sequence of ages from birth to death; infancy, youth, marriage, parenthood, grandparenthood, in some form or another family life cycle stages are universally used in human cultures. Parenthood, unlike marriage, is never reversed; once a parent, the status cannot be changed, though the obligations of that status may alter. Generation as a network, then, combines all members of a society who are related by kinship. Kinship sets up a succession of generations relative to each other. Its basic comparison is between parents and children, whatever their dates of birth (Acock & Bengston, 1980; Bengston, 1975; Bettleheim, 1962; Faris, 1947).

Interaction between members in separate generations should proceed on the assumption that the generations form a hierarchy of different ranks or strata. In modern societies, social theory states that exchanges between age cohorts of citizens will be explained by referring to norms different from those used for acts between generations of persons. This is because in the public sector, intergenerational exchanges of goods and services will be organized by bureaucratic agencies. When the context of the exchange is power the norm has been called civility (Elias, 1982). Applied to intergenerational relations this norm results in official actions called entitlements. In these actions, eligibility is determined by formal rules. Today these intergenerational transfers redistribute goods and services between the old and the young, the employed and the unemployed, the handicapped and the fit. Bargaining over the terms of exchange takes place between professionals in the political arena. When the rules apply to all members of an age generation, the stigma of dependency is avoided. The calculations involved in the terms of the exchange, fairness between those equal in eligibility, efficiency and conformity to rules, separate this social process from altruism. The norms of altruism still operate between citizens to motivate individuals to respond to sudden and unanticipated events.

By contrast, intergenerational transfers between parents and children follow a different combination of norms. Between generations as networks there is some bargaining, but the regularity and continuity of these relations has been distinguised from altruism by a new term, amity (Fortes, 1969; Farber, 1981). Goods and services, money and loving, flow from those who control these resources to those who have need of them. Those responding do so to the implicit demands of significant others, not to commands from superiors, nor as a result of bargains that are negotiated between status equals (Sahlins, 1965). This form of unbalanced reciprocity could be called altruism or generosity, if it were sporadic and episodic. All the evidence to be quoted later, is that this self-regulating behavior is continuous between members of different generations and remains an important and essential form of social behavior in all modern societies. It has been estimated that the value of these intergenerational transfers between family members is as much as all political entitlements transferred in the public sector of any modern welfare state (Bowles, 1988).

COHORT GENERATIONS AND SOCIAL POLICY

It has been argued persuasively that citizenship, the separation of administration into public and private sectors, marks the beginning of the modern nation state (Eisenstadt, 1956). This argument can be expanded plausibly by noting that childhood, as a culturally recognized and separate stage of the lifecourse, began at about the same period (Aries, 1962). We may say that citizenship created childhood, because as the nation state evolved there emerged schooling for all, the expectation of a neolocal household as a norm for married couples, and as noted above the legal expectation that those about to marry will bargain freely over that decision, and cannot be forced to marry someone chosen by their parents.

In the nation state, public responsibility turns age mobility into social mobility. Bureaucracies address the problems of individuals by using eligibility rules that apply equally to all members of a class, or cohort. Sudden demographic events, wars, plagues, famines, alter the lifetime prospects for social mobility for all existing cohorts. For example, the unpredicted increase in births in the USA after 1947, the 'baby boom' cohort, led firstly to formal administrative changes in home building by local governments and in its financing by state or federal regulations. Later came changes in schools and universities, and later still, a generation and a decade later, in social security, medical care, and social services to supplement the personal care for older parents by the current generation of child rearers.

Recent public changes in the distribution of resources come about because governments through laws, justified by the norm of civility, command their officials to make them. The top ranks in government agencies prepare rules that transfer goods or services to all eligible individuals in a cohort. Intergenerational transfers of goods or services that are legal and apply equally and efficiently to all members of a class of individuals would be described by social theorists as action with a collectivity orientation. Citizens could try to modify this activity by banding together into associations and petitioning for their view of the situation.

The literature on this period is enormous and expanding. It ap-

pears in economics, administration, law, cultural attitudes as between cohorts, and social policies as well as in family studies, psychology and sociology (Anon., 1987; Binney, 1987; Feuer, 1969;
Foner, 1974; Havlik, 1986; Kertzer & Keith, 1984; Kovar, 1986 (a)
and (b); Lyons, 1986; Mead, 1970; Ray, 1987; Slater, 1976; Smith,
1987; Stone, 1986; Wenger, 1984; Wynne, 1986).

A special element in this stream of research concentrates on social mobility between cohort generations. These publications document changes in social class between parents and children that may
be attributed to structural changes in norms. This sort of change is
called modernization for residents, or acculturation for migrants.
One section of this stream is about the 'three generations hypothesis.' Although much of this literature describes American experiences, this hypothesis was most economically stated in Lancashire
during the first industrial revolution in England. Looking at the
newly rich and powerful mill owners and the new professionals who
served them, the general public predicted these people would go
from '*clogs to clogs in three generations.*' This hypothesis has been
used more often to explain the differences in attitudes between immigrant parents and their American born children; but that literature
belongs more to intergenerational connections between networks
than between cohorts. It comes in the next section of this paper
(Andersson, 1973; Bowers, 1987; Bytheway, 1977; Connor, 1974;
Duncan & Morgan, 1983; Francesca, 1958; Gilmore, 1932; Hill et
al., 1970; Hofstee & Kooy, 1956; Jennings, 1981; Kitano, 1961;
Klatzky, 1972; Kobayashi, 1956; Knight & Kagan, 1978; Kovar,
1986 (b); 1988; Lazerwitz & Rowitz, 1964; Roher & Edmunson,
1960; Segalen, 1977; Sharot, 1973; Thomas, 1974; Thrall, 1978;
Wenger, 1984; Wisler & Eklund, 1986; Wynne, 1986).

NETWORK GENERATIONS
AND SOCIAL ATTITUDES

Studies of generations as networks turn the three generation hypothesis around by asking how do these collective norms come to
affect persons? In theory terms this is a self orientation approach, to
contrast with the collective orientation in the discussion of genera-

tions as cohorts. Papers on the three generation hypothesis in this literature often focus on custom or tradition in place of formal arguments using rationality or due process. The concern of these scholars is with explaining how social attitudes, or norms, or expectations, are transferred between members of different generations. Instead of members being considered as persons or as individuals, this is the research world of the self as a crucial part of modern society.

The foundations of self identity are laid down during caregiving between a specific mother and her child. This process of taking turns might be stated more generally as between adults of one generation and the newborns who will succeed them. Against this statement, success in the transformation of a newborn into a self-regulating person seems to depend on continuous interaction for a number of years between a specific adult and a newborn. This continuity, in its turn, depends on the difference in status of the two generations. Such a hierarchical structure depends for its permanence on the inability of the members to change the status structure. The newborn cannot take commands, nor can they bargain, nor keep a contract, so they are dependent on the normative propensity of the adult to meet their demands for goods (food) and services (loving care). In this structure taking turns depends on the norm of amity. Neither exchange theory whose process is bargaining, nor organization theory, where behavior follows commands from those higher in status, has had much success in interpretating data in this area of family sociology (Furstenburg et al., 1987; Johnson & Stokes, 1976; Johnson & Barer, 1987; Kivnik, 1982; Klein & Aldous, 1987; Peterson & Rollins, 1987; Powell & Arquitt, 1978; Sussman, 1955).

In the beginning of this paper I made two summary theory statements: (1) feelings of solidarity or attachment between parent and child still persist between American generations; (2) that this continuing relationship is not adequately explained by any current social theory. A more recent publication about the problem of explaining solidarity allows me to add new detail to this discussion. Using about 250 sets of three generation lineages containing over 2000 respondents, thirteen significantly different patterns of solidarity among lineages are recognized. By solidarity these researchers mean similarities between members of the same kin network in attitudes and behaviors (Mangan et al., 1988).

From this report, solidarity between generational networks can be said to be related to two major variables, the proximity of the households, and the affect felt in the bond between the persons. When households live close-by, interaction is easier and more frequent, and this in turn enables persons to care for each other through the exchanges of services and gifts. This is the basic thesis of exchange theory; it says that proximity leads to interaction, that interaction leads to feelings of closeness, and that this friendly feeling leads to generosity in the exchanges. Unfortunately only 13% of lineage exchanges follows this pattern. Among the geographically distant kin, more than half continue to feel close, though the frequency of interaction is low. For proximity, the unit of analysis is the household.

The second major variable, affect, comes through the analysis most clearly when it is negative. Those individuals who feel socially distant, though they live close-by, have little interaction and fewer exchanges of services. Some 18% of grandparents, parents and children behave as if they were neighbors and follow this pattern. For the rest, 69% of the sets, using the proximity variable explains as much of the variance in the data as the affect variable does. Consequently, the linear models of exchange theory do explain more of the behavior than any other. It remains difficult to tell whether the explanation is based on residential choice or on affect, the inner feelings.

All the persons in this study are related by kinship. If kinship was a single variable it could not be used to explain differences in the feelings that relatives have for one another. However, kinship is complex and any explanation for the strength of feelings in kin networks will use more than one variable. Within the kinship network, obligations felt towards ancestors can differ from those felt towards children or grandchildren, and from those felt towards aunts, cousins or uncles or towards more distant relatives. The norm of amity, the expectation that relatives should get treated more generously than non-relatives, allows for differences in attitudes and behavior between generations. The 'three generations hypothesis' explains these variations by pointing to changes in the economy or in national political institutions. Exchange theories explain them by variations in interaction frequency. Such explanations rest either on the norm of civility, the response of command systems such as organizations, or alternatively on the norm of the market and that is to bargain over the outcome of the interaction. The norm of amity, that the demands of kin take priority, provides a third possibility for an explanation. This normative response begins with filiation, the self identity established in infancy before other skills in interaction are learned.

Kinship combines three independent dimensions: marriage which is a bargain or market type relation, residence which is an achievement or performance type relation, and generation which through amity gives generosity to the responses that relatives give to the demands of other relatives. Kinship structures are informal and self-regulating. Because this sense of identity represents the filiation of the self to the collective kin network, obligations between members are not easily changed. For the same reason, these obligations give rise to feelings of personal guilt and so can never be entirely passed over to public agencies, or to the marketplace. In the choice of friends among members of voluntary networks, age and sex are important variables, but kinship positions which use distance from an ancestor as well as age and sex, have an extra specificity that seems to be related to the extent of the claims that can be made on others of a different generation (Davis, 1985; McPherson & Smith-Lovin, 1987; Sprey & Matthews, 1985).

The evidence for modern changes in intergenerational relations is voluminous. On a national scale since 1900, the rise of social work as a new profession and the increase in the number of its practitioners in both public and private practice, marks a fundamental change in the demands that persons belonging to current generations make on their communities of residence. The self-regulating, private, world in which family tradition saw that basic moral values continued for another generation, now requires guidance from other institutions of society (Kaslow, 1980).

Using the concepts of this essay, we might interpret these changes as the transfer of normative control over response patterns from demand based amity structures to two other social structures.

One would be the market, in that persons now exercise new choices in free bargaining. Second would be political command structures, where individuals use citizenship, rather than kinship or ethnicity, to claim an entitlement to public support. As these changes occur, relations between family members and other relatives are becoming more and more like those between friends, neighbors, or associates in voluntary groups. This transformation is undoubtedly happening: records show that more and more marriages end in divorce and remarriage is common. So is living together without marriage.

The family household has also changed composition in that homes with two parents living with their own children are only about 30% of all households and the numbers of one parent households, mostly mothers and children, are increasing. In the 1980 Census they amounted to 7% of all 81 million households. Yet, from another standpoint, family and kinship continue to explain the composition of households. Between 1960 and 1976, children under 18 living with a non-relative fell from 1% to 0.7% and in 1980 parents and children living with a non-relative made up less than 0.7% of all family households (Glick, 1977; Kovar, 1986 (a); Minkler, M. & Stone, R. 1985; Mogey, 1988; Sweet & Bumpass, 1987).

Further, those who live alone, 23% of all households in 1980, are helped with the activities of daily living and receive most gifts of money or goods from kin (Cheal, 1983; Mogey, 1988; Sussman et al., 1970). Disinheriting a relative is a rare event. Survey records show that only 5% or 6% of wills disbar legal heirs from inheriting (Rosenfeld, 1982; Cates & Sussman, 1983). Intergenerational caregiving for the elderly, studied by many careful researchers over the past twenty years, involves public agencies, the purchase of services, informal support groups, and relatives. Kinship dominates these networks. The most frequent and reliable help is exchanged between parents and children. When this fails, other close relatives take over; when these fail more distant relatives are called upon. Few persons turn for care to non-kin individuals like friends, neighbors, or associates such as fellow church members, but some do (Landsberger, 1985; Litwak, 1985; Riley et al., 1972; Shanas & Streib, 1965; Steinmetz, 1988; Sussman, 1979; Wenger, 1984).

In this hierarchy of intergenerational interactions, the specificity or diffuseness of the relationship can be used to explain how certain changes occur. Diffuse statuses, those that are achieved through performance, require separate physical spaces for their action (Sommer, 1969). If household members are related to each other by kinship statuses, that are ascribed and not achieved, then family households can share a common physical space. Relatives value each other for their own sake and not for their performance alone.

SUMMARY

In this essay, statements used in the research literature about relations between the generations are examined to discover how theories are being used. It is a murky area but continuity for longer than a single lifespan seems clearly to be associated with a hierarchy social structure. Hierarchies, based on inequalities in status that are difficult to change, are contrasted to markets, where those who interact behave as if they were equals in the processes of exchange.

Ascribed status is difficult to change and age, a crucial basis for generational classes, is an ascribed status. However, age can be measured either on an absolute scale, or on a relative one. For absolute age, there must be a political decision to apply the same time scale to all citizens. Alternatively, age may compare each member of a set to a common ancestor; these groups are kin or ethnic groups, depending on the way that membership in the networks is defined.

It would seem that differences in the norms for entry into these two sorts of age-based hierarchy generate distinct sorts of response from the members of a society. Professionals in government offices count citizens in cohorts and, responding to commands that are made legitimate by shared expectations, generate entitlements for those eligible. These expectations lead to intergenerational transfers as citizenship tries to correct abuses or to respond to conflicts in other parts of the society. Of course, some bureaucrats are incompetent, and some citizens are greedy, so the norm of civility needs to be moderated by other norms from the wider context of the societal community.

The second form of age-based hierarchy is self directing and follows the norms of amity and altruism. Amity is the norm of kinship, while altruism is the norm of friendship. Following marriage which is the result of bargaining and agreement between the two partners, the norm of kinship sets obligations to respond, not to commands, but to demands made by members of the network. Kinship functions through marriages, parenthood, grandparenthood, close and distant relatives. Interactions between kin become apparent through observations about household composition, and inter-household exchanges of goods and services. This private intergenerational connection continues to transfer as much resources between the generations as do public sector entitlements in all modern industrial societies. When amity expectations are not met, as in abandonment of kin, child abuse, or distortion of self identity, neither the norm of civility, nor that of altruism can easily correct the problem. Altruism describes the exchanges between friends, neighbors, or associates in the society; it is based on balanced reciprocity and so is episodic and activated most often in exceptional rather than repetitive situations.

The essay raised the issue of the continuity of intergenerational transfers between kin while at the same time noting the evidence of a breakdown in domestic relations. Kinship creates self and maintains the capacity of the self to choose a personal lifestyle. No society can be understood as authority or as contract relations without an exploration of the conceptual base for kinship, or to use a term of this essay, demand structures. A similar conclusion is reached in a broader review of theory for social support; in it, demands are conceived as the source of conflicts, and support as the affective aspect of processes that produce and reproduce integration, or continuity, in social structures (House et al., 1988).

Intergenerational connections between citizens set the conditions from which lifestyles can be chosen. Kinship networks and households are units where individuals can forge a shared lifestyle. They are maintained by a complex set of transfers, from kin, from markets, and from public treasuries. In turn, households and kinship networks turn newborns into persons who can participate in the public life of their society first as children and later as citizens.

REFERENCES

Acock, A. C. & Bengston, V. L. (1980). Socialization and attribution processes: Actual versus perceived similarity among parents and youth. *Journal of Marriage and the Family, 42,* 501-515.

Anonymous. (1987). Intergenerational programs in the 'Youth 2000' Campaign. *Aging,* 356, 17-20.

Andersson, B. E. (1973). Misunderstandings between generations. A general phenomenon. *Scandinavian Journal of Educational Resources,* 1-10.

Aries, P. (1962). *Centuries of childhood: A social history of family life.* New York: Vintage Books.

Bengtson, V. L. (1975). Generation and family effects in value socialization. *American Sociological Review, 40*(3), 358-371.

Bettleheim, B. (1962). The problem of generations. *Daedalus, 91,* 68-96.

Binney, E. A. (1987). The retreat of the State and its transfer of responsibility: The intergenerational war. *International Journal of Health Services,* 18(1), 83-96.

Bowers, B. J. (1987). Intergenerational caregiving: Adult caregivers and their aging parents. *Adv. Nurs. S., 9*(2), 20-31.

Bowles, S. (1988, November 6). Set a Moral Agenda for the Economy. *New York Times,* Business Section.

Burgess, E. W. (1957). The older generation and the family. In W. Donahue & C. Tibbetts (Eds.), *The new frontiers of aging* (pp. 158-171). Ann Arbor: Univ. Michigan Press.

Burr, W. R., Hill, R., Nye, F. I., & Reiss, I. L. (Eds.). (1979). *Contemporary theories about the family* (Vols. 1 & 1). New York: Free Press.

Bytheway, W. (1977). Problems of representation in the three generation family. *Journal of Marriage and the Family, 39*(2), 243-250.

Cates, J. & Sussman, M. B. (1983). *Family systems and inheritance.* New York: Haworth Press.

Cheal, D. J. (1983). Intergenerational family transfers. *Journal of Marriage and the Family, 45*(4), 805-813.

Connor, J. W. (1974). Acculturation and family continuities in three generations of Japanese Americans. *Journal of Marriage and the Family, 36*(1), 159-165.

Cutler, N. E. & Bengston, V. L. (1974). Age and political alienation; maturation, generation and period effects. *American Academy of Political and Social Sciences Annals,* 415, 160-175.

Davis, R. A. (1985). Social structure, belief, attitude, intention, and behavior: A partial test of Liska's revisions. *Social Psychology Quarterly, 48*(1), 89-93.

Dumont, L. (1980). *Homo hierarchicus: An essay on the caste system and its implications.* Chicago: Univ. of Chicago Press.

Duncan, G. J. & Morgan, J. N. (1983). Five thousand American families: Patterns of economic progress. Ann Arbor: Institution of Social Research.

Eisenstadt, S. (1956). From generation to generation: Age groups and social structure. Glencoe: Free Press.

Elias, N. (1982). *Power and civility—The civilizing process (Vol. 2)*. New York: Pantheon Books.

Farber, B. (1977). Social context, kinship mapping and family norms. *Journal of Marriage and the Family, 33*(2), 227-240.

Farber, B. (1975). Bilateral kinship: centripetal and centrifugal types of organization. *Journal of Marriage and the Family, 37*(4), 871-888.

Farber, B. (1981). *Conceptions of kinship*. New York: Elsevier.

Faris, R. E. (1947). Interaction of generations and family stability. *American Sociological Review, 12*, 159-164.

Feather, N. T. & Cross, D. G. (1975). Value systems and delinquency: Parental and generational discrepancies in value systems for delinquent and non-delinquent boys. *British Journal of Social and Clinical Psychology, 14*(2), 117-129.

Feuer, L. S. (1969). *The conflict of generations: The character and significance of student movements*. New York: Basic Books.

Foner, N. (1984). *Ages in conflict: A cross cultural perspective on inequality between old and young*. New York: Columbia University Press.

Fortes, M. (1969). *Kinship and the social order*. Chicago: Aldine.

Francesca, S. M. (1958). Variations of selected cultural patterns among three generations of Mexicans in San Antonio, Texas. *American Catholic Sociological Review, 19*, 24-34.

Furstenburg, F. F., Brooks-Gunn, J., Morgan, S. P. (1987). *Adolescent mothers in later life*. New York: Cambridge University Press.

Gallaher, B. J. (1974). An empirical analysis of attitude differences between three kin related generations. *Youth and Society, 5*(3), 327-349.

Gilmore, H. W. (1932). Five generations of a begging family. *American Journal of Sociology, 37*, 768-774.

Glick, P. (1977). Marrying, divorcing and living together in the U.S. today. *Population Bulletin, 32*(5), 1-41.

Goode, W. J. (1963). *World revolution and family patterns*. New York: Macmillan.

Havlik, R. J. (1986). Impaired senses for sound and light in persons age 65 years and over. In *Aging in the eighties. Advance Data from Vital and Health Statistics No. 125* (DHHS Pub. No. (PHS) 86-1250). Washington, DC: National Center for Health Statistics.

Hill, R., Foote, N., Aldous, J., Carlson, R., Macdonald, R. (1970). *Family development in three generations*. Cambridge, MA: Schenkman.

Hofstee, E. W. & Kooy, G. A. (1956). Traditional households and neighborhood group: Survival of the genealogical territorial societal patterns in eastern parts of the Netherlands. *Transcripts of the 3rd World Congress of Sociology, 4*, 75-79.

House, J. S., Umberson, D., Landis, K. R. (1988). Structures and processes of social support. In W. R. Scott & J. Blake (Eds.), *Annual review of sociology: Vol. 14* (pp. 291-318). Palo Alto: Annual Reviews Inc.

Hoyt, D. R. & Babchuk, N. (1983). The selective formation of intimate ties with kin. *Social Forces, 62*(1), 84-101.

Jennings, M. K. (1981). *Generations and politics: A panel study of young adults and their parents.* Princeton: Princeton Univ. Press.

Johnson, C. L. & Barer, B. M. (1987). Marital instability and the changing kinship networks of grandparents. *The Gerontologist, 27,* 330-335.

Johnson, N. E. & Stokes, C. S. (1976). Family size in successive generations: The effects of birth order, intergenerational change in life style, and familial satisfaction. *Demography, 13*(2), 175-187.

Kaslow, F. W. (1980). History of family therapy in the United States: A kaleidoscopic overview. *Marriage and Family Review, 13,* 77-111.

Kell, L. & Aldous, J. (1960). Trends in child care over three generations. *Marriage and Family Living, 22,* 176-177.

Kertzer, D. J. & Keith, J. (Eds.). (1984). *Age and anthropological theory.* Ithaca: Cornell University Press.

Kitano, H. (1961). Differential child rearing attitudes between first and second generation Japanese in the United States. *Journal of Social Psychology, 53,* 13-19.

Kivnick, H. Q. (1982). Grandparenthood: An overview of meaning and mental health. *The Gerontologist, 22,* 59-66.

Klatzky, S. R. (1972). *Patterns of contact with relatives.* Washington, DC: American Sociological Association.

Klein, D. M. & Aldous, J. (Eds.). (1988). *Social stress and family development.* New York: Guilford Press.

Knight, G. P. & Kagan, S. (1977). Development of prosocial and competitive behaviors in Anglo-American and Mexican-American children. *Child Development, 48,* 1385-1394.

Kobayashi, K. (1956). A statistical study of the generation composition of farm households. *Juik Omondai Kenkyu-10-Kenkyushirio,* 113 (Japanese).

Kovar, M.G. (1986a). Preliminary data from the supplement on aging to the National Health Interview Survey—National Center for Health Statistics. In *Aging in the eighties. Vital and Health Statistics No. 115* (DHHS Pub. No. 86-1250). Washington, DC: 1986 National Center for Health Statistics.

Kovar, M. G. (1986b). Age 65 Years and over and living alone: Contacts with family, friends, and neighbors. In *Aging in the eighties. Vital and Health Statistics No. 116* (DHHS Pub. No. 86-1250). Washington, DC: National Center for Health Statistics.

Kovar, M. G. (1988). People living alone—Two years later. In *Aging in the eighties. Vital and Health Statistics No. 149* (DHHS Pub. No. 88-1250). Washington, DC: National Center for Health Statistics.

Landsberger, B. H. (1985). *Long term care of the elderly: A comparative view of layers of care.* New York: St. Martins.

Lazerwitz, B. & Rowitz, L. (1964). The three generations hypothesis. *American Journal of Sociology*, *69*(5), 529-538.

Litwak, E. (1985). *Helping the elderly: The complimentary roles of informal networks and formal systems*. New York: Guilford.

Litwak, E. & Kulis, S. (1987). Technology, proximity and measures of kin support. *Journal of Marriage and the Family*, *49*(3), 649-661.

Lyons, C. W. (1986). Generations together. *Children Today*, *15*, 21-26.

MacFarlane, A. (1985). *Marriage and love in England: Modes of reproduction, 1300-1840*. New York: Basil Blackwell.

Mangan, D. J. (1987). Measuring intergenerational family relations. *Research In Aging*, *8*(4), 515-535.

Mangan, D. J., Bengston, V. L., Landry, P. H. (Eds.). (1988). *Measurement of intergenerational relations*. Newbury Park, CA: Sage Publications.

Mannheim, K. (1952). *Essays on the sociology of knowledge*. London: Routledge & Kegan Paul.

Marshall, T. (1950). *Citizenship and social class*. London: University Press.

McPherson, J. M. & Smith-Lovin, L. (1987). Homophily in voluntary organizations: Status distance and the composition of face-to-face groups. *American Sociological Review*, *52*, 370-379.

Mead, M. (1970). *Culture and commitment: A Study of the generation gap*. Garden City: National History Press.

Minkler, M. & Stone, R. (1985). The feminization of poverty and older women. *The Gerontologist*, *25*, 351-357.

Mogey, J. (1988). Households of the elders. In S. K. Steinmetz (Ed.), *Family and support systems across the lifespan* (pp. 213-224). New York: Plenum Press.

Palmore, E. (1981). *Social patterns in normal aging: Findings from the Duke longitudinal study*. Durham, NC: Duke University Press.

Parsons, T. (1971). *The system of modern societies*. Englewood Cliffs: Prentice-Hall.

Peterson, G. W. & Rollins, B. C. (1987). Parent-child socialization. In M. B. Sussman & S. K. Steinmetz (Eds.), *Handbook of marriage and the family* (pp. 471-507). New York: Plenum Press.

Powell, J. A. & Arquitt, G. E. (1978). Getting the generations back together: A rationale for the development of community based intergenerational programs. *The Family Coordinator*, *27*(4), 421-426.

Ray, D. (1987). Economic growth and intergenerational altruism. *Review of Economic Sciences*, *54*(2), 227-234.

Riley, M. W., Johnson, M., Foner, A. (1972). *Aging and society, Vol. 3, A sociology of age stratification*. New York: Russell Sage.

Robertson, J. F. (1975). Interaction in three generation families: Parents as mediators. Towards a theoretical perspective. *International Journal of Aging & Human Development*, *6*(2), 103-110.

Robertson, J. F. (1977). Grandmotherhood. *Journal of Marriage and the Family*, *39*(1), 165-174.

Rosenfeld, J. P. (1982). Disinheritance and will contests. *Marriage and Family Review*, 5(3), 75-86.

Sahlins, M. D. (1965). On the sociology of primitive exchange. In M. Gluckman & F. Eggan (Eds.), *The relevance of models for social anthropology*. New York: Barnes and Noble.

Segalen, M. (1977). The family life cycle and household structure: Five generations in a French village. *Journal of Family History*, 2(3), 223-236.

Shanas, E. & Streib, G. (Eds.). (1965). *Social structure and the family: Intergenerational relations*. Englewood Cliffs: Prentice Hall.

Sharot, S. (1973). The three generations thesis and the American Jews. *British Journal of Sociology*, 24(2), 151-164.

Shock, N. W., Andres, R., Arensberg, D., Costa, P. J. Jr., Greulich, R. C., Tobin, J. D. (1984). *Normal human aging: The Baltimore longitudinal study of aging* (N.I.H. Publ. No. 84-2450). Washington, DC: U.S. Government, Department of Health and Human Services.

Slater, P. E. (1976). *The pursuit of loneliness: American culture at the breaking point*. Boston: Beacon Press.

Smith, L. (1987). The war between the generations. *Fortune*, 116, 78-80.

Sommer, R. (1969). *Personal space: The behavioral basis of design*. Englewood Cliffs: Prentice Hall.

Sprey, J. & Matthews, S. H. (1985). Adolescents relationships with grandparents: An empirical contribution to conceptual clarification. *Journal of Gerontology*, 40, 621-626.

Steinmetz, S. K. (Ed.). (1988). *Family and support systems across the life span*. New York: Plenum.

Stone, R. (1986). Age 65 Years and over — Use of community services. *Aging in the Eighties: Vital and Health Statistics No. 124* (DHHS Pub. No. (PHS) 86-1250). Washington, DC: National Center for Health Statistics.

Sussman, M. B. (1955). Family continuity: Selective factors which affect relationships between families at generational levels. *Marriage and Family Living*, 16, 112-120.

Sussman, M. B. & Jeter, K. (1979). *Social and economic supports and family environments for the elderly*. (Final Report — Grant #90-A-316(03). Washington, DC: Administration on Aging.

Sussman, M. B., Cates, J. N., Smith, D. T. (1970). *The family and inheritance*. New York: Russell Sage.

Sussman, M. B. & Steinmetz, S. K., (Eds.). (1987). *Handbook of marriage and the family*. New York: Plenum.

Sweet, J. A. & Bumpass, L. L. (1987). *American families and households*. New York: Russell Sage.

Thomas, L. E. (1974). Generational discontinuity in beliefs: An exploration of the generation gap. *Journal of Social Issues*, 30(3), 1-22.

Thrall, C. A. (1978). Who does what? Role stereotypy, children's work and continuity between the generations in household divisions. *Human Relations, 31*(3), 249-266.

Troll, L. & Bengston, V. L. (1979). Generations in the family. In W. R. Burr, R. Hill, F. I. Nye, I. L. Reiss (Eds.), *Contemporary theories about the family* (pp. 127-161). New York: Free Press.

Wellman, B. (1979). The community question. *American Journal of Sociology, 84*, 1201-1231.

Wenger, G. C. (1984). *The supportive network: Coping with old age*. London: Allen & Unwin.

Wisler, S. C. & Eklund, S. J. (1986). Women's ambitions: A three generation study. *Psychological Women Quarterly, 10*, 353-362.

Wynne, E. A. (1986). Will the Young support the old? *Society, 23*(6), 40-47.

Life Course Perspectives on Intergenerational and Generational Connections

Linda K. George
Deborah T. Gold

Life course perspectives are recent additions to the conceptual armamentarium of the social sciences. Nonetheless, they already have demonstrated their value for understanding temporal aspects of life patterns. At the individual level, life course perspectives have proven to be especially important in highlighting the ways that events and decisions that occur earlier in life can have persistent effects on the structure and quality of life at later points in time. At the macro, population-based level, life course perspectives have been useful in highlighting the ways in which social change generates different patterns of social structure and personal biography across cohorts.

In this paper, we examine the contributions and limitations of life course perspectives as conceptual tools for understanding generational and intergenerational connections in the family. The family is an ideal context for application of life course perspectives. Several authors have noted that it is the "middle ground" (Hagestad, 1990) of primary groups such as the family that hold the most promise for

Linda K. George is Professor, Departments of Psychiatry and Sociology, Duke University, and Associate Director, Duke University Center for the Study of Aging and Human Development. Deborah T. Gold is Assistant Professor, Departments of Psychiatry and Sociology, Duke University, and Senior Fellow, Duke University Center for the Study of Aging and Human Development.

Preparation of this paper was supported by two grants from the National Institute on Aging (AG00371 and AG05462) and a grant from the NIH Division of Research Resources (BSRG SO7 RR 05405).

explicating the links between the individual and society and between history and biography. Similarly, Elder has consistently urged investigators to explore the meanings of historical and social changes via their effects on the primary environments of family, work, and friends (e.g., Elder, 1974; 1985a; Elder & Clipp, 1988). We believe that the extant knowledge base supports these hypotheses regarding natural and useful links between life course perspectives and family relationships within and across cohorts and generations.

This paper is organized into three major sections. In the first, general principles of life course perspectives that are particularly relevant to generational and intergenerational connections are briefly reviewed. In the second and major section, the impact of social change on family life course patterns during the past century is examined. Evidence is presented that demographic and other changes have both generated new family forms and transformed the parameters of family relationships. In the final section, the contributions and limitations of life course perspectives are briefly discussed in broader context. Because of space limitations this review is necessarily selective rather than comprehensive.

LIFE COURSE PERSPECTIVES: GENERAL PRINCIPLES

There is no systematic, unified theory of the life course. Instead, it is appropriate to discuss *life course perspectives*. Two aspects of this phrase merit attention: (1) use of the term "perspectives" rather than "theory" and (2) use of the plural (i.e., perspectives) rather than the singular (i.e., perspective). These characteristics highlight the fluid and heterogeneous nature of life course perspectives in the social sciences. Nonetheless, life course perspectives also share important general principles. Four of these principles are particularly relevant to understanding intergenerational and generational connections in the family.

The life course is a social phenomenon, distinct from the life span (e.g., Clausen, 1986; George, 1982; Hagestad & Neugarten, 1985). Most scholars agree that life span refers to duration of life and that life-span characteristics are closely related to age and relatively invariant across time and place. In contrast, the life course reflects the intersection of social and historical factors with personal biography. Moreover, heterogeneity of life course patterns is expected within and across time and space. In our later discussions of generational and intergenerational connections, special attention is paid to cohort differences in life patterns and to gender and race as important sources of variability in life course patterns.

Life course perspectives focus on the "age-differentiated, socially-recognized sequences of transitions" (Rossi, 1980) that characterize the lives of individuals, population subgroups, and populations. Within this rubric, investigators examine a variety of life course issues. Some scholars focus on one or more characteristics of life course transitions, such as prevalence, duration, timing, and sequencing. Other investigators focus on the antecedents and consequences of life course transitions. Also, life course patterns are examined at multiple levels, though integration of findings from macro- and micro-levels has yet to be successfully achieved (Bengtson, 1986).

The concepts of transitions and trajectories are particularly important in life course perspectives (Elder, 1985a; Hagestad, 1990). Transitions refer to changes in status (sometimes called changes in role states, e.g., Nydegger, 1986) that are discrete and relatively bounded in duration (although their consequences may be observed over long periods of time). Trajectories refer to long-term patterns of stability and change, often including multiple transitions, that can be reliably differentiated from alternate patterns. Transitions and trajectories are inherently interrelated. As Elder notes, "transitions are always embedded in trajectories that give them distinctive form and meaning" (1985a, p. 31). It is tempting, but inappropriate, to view trajectories as synonomous with the more familiar concept of career. There are two major differences between trajectories and careers. First, unlike careers, trajectories are not assumed to involve specific stages or steps toward a predetermined outcome. Second, the term career typically is applied to a single life domain, e.g., occupational careers, family careers. In contrast, trajectories often include the intersections and joint effects of multiple life domains. Family life is characterized by both transitions and trajectories. Examples of family transitions include marriage, parenthood, and widowhood. Trajectories also are applicable to family relationships. For example, one may occupy the status of child for fifty years or more, but the role of child changes with time and differs across status occupants, yielding multiple trajectories. Other trajectories may involve multiple domains, such as family and work. Thus, investigators may examine the impact of family transitions on women's work trajectories.

As implied by previous principles, life course analysis requires a dynamic, longitudinal perspective. This dynamic orientation is critical for both population and individual studies. Unfortunately, longitudinal data spanning long periods of time are very scarce. Consequently, the vast majority of research informed by life course perspectives examines transitions rather than trajectories. (For an exception, however, see the edited volume by Elder, 1985b.) As further described in a later section, most extant research examining trajectories is based on simulated cohorts and retrospective life accounts rather than on longitudinal data. The study of life course trajectories also is hindered by statistical methods. Although hazard models in general and event history analysis in particular have advanced our understanding of life course transitions, such models are quite limited in terms of the ability to link multiple transitions in a way suitable for identification of long-term patterns (Allison, 1984; Winship, 1986).

Life course studies are relatively recent additions to the social sciences, though research in developmental psychology and the social aspects of aging was important in fostering the development of life course perspectives. In the United States, Elder's study of *Children of the Great Depression* (1974) is widely recognized as a critical catalyst in the development of life course perspectives. Following his lead, most U.S. investigators using life course perspectives have focused on transitions, their characteristics, and their consequences. Though these studies are more historical—in the sense of identifying historical conditions that generate cohort differences—than much previous research that examined transitions and other life events, the focus has remained fixed largely on life course patterns for cohorts born in the 20th century.

Other scholars, often European rather than North American, have examined the historical conditions—including demographic, structural, and cultural changes—that set the stage for emergence of the life course as a concept that is meaningful to both social scientists and their study participants (e.g., Anderson, 1985; Kohli, 1986; Kohli & Meyer, 1986; Meyer, 1988). It is generally agreed that the dramatic increase in life expectancy during the past 100 years or so—with the result that a majority of persons born now survive to late adulthood—was a necessary prerequisite for emergence of the life course as a meaningful cultural construct (e.g., Watkins, Menken, & Bongaarts, 1987; Riley, 1986). In addition, social differentiation resulting from industrialization, urbanization, and the rise of the modern nation state generated the heterogeneity of life patterns, as well as a mode of consciousness based on the individual rather than the collectivity and a "temporalized" view of life, that facilitated social construction of concepts such as life course, personal biography, and "social clocks" (Mayer & Muller, 1986; Roth, 1983).

Ironically, just as social change set the stage for the emergence of life course as a meaningful concept, social change may render it obsolete. During the past decade, scholars have come to recognize that the life course is both less predictable and more heterogeneous than was initially imagined. Earlier depictions of the life course emphasized the existence of age norms, relative consensus concerning the preferred sequencing of life course transitions, and similarities in the timing of transitions both within and across cohorts (e.g., Clausen, 1986; Neugarten & Hagestad, 1976; Hogan, 1981). Recent writings emphasize the modest to weak associations between age and many life course transitions, the modest relationships between preferred and actual sequencing of life course transitions, and the tremendous variability of transitions and trajectories within and across cohorts (e.g., Hagestad, 1990; O'Rand, 1990; Kertzer & Hogan, 1988). In these later writings, scholars attribute much of the variability to social change. For example, as discussed in greater detail in the next section, it now appears that the diversity of family forms characteristic of modern U.S. society in large part reflects the joint effects of dramatic increases in life expectancy and greatly increased personal choice in the areas of marriage and parenthood. Though less often noted in explicit terms, the *rate* of social change also appears to affect life course heterogeneity. Rapid rates of social change increase differences between and within cohorts. Thus, one might speculate that, if rates of social change continue to escalate, it may become more difficult to incorporate the resulting diversity of transitions and trajectories under the umbrella of a single concept such as the life course.

IMPACT OF SOCIAL CHANGE ON INTERGENERATIONAL AND GENERATIONAL FAMILY CONNECTIONS

During the past century, family life in Western, particularly North American societies has been dramatically affected by two major types of social change (Bengtson, Rosenthal, & Burton, 1990). First, a number of demographic shifts—primarily dramatic increases in life expectancy and concomitant decreases in fertility—have changed the structure of families and, hence, family roles. Second, there has been increased diversity in family forms, behaviors, and norms. The traditional nuclear family, consisting of a once-married couple and their minor children, has become less prevalent—though it appears that, despite its waning prevalence, this family form remains a cultural ideal (Sweet & Bumpass, 1987). In this section, we examine several family forms of increasing prevalence in North American society. For each family form described, implications for generational and intergenerational connections also are discussed. Decreasing family involvement by men, changes in the predictability of family transitions, and marital quality also are discussed.

Verticalization of the Family

A major change in family structure during the past century is the "verticalization" of the family—a pattern also described as emergence of the "beanpole family structure" (Bengtson et al., 1990; Hagestad, 1988; Knipscheer, 1988). Verticalization refers to an increase in the number of generations in a family accompanied by a decrease in the number of family members within generations. Emergence of this family form is a direct result of increased longevity and decreased fertility. Verticalization is probably the most consistent and important change in family structure during the past century.

Verticalization of the family has a number of potentially consequential implications for family roles, transitions, and trajectories. For example, verticalization has altered the length of time spent in specific family roles. Using simulated cohort data from census records, Gee (1986) compared time spent in specific family roles by Canadian women in the 1830s and the 1950s. She estimates that, during the 1830s, married women spent fully 90% of their married years rearing minor children. By the 1950s, this percentage had dropped to 40%. In another study of Canadian adults, Gee (1987) estimated that in 1860, 16% of 50 year old Canadians still had living parents. By 1960, this proportion had increased to 60%. Watkins et al. (1987) report similar results for three simulated cohorts of U.S. adults in 1800, 1900, and 1980. They estimate that the number of years that an American woman could expect to have living parents nearly tripled between 1800 and 1980. Thus, emergence of adult children as the "generational bridge" between grandchild and grandparent generations (Knipscheer, 1988) is a recent phenomenon — and represents a status that most North American adults occupy for a significant length of time. Verticalization of the family also underlies, in part, the emergence of scientific and policy interest in middle-aged adults as caregivers of impaired older parents (e.g., Brody, 1981).

Because of sex differences in longevity, verticalization has had stronger effects on the family lives of women than of men (Bengtson et al., 1990; Treas & Bengtson, 1987). Although the proportion of adulthood spent as parents of minor children has decreased and the proportion of time spent as adult children of surviving parents has increased for both sexes, differences across time and cohorts have been greater for women. Thus, even widespread patterns of change can have differential effects for population subgroups.

It is likely that verticalization has other important consequences for family relationships. For example, patterns of interaction, value congruence, and exchange of instrumental support across and within generations may be affected by the extent to which family linkages are vertical vs. horizontal (Bengtson et al., 1990). At this point, there are no data that permit comparison of the more horizontal families of earlier decades with the more vertical families of recent history. It would be possible, however, to compare current families that differ in degree of verticalization in terms of these kinds of family characteristics. Though such comparisons could not be used to generalize about historical changes in family characteristics, they would highlight differences that may be associated with vertical vs. horizontal family structures.

Age-Condensed and Age-Gapped Family Structures

During the past three decades, timing of the transition to parenthood has become less predictable. For the population as a whole, age at birth of first child has increased for women. However, this population trend masks distinctive patterns of family structure (Baldwin & Nord, 1984). Bengtson et al. (1990) describe two increasingly common family patterns based on timing of fertility: age-condensed family structure and age-gapped family structure.

The age-condensed family form results from early fertility, especially teenage pregnancy. Early fertility results in small age distances between generations. Specifically, early fertility results in not only a young mother, but also in young grandparents and, perhaps in young great-grandparents. In age-condensed families, boundaries between generations are likely to blur because of the narrow age gap between them (Bengtson et al., 1990). This is especially likely when early fertility occurs across multiple generations of family members.

There are few empirical studies of age-condensed families and their implications for generational and intergenerational relationships. An important exception to this pattern, however, is the work of Burton (1985; 1990; Burton & Bengtson, 1985; Hagestad & Burton, 1985). Burton studied intergenerational relationships in multi-generational black families, many of which displayed age-condensed family structures. Her findings suggest that age-condensed family structure is associated with characteristic patterns of family relationships and strains. Most of the young grandmothers in these families resisted participation in active grandparenting and were especially unlikely to participate in direct care of the infant and the teenage mother (Burton & Bengtson, 1985). In turn, this pattern resulted in increased responsibilities for the infants' great-grand-mothers — many of whom provided direct care for their infant great-grandchildren and their teenage grandchildren. In addition, these relatively young great-grandmothers often provided care to their own aging parents. Burton also observed the expected blurring of intergenerational lines between teenage mothers and their own mothers. She notes that these mothers and daughters perceived themselves as being more like siblings than like parents and children.

An additional offshoot of this age-condensed family form was a matrilineal intergenerational structure, with the primary family figures being teenage mothers, their own mothers, and their grand-mothers (Burton, 1990). In 1986, approximately half of all births to black women involved unmarried mothers (U.S. Bureau of the Census, 1987). Matrilineal family forms are especially likely under these conditions. And, when the births are experienced by unmarried teenagers, the matrilineal family form is likely to exhibit age-condensed generational structure.

Age-condensed families undoubtedly are more prevalent among black than white families in the U.S. Nonetheless, the implications of age-condensed family structure merit increased attention among all population subgroups. For example, tendencies toward matrilineal family forms among American blacks have been observed for several decades. It is not clear whether age-condensed family structure increases the likelihood of matrilineal family forms among other segments of the population, for whom matrilineal families have more limited historical precedence.

In contrast to age-condensed family structure, age-gapped family structure results from delayed childbearing, i.e., first child born at age 30 or later, and is especially likely if delayed fertility has been a family pattern, affecting multiple generations (Bengtson et al., 1990). A central characteristic of age-gapped family structure is increased age differences between generations. Boundaries between generations are clear-cut, but large age differences may hinder the development of affective bonds and value congruence across generations (Rossi, 1987). Given the large age gaps between generations, it is unlikely that the number of living generations in age-gapped families will exceed three. Census data suggest that age-gapped families are more likely among white Americans than among minority groups (U.S. Bureau of the Census, 1987)—and there is reason to believe that, among whites, ethnic background is related to the age boundaries among generations (Hogan, 1981).

With regard to the provision of family care to aging parents, age-gapped families appear to be especially likely to face two specific strains. First, middle-aged adults are especially likely to face the demands of childrearing responsibilities and the need to provide assistance to aging parents at the same time (Brody, 1981; Rossi, 1987). Second, because of the distance between generations, the pool of potential caregivers is likely to be small and restricted to members of the middle generation.

We are aware of no empirical studies of age-gapped families. Such studies are badly needed. It is likely that an age-gapped family structure has implications for generational and intergenerational relationships beyond those speculated about above. Studies that compare age-condensed and age-gapped families would be especially valuable; comparisons of distinctly different family forms are particularly useful for highlighting the implications of family structure for generational and intergenerational relationships.

Truncated Family Structure

One result of the decline of fertility that has occurred since the end of the Baby Boom is a dramatic increase in the proportion of American adults who remain childless (U.S. Bureau of the Census, 1987). Indeed, in the next 30-40 years, an unprecedented number and proportion of adults will enter old age having remained childless. It is possible that generational ties among siblings will be especially important for childless older people (Gold, 1987). Intergenerational relationships within the family will be restricted to those involving extended kin, such as nieces and nephews—provided that childless older adults have extended kin. It also is likely that childless older adults will make greater intragenerational investments in relationships with non-kin age peers and stronger intergenerational investments in fictive kin.

Caregiving may be especially problematic for aging members of truncated families. Evidence suggests that childless older persons in current cohorts are less likely to have family members to whom they can turn for caregiving assistance (e.g., Chapman, 1989). Moreover, even when age peers and/or extended kin are willing to provide caregiving assistance, there are more stringent limits on the duration and intensity of that assistance than are characteristic of situations in which caregiving is provided by a spouse or adult child (Johnson & Catalano, 1981).

The family relationships of childless adults have received little attention in previous research. The limited evidence available is restricted almost entirely to the implications of childlessness for caregiving during later life. This important issue clearly merits increased attention.

Reconstituted Families

Rates of divorce among young and middle-aged adults increased substantially during the past quarter century. Fortunately, in terms of family stability, divorce rates appear to have leveled off during the past five years, though they remain high in absolute terms (Sweet & Bumpass, 1987). A corollary of the high divorce rate has been an unprecedented increase in the prevalence of "reconstituted families" (i.e., families formed by the marriages of previously divorced persons). In terms of family relationships, the most important reconstituted families are those that involve intergenerational bonds (i.e., step-parents and step-grandparents).

Reconstituted families are at considerable risk of disruptions and strains in intergenerational bonds (Aldous, 1987; Hagestad, 1988). Divorce itself regardless of whether one or both parents remarry may result in the children experiencing strained relationships with the custodial parent, the non-custodial parent, or both. When parents remarry, especially the custodial parent, family formation and adjustment may be difficult for children, their parents, and their step-parents. Grandparents also face potential relationship strains when their children divorce (Gladstone, 1987; Johnson, 1985). Grandparents on both sides of the divorce typically must change their relationships with their former sons- and daughters-in-law. If their children remarry, members of the grandparent generation must negotiate the establishment of relationships with the new child-in-law—and perhaps with step-grandchildren. Grandparents whose children did not receive custody of their grandchildren also may be forced to accept less interaction with and active grandparenting of their grandchildren than they prefer or than was the case prior to their children's divorces. Thus, both divorce and, especially, reconstituted families often pose special problems and adjustments for members of all family generations.

Decreased Family Involvement of Men

Available evidence suggests that men typically are less intensely involved in family relationships than women. For example, numerous studies indicate that women report larger, denser support networks than men and higher levels of interaction with non-resident family members than men (e.g., Antonucci, 1985; 1990; Buhrke & Fuqua, 1987). Similarly, in a study of older siblings, Gold (1987; 1989a; 1989b) reports that highest levels of interaction and intensity were reported for sister-sister relationships, followed by sister-brother relationships, with brother-brother relationships being least intense and exhibiting lowest levels of interaction. The caregiving literature also testifies to women's greater investments in family relationships (e.g., George & Gwyther, 1986). When a spouse is available, sex is unrelated to caregiver selection—both husbands and wives take responsibility for care of their impaired mates. When the impaired older adult is unmarried and caregiving responsibilities fall upon the shoulders of relatives other than spouses, however, women are much more likely to take on the role of caregiver (e.g., daughters rather than sons, sisters rather than brothers).

A number of social trends related to the increasingly prevalent family forms described above suggest that men are even less intensely involved in family relationships than previously. For example, the link between age-condensed family structure and matrilineal intergenerational involvements was noted. High divorce rates also tend to reduce many men's involvement in childrearing because mothers are much more likely than fathers to receive custody of minor children. Limited but important empirical data support the hypothesis of decreased family involvement among recent cohorts of American men. Eggebeen and Uhlenberg (1985) examined historical changes in the average number of years that American men from different birth cohorts spent in various family roles. During the past 50 years, there has been a precipitous decrease in the number of years, on average, that men spend living with minor children. Three social trends appear to account for this decrease: a higher proportion of never-married men in recent cohorts, decreased fertility among married couples in recent cohorts, and, especially, the increased divorce rate among recent cohorts. The authors suggest that the decreased investment of men in families with minor children may have serious and socially dysfunctional implications for men's commitments to family members and to the welfare of others in general. The high rates of divorced fathers' failures to pay child support for their minor children may be related to this larger picture of men's lessened commitments to their children (Preston, 1984). Clearly, this issue merits additional research.

Predictability of Family Transitions

Issues discussed above included limited attention to the predictability of family transitions. At this point, we focus specifically on cohort differences and historical changes in the predictability of family transitions across the adult life course. Interestingly, some family transitions have become more predictable in their timing than was true earlier in the century; others have become less predictable.

Most of the family transitions that now are less predictable than in the late 1800s and early 1900s are concentrated in the early adult years. In particular, the timing of marriage and parenthood exhibits greater heterogeneity among younger than older cohorts (Baldwin & Nord, 1984; Modell, 1980). In addition, the occurrence of these transitions is less predictable than earlier in the century. For example, greater proportions of recent cohorts do not marry and/or do not have children (Hogan & Astone, 1986). In part, the less predictable timing of marriage and parenthood is due to greater variability in the levels of education characteristic of recent cohorts. Hogan (1981; 1985) notes that recent cohorts of American men have exhibited increased disorderliness in the sequencing of events that mark the transition to adulthood, with an orderly sequence consisting of completing school, followed by obtaining first full-time job, followed by marriage. In addition, recent cohorts of men experienced multiple transitions in a shorter period of time than was characteristic of older cohorts, suggesting compression of the transition from adolescence to early adulthood. Similarly, using data from a sample of Norwegian men from the 1921, 1931, and 1941 birth cohorts, Featherman and Sorensen (1983) conclude that later cohorts of men exhibited more complex configurations of work and family roles during early adulthood than their predecessors. A final family transition that has become less common and less predictable during early adulthood is death of a minor child (Anderson, 1985; Uhlenberg, 1980; Watkins et al., 1987). As Uhlenberg (1980) notes, early in this century parents had a 62% chance of losing at least one minor child; in 1980, the probability of experiencing death of a minor child had dropped to 4%.

In contrast to the pattern for early adulthood, several transitions characteristic of middle-age and later life have become more predictable during this century. Winsborough (1980) compared more distant and recent cohorts with regard to the experience of death of a parent. For recent cohorts, death of a parent occurs at older ages than for previous cohorts. In addition, parental death has become a more predictable event; that is, it is experienced by a majority of cohort members over a shorter interval than previously. Winsborough argues that because parental death is now more strongly linked to children's ages, it has become a more publicly recognized life course marker. Using data from both the U.S. and Canada, Martin Matthews (1987) demonstrates that widowhood has become more closely related to both sex and age during the past century. She argues that the increased predictability of widowhood has helped recent cohorts of older women to better prepare themselves psychologically for the deaths of their husbands and has provided natural support groups of age peers experiencing the transition to widowhood.

Marital Quality

Thus far, discussion has focused primarily on intergenerational relationships, i.e., between parents and minor children, adult children and aging parents, grandchildren and grandparents. Life course perspectives also contribute to our understanding of intra-generational relationships. Marital satisfaction is a case in point.

Numerous studies, spanning almost two decades, suggest that marital satisfaction follows an identifiable course across the adult years. The form of this pattern is a u-shaped curve (Campbell, Converse, & Rodgers, 1976; Lupri & Frideres, 1981; Rollins & Feldman, 1970; Spanier, Lewis, & Coles, 1975). Levels of marital satisfaction are high during the early years of marriage; then decline, reaching their lowest point during middle-age; after which they increase and peak again during old age. Two methodological cautions should be noted. First, these studies are based on cross-sectional data; therefore, this pattern could reflect cohort differences rather than changes across age or duration of marriage. Second, very unhappy marriages are likely to end in divorce, thus leaving the more satisfying, intact marriages available to be sampled and studied (George, 1980).

Several scholars note that the u-shaped curve of marital satisfaction tends to coincide with the timing of childrearing responsibilities (e.g., Rollins & Feldman, 1970; Lupri & Frideres, 1981). After the birth of children and especially during children's teenage years, marital satisfaction tends to decrease until the departure of children from the parental home. After the "launching stage," marital satisfaction increases again. This line of reasoning is buttressed by two additional research findings. First, available evidence suggests that the u-shaped curve dips more deeply for women than for men (e.g., Campbell et al., 1976; Rollins & Feldman, 1970). This finding is compatible with life course perspectives because mothers have traditionally been more involved in childrearing than fathers. Second, the u-shaped curve is much less distinctive for married couples without children (Campbell et al., 1976).

It is possible that responsibility for the care of aging parents and the grief that accompanies parental death during adulthood also contribute to this u-shaped curve of marital satisfaction. At this point, there is limited evidence that caregiving responsibilities can lead to conflict between spouses and between middle-aged spouses and their minor children (e.g., Brody, 1981; George, 1986). Given the increased probability that caregiving responsibilities fall on adult daughters rather than sons, the greater dip in the u-shaped curve for women is compatible with caregiving to parents as well as with greater involvement in childrearing. The implications of caring for older parents and parental death for marital quality merit further inquiry.

CONTRIBUTIONS AND LIMITATIONS OF LIFE COURSE PERSPECTIVES

Today's families are participants in a "quiet revolution" (Bengtson et al., 1990) that is transforming multiple facets of family life. Widespread demographic changes have led to verticalization of the family, resulting in an increase in the number of generations in most families, but also decreasing the numbers of family members within generations. This broad pattern of verticalization has been accompanied by unprecedented choices about whether and when to marry and about whether and when to have children. Adults—and, frequently, teenagers—have exercised their personal choices with regard to family transitions, resulting in a previously unobserved diversity of family forms. Family transitions that once were predictable markers of entry into adulthood have become less predictable. But increased longevity has generated predictable new transitions that have become characteristic of middle and later life. The quality of family life is undoubtedly affected by these transitions. Families are formed, disbanded, and reconstituted, requiring negotiations and adaptations within and across generations. Young grandmothers in age-condensed families may not welcome grandparenthood, sometimes pushing their responsibilities as mothers and grandmothers onto their own mothers. Generations in age-gapped families may be so chronologically distant that it is difficult to build intergenerational solidarity, although some forms of generational solidarity may be facilitated. Dual responsibilities to children and aging parents can place strains on the quality of stable, intact marriages. Life course perspectives, with their emphasis on transitions that mark change and on trajectories that trace more fundamental, long-term life patterns, help to identify the nature, antecedents, and consequences of this quiet revolution—both within individual lives and across cohorts and time.

Ironically, though life course perspectives have been valuable for making sense of the diversity of family patterns within and across cohorts, the major limitation of life course perspectives may be the inability to reveal and make sense of the even greater diversity that apparently exists with regard to family patterns and the intersections of family and other life domains. As noted by Featherman (1986) and Dannefer (1988), most research using life course perspectives continues to focus on modal transition patterns and/or statistical averages (e.g., in the timing of transitions), without fully acknowledging that large proportions of individuals do not fit those patterns.

An important study by Rindfuss, Swicegood, and Rosenfeld (1987) illustrates this point. Using data from the National Longitudinal Survey of the High School Class of 1972, these authors coded study participants' role sequences over an eight-year interval following high school graduation. They examined five types of roles: work, education, homemaker, military, and other. Rindfuss et al. report that 1,100 distinct sequences were needed to describe the experiences of the 6,700 men in their sample. Similarly, 1,800 separate sequences were required to characterize the patterns of the 7,000 women in their sample. Even when focusing on a simple, two-event sequence of education followed by work, these authors found that only slightly more than half the men, and less than half the women, fit that transition sequence. Clearly, this level of heterogeneity poses a major challenge to life course perspectives — indeed, to any perspectives based on the assumption that there are underlying patterns to life transitions.

Despite the challenges posed by heterogeneity, life course perspectives remain important conceptual tools in efforts to understand generational and intergenerational connections. Relative to other conceptual orientations, life course perspectives encourage greater attention to historical and social change, to the interrelationships among transitions, to the intersections among life domains (e.g., work and family), and to major sources of variability within and across cohorts. Perhaps most importantly, life course perspectives encourage a balanced view of the dynamics of life patterns, incorporating not only discrete transitions, but also, through the concept of trajectories, the social, historical, and personal contexts that render life patterns meaningful.

REFERENCES

Aldous, J. (1987). Family life of the elderly and near elderly. *Journal of Marriage and the Family, 49*, 227-234.

Allison, P.D. (1984). *Event history analysis*. Beverly Hills, CA: Sage.

Anderson, M. (1985). The emergence of the modern life cycle in Britain. *Social History, 10*, 69-87.

Antonucci, T.C. (1985). Personal characteristics, social support and social behavior. In R.H. Binstock & E. Shanas (Eds.), *Handbook of aging and the social sciences* 2nd edition (pp. 94-128). New York: Van Nostrand Reinhold.

Antonucci, T.C. (1990). Social supports and social relationships. In R.H. Binstock & L.K. George (Eds.), *Handbook of aging and the social sciences* 3rd edition (pp. 205-227). New York: Academic Press.

Baldwin, W.H. & Nord, C.W. (1984). Delayed childbearing in the U.S.: Facts and fictions. *Population Bulletin, 39*, 1-42.

Bengtson, V.L. (1986). Comparative perspectives on the microsociology of aging: Methodological problems and theoretical issues. In V.W. Marshall (Ed.), *Late life: The social psychology of aging* (pp. 304-336). Beverly Hills, CA: Sage.

Bengtson, V.L., Rosenthal, C. & Burton, L. (1990). Families and aging: Diversity and heterogeneity. In R.H. Binstock & L.K. George (Eds.), *Handbook of aging and the social sciences* 3rd edition, (pp. 263-287). New York: Academic Press.

Brody, E.M. (1981). Women in the middle and family help to older people. *The Gerontologist, 21*, 471-480.

Buhrke, R.A. & Fuqua, D.R. (1987). Sex differences in same- and cross-sex supportive relationships. *Sex Roles, 17*, 339-352.

Burton, L.M. (1985). *Early and on-time grandmotherhood in multigeneration black families*. Unpublished doctoral dissertation. University of Southern California.

Burton, L.M. (1990). Adolescent childbearing as an alternative life course strategy in multigeneration black families. *Human Nature, 1*, 123-143.

Burton, L.M. & Bengtson, V.L. (1985). Black grandmothers: Issues of timing and continuity of roles. In V.L. Bengtson & J. Robertson (Eds.), *Grandparenthood* (pp. 61-77). Beverly Hills, CA: Sage.

Campbell, A., Converse, P.E., & Rodgers, W.L. (1976). *The quality of American life*. New York: Russell Sage Foundation.

Chapman, N.J. (1989). Gender, marital status, and childlessness of older persons and the availability of informal assistance. In M.D. Petersen & D.L. White (Eds.), *Health care for the elderly: An information source book* (pp. 102-120). Newbury Park, CA: Sage.

Clausen, J.A. (1986). *The life course*. Englewood Cliffs, NJ: Prentice-Hall.

Dannefer, D. (1988). What's in a name? An account of the neglect of variability in the study of aging. In J.E. Birren & V.L. Bengtson (Eds.), *Emergent theories of aging* (pp. 356-384). New York: Springer.

Eggebeen, D. & Uhlenberg, P. (1985). Changes in the organization of men's lives: 1960-1980. *Family Relations, 34,* 251-257.

Elder, G.H. Jr. (1974). *Children of the Great Depression.* Chicago: University of Chicago Press.

Elder, G.H. Jr. (1985a). Perspectives on the life course. In G.H. Elder, Jr. (Ed.), *Life course dynamics: Trajectories and transitions, 1968-1980* (pp. 23-49). Ithaca, NY: Cornell University Press.

Elder G.H. Jr. (Ed.). (1985b). *Life Course dynamics: Trajectories and transitions, 1968-1980.* Ithaca, NY: Cornell University Press.

Elder, G.H. Jr. & Clipp, E. (1988). War experience and social ties: Influences across 40 years in men's lives. In M.W. Riley (Ed.), *Social structures and human lives* (pp. 306-327). Newbury Park, CA: Sage.

Featherman, D.L. (1986). Biography, society, and history: Individual development as a population process. In A.G. Sorensen, F.E. Weinert, & L.R. Sherrod (Eds.), *Human development and the life course: Multidisciplinary perspectives* (pp. 99-149). Hillsdale, NJ: Erlbaum.

Featherman, D.L. & Sorensen, A. (1983). Societal transformation in Norway and change in the life course transition into adulthood. *Acta Sociologica, 26,* 105-126.

Gee, E.M. (1986). The life course of Canadian women: A historical and demographic analysis. *Social Indicators Research, 18,* 263-283.

Gee, E.M. (1987). Historical change in the family life course of Canadian men and women. In V.W. Marshall (Ed.), *Aging in Canada* 2nd edition (pp. 265-287). Markham, Ontario: Fitzhenry and Whiteside.

George, L.K. (1980). *Role transitions in later life.* Belmont, CA: Wadsworth.

George, L.K. (1982). Models of transitions in middle and later life. *Annals of the Academy of Political and Social Science, 464,* 22-37.

George, L.K. (1986). Caregiver burden: Conflict between norms of reciprocity and solidarity. In K. Pillemer & R. Wolf (Eds.), *Conflict and abuse in families of the elderly: Theory, research, and intervention* (pp. 67-92). Boston: Auburn House.

George, L.K. & Gwyther, L.P. (1986). Caregiver well-being: A multidimensional examination of family caregivers of demented adults. *The Gerontologist, 34,* 253-259.

Gladstone, J.W. (1987). Factors associated with changes in visiting between grandmothers and grandchildren following an adult child's marriage breakdown. *Canadian Journal on Aging, 6,* 117-126.

Gold, D.T. (1987). Siblings in old age: Something special. *Canadian Journal on Aging, 6,* 199-215.

Gold, D.T. (1989a). Sibling relations in old age: A typology. *International Journal of Aging and Human Development, 28,* 37-51.

Gold, D.T. (1989b). Generational solidarity: Conceptual antecedents and consequences. In V.H. Bedford & D.T. Gold (Eds.), *American Behavioral Scientist, 33,* 19-32.

Hagestad, G.O. (1988). Demographic change and the life course: Some emerging trends in the family realm. *Family Relations, 37,* 405-410.

Hagestad, G.O. (1990). Social perspectives on the life course. In R.H. Binstock & L.K. George (Eds.), *Handbook of aging and the social sciences* 3rd edition (pp. 151-168). New York: Academic Press.

Hagestad, G.O. & Burton, L. (1986). Grandparenthood, life context, and family development. *American Behavioral Scientist, 29,* 471-484.

Hagestad, G.O. & Neugarten, B.L. (1985). Aging and the life course. In R.H. Binstock & E. Shanas (Eds.), *Handbook of aging and the social sciences* 2nd edition (pp. 36-61). New York: Van Nostrand Reinhold.

Hogan, D.P. (1981). *Transitions and social change: The early lives of American men.* New York: Academic Press.

Hogan, D.P. (1985). The demography of life-span transitions: Temporal and gender comparisons. In A. Rossi (Ed.), *Gender and the life course* (pp. 65-78). New York: Aldine.

Hogan, D.P. & Astone, N.M. (1986). The transition to adulthood. *Annual Review of Sociology, 12,* 109-130.

Johnson, C.L. (1985). Grandparenting options in divorcing families: An anthropological perspective. In. V.L. Bengtson & J. Robertson (Eds.), *Grandparenthood* (pp. 81-96). Beverly Hills, CA: Sage.

Johnson, C.L. & Catalano, D.H. (1981). Childless elderly and their family supports. *The Gerontologist, 21,* 610-618.

Kertzer, D.I. & Hogan, D.P. (1988). Family structure, individual lives, and societal change. In M.W. Riley (Ed.), *Social structure and human lives.* (pp. 83-100). Newbury Park, CA: Sage.

Knipscheer, C.P.M. (1988). Temporal embeddedness and aging within the multigenerational family: The case of grandparenting. In J.E. Birren & V.L. Bengtson (Eds.), *Emergent theories of aging* (pp. 426-446). New York: Springer.

Kohli, M. (1986). The world we forgot: A historical review of the life course. In V.W. Marshall (Ed.), *Later life: The social psychology of aging* (pp. 271-303). Beverly Hills, CA: Sage.

Kohli, M. & Meyer, J.W. (1986). Social structure and social construction of life stages. *Human Development, 29,* 145-180.

Lupri, E. & Frideres, J. (1981). The quality of marriage and the passage of time: Marital satisfaction over the family life cycle. *Canadian Journal of Sociology, 6,* 283-305.

Martin Matthews, A. (1987). Widowhood as an expectable life event. In V.W. Marshall (Ed.), *Aging in Canada: Social perspectives* 2nd edition (pp. 343-366). Markham, Ontario: Fitzhenry and Whiteside.

Mayer, K.U. & Muller, W. (1986). The state and the structure of the life course. In A.G. Sorensen, F.E. Weinert, & L.R. Sherrod (Eds.), *Human development and the life course: Multidisciplinary perspectives* (pp. 217-245). Hillsdale, NJ: Erlbaum.

Meyer, J.W. (1988). Levels of analysis: The life course as a cultural construction.

In M.W. Riley (Ed.), *Social structure and human lives* (pp. 49-62). Newbury Park, CA: Sage.

Modell, J. (1980). Normative aspects of American marriage timing since World War II. *Journal of Family History*, *5*, 210-234.

Neugarten, B.L. & Hagestad, G.O. (1976). Age and the life course. In R.H. Binstock & E. Shanas (Eds.), *Handbook of aging and the social sciences* (pp. 35-55). New York: Van Nostrand Reinhold.

Nydegger, C. (1986). Age and life course transitions. In C.L. Fry & J. Keith (Eds.), *New methods for old age research* (pp. 131-161). South Hadley: Bergin and Garvey.

O'Rand, A.M. (1990). Stratification and the life course. In R.H. Binstock & L.K. George (Eds.), *Handbook of aging and the social sciences* 3rd edition (pp. 130-150). New York: Academic Press.

Preston, S.H. (1984). Children and the elderly: Divergent paths for America's dependents. *Demography*, *21*, 435-457.

Riley, M.W. (1986). Overview and highlights of a sociological perspective. In A.G. Sorensen, F.E. Weinert, & L.R. Sherrod (Eds.), *Human development and the life course: Multidisciplinary perspectives* (pp. 153-175). Hillsdale, NJ: Erlbaum.

Rindfuss, R.R. Swicegood, C.G., & Rosenfeld, R.A. (1987). Disorder in the life course: How common and does it matter? *American Sociological Review*, *52*, 785-801.

Rollins, B.C. & Feldman, H. (1970). Marital satisfaction over the family life cycle. *Journal of Marriage and the Family*, *32*, 20-28.

Rossi, A.S. (1980). Life-span theories and women's lives. *Signs*, *6*, 4-32.

Rossi, A.S. (1987). Parenthood in transition: From lineage to child to self-orientation. In J. Lancaster, J. Altman, A. Rossi, & L. Sherrod (Eds.), *Parenting across the life span: Biosocial dimensions* (pp. 435-456). Hawthorne, NY: Aldine de Gruyter.

Roth, J.A. (1983). Timetables and the lifecourse in post-industrial society. In D.W. Plath (Ed.), *Work and the lifecourse in Japan* (pp. 248-260). Albany: State University of New York Press.

Spanier, G.B., Lewis, R.A. & Coles, C.L. (1975). Marital adjustment over the family life cycle: The issue of curvilinearity. *Journal of Marriage and the Family*, *37*, 263-275.

Sweet, J.A. & Bumpass, L.L. (1987). *American families and households*. New York: Russell Sage Foundation.

Treas, J. & Bengtson, V.L. (1987). Family in later years. In M. Sussman & S. Steinmetz (Eds.), *Handbook on marriage and the family* (pp. 625-648). New York: Plenum.

Uhlenberg, P. (1980). Death and the family. *Journal of Family History*, *5*, 313-320.

U.S. Bureau of the Census. (1987). Fertility of American women: June 1986. *Current Population Reports* (Series P-20, No. 421). Washington, D.C.: U.S. Government Printing Office.

Watkins, S.C., Menken, J.A., & Bongaarts, J. (1987). Demographic foundations of family change. *American Sociological Review, 52,* 346-358.

Winsborough, H.H. (1980). A demographic approach to the life-cycle. In K.W. Back (Ed.), *Life course: Integrative theories and exemplary populations.* Boulder, CO: Westview Press.

Winship, C. (1986). Heterogeneity and interdependence: A test using survival models. In N. Tuma (Ed.), *Sociological methodology, 1986* (pp. 250-282). Washington, D.C.: American Sociological Association.

Small Worlds
and Intergenerational Relationships

Jaber F. Gubrium
Maude R. Rittman

The purpose of this paper is to critically review and broaden the concept of intergenerational relationships, in particular, intergenerational responsibility. First, an existing global orientation to intergenerational relationships is described, providing a basis for considering the lack of concern for the relationships' interpersonally coincidental and circumstantial features. Second, the concept of "small worlds" is introduced in order to capture what is lacking. Third, ethnographic data are used to illustrate the concept. And fourth, suggestions are offered for extending the conceptual purview of intergenerational relationships.

Data are drawn from a field study of two family-oriented treatment programs, one located in an outpatient, family counseling center and the other in a private psychiatric hospital. The programs treat common problems such as substance abuse, domestic troubles, truancy, and general misbehavior. The settings provide important contexts for demonstrating how both chance encounters and the application of contrasting institutional views of domestic order generate diverse senses of the intergenerational relationship.

THE GLOBAL ORIENTATION

Mannheim (1952) and Eisenstadt (1956) teach meanings of generation that students of intergenerational relationships seem to have forgotten. Mannheim points out that a generation is as much a set of

Jaber F. Gubrium is Professor of Sociology, University of Florida, Gainesville, FL 32611. Maude R. Rittman is Nurse Researcher/Educator, VA Medical Center, Gainesville, FL 32602.

experiences as it is a range of years. When social change is rapid, there are likely to be more generations than when the passing years are undistinguished. A relative lack of change homogenizes the lives of grandparent, parent, and child; social change distinguishes them, causing an experience of separateness. Eisenstadt examines kinship in relation to the division of labor. He argues that in societies where kinship is the primary unit of the division of labor, age-heterogenous groupings are prevalent and mix the generations; where the division of labor is organized by market relations, age-homogeneous groupings are predominant and distinguish generations. Both remind us that intergenerational relations are not simply global characteristics of populations, but take on their meaning in diverse circumstances.

In contrast to Mannheim's attempt to embed generational differences in the experience of change, and Eisenstadt's linkage of generational age-homogeneity with the division of labor, recent and current debates over the status of intergenerational relationships decontextualize the generational experience. A global orientation animates public debate over generational relations. In the global orientation, the generational experience and intergenerational boundaries are separated from the concrete social relationships of everyday life. Typically, decontextualized generational variables are examined for their impact on a range of social psychological factors. For example, members of different generations are asked to specify their attitudes toward ostensibly traditional family values. The attitudes might be compared to hostility or empathy, or explored for whether generational differences explain them. The question of how the distinct variables are linked with everyday life is overshadowed by statistical generalizations.

Politics and the Generation Gap

Globally-oriented studies have two phases. The first phase, from the sixties through the early seventies, centered on a widely-presumed "generation gap." The focus was mainly political. Student involvement in the civil rights movement, resistance to the Vietnam War, and the counter-cultural sentiments suggested that youth were experiencing life in an entirely different way than older adults. It was noted that the resulting generation gap fueled intergenerational conflict. The question of what the generations owed to each other — intergenerational responsibility — took a backseat to differential world views and personal independence.

The political debate led to research examining the extent and character of the gap. Some, like Bengtson (1971), concentrated on perceptions. Bengtson examined three-generation families and found that while there was agreement over a generation gap, the gap within respondents' own families was not perceived to be as wide as among others. Moreover, the older generation was less likely than the grandchildren to see a gap in the family. Other studies considered age variations in values and attitudes. Hill (1970) found that generations differed in the relative value they placed on parenthood. The younger generation stressed independence in making life choices while the older generation favored obedience and respect. With caution for possible cohort effects, Riley and Foner (1968) noted that the evidence suggested that, generally, older persons are more conservative than younger ones. The older generation was more resistant to change and less tolerant of nonconformity. The evidence for differences in conservatism, however, was less clear for policies that specifically benefitted an age-group.

Yet the overall findings regarding generational differences were inconsistent. For example, Thomas (1974) found similarity from one generation to another on attitudes toward politics and business. Bengtson, Furlong, and Laufer (1974) pointed out that student activists might not only be reflecting their parents' attitudes but actually carrying out the parents' sentiments. Still, as Thomas (1974) indicated, similarities in attitudes may hide value differences such as present- versus future-orientation.

In terms of intergenerational responsibility, the first phase of research implied that generations owed very little to each other. Although the data were inconsistent, the surrounding ideological aura was rooted in sentiments toward renewal and the view that the change was the bailiwick of the young. Social problems were believed to originate in the historical foibles of the older generation. Ideology, public sentiment, and attitudes combined to widen the public image of the generation gap despite the lack of clear statistical evidence for intergenerational differences. While Neugarten and

Neugarten (1986, p. 42) recently have suggested that the generation gap is probably more image than reality, it is important to add that, in the realm of experience, reality is as much image as image is reality. Image or not, the generation gap was taken to be reality.

Intergenerational Equity

The second phase of research from a global orientation occurred during the late seventies into the eighties. It was as economically as politically focused. The issue of intergenerational responsibility centered on the question of who, among the needy in various age-groups, most deserved public funds. This reflected the demise of political optimism, which was tied to an economic downturn resulting from the international oil crisis. Neugarten and Neugarten (1986) indicate that there was increasing fear that intergenerational conflict would center on the Social Security program. A major worry was that those of working age would resist increasing Social Security taxes to support a growing proportion of retirees.

The issue was called "intergenerational equity," or as Pifer (1986, p. 409) puts it, "more precisely, intergenerational inequity." In contrast to the more neutral phrase "generation gap," differences in the distribution of resources were emphasized. As Pifer adds, "The general tenor of the discussion, the thrust of which is that younger age groups have been unfairly treated by older groups, has been marked by a language of conflict and retaliation, and the use of such terms as 'intergenerational rivalry' or even 'the war between the generations'" (1986, p. 409).

Pifer (1986) and Neugarten and Neugarten (1986) have questioned the extent of generation disparity. Even while there have been increasing generational differences in federal budget allocations, Pifer believes that the argument that one generation cynically acts to benefit itself at the expense of others is dubious. Neugarten and Neugarten, who prefer to use the term "age-groups," not "generations," indicate that there is a large body of research which shows that parents "remain invested in the welfare of their offspring, and that ties of obligation, whether or not they are also ties of affection, remain strong in offspring" (1986, p. 43). They marshal extensive evidence against the intergenerational (in)equity argument: surveys which show that workers in the United States are not acting against rising Social Security taxes (National Council on the Aging, 1975, 1981); studies of intergenerational support (Shanas, 1979; Brody, 1985); and historical research indicating that in the postwar period, labor unions, not a "gray lobby," were the prime advocates of increasing Social Security benefits (Pratt, 1976, 1982).

More recently, the possibility that the debate over intergenerational equity would lead to a backlash against the elderly has prompted attempts to broaden the politics of aging (Kingson, 1988). For example, it has been argued that the interests of the aged, for example, would be best served by advocating benefits for the needy of all age-groups (Kingson, Hirshorn, & Cornman, 1986).

The issue of intergenerational responsibility continues to be posed in terms of "either/or"—either there is a generation gap or there is not; either there is a generational inequity or there is not. While there always has been provision for answering related questions in terms of more-or-less, for example, less of a gap in reality than the public image conveys, and in terms of multivariate complications, for instance, less of a gap among the working class than among professional families, the subtleties end there. The global orientation to intergenerational relationships still ignores the place of everyday social relations, the dynamics of happenstance, and the effect of circumstance on its interpretation.

SMALL WORLDS

In considering the concrete experiences of intergenerational relations, a number of questions arise. How do we perceive and engage intergenerational responsibility in everyday life? Is it something separate from our daily affairs with age-peers, older, and younger persons? Can we imagine what we think and feel about the aged and the young without attending to how we concretely know in relation to others? When we are asked, in survey after survey, what our attitudes are—"in general" or "overall"— what are we being asked about? Can the responses possibly be about us, who live our lives, day in and day out, within the purview of actual relations with others, none of which are "overall" but, rather, concretely inter-personal?

The answers to these questions bear on how we conceptualize intergenerational relations and responsibility. It is in this connection that we introduce the concept "small worlds" as a way of con-cretely specifying the everyday meaning of "gaps" and "equity," among other terms of reference to intergenerational relations. The global orientation has produced aggregate (statistical) knowledge; the "small worlds" concept captures social detail.

A small world is an interpersonal domain of understanding. It is about what we happen to think, feel, and do about something in particular situations. A small world has experiential boundaries. Regarding filial obligations, for example, we might feel one way at home in the unexpected company of a health visitor and quite dif-ferently at work in sharing thoughts with a new employee. The two small worlds cast a different light on obligations. Should we be asked in a formal interview for our opinion "in general" or "over-all" about responsibility to frail, elderly parents, the interview situ-ation (another small world) elicits its particular opinions. Regard-less of what is ultimately found in each case, it is methodologically important to allow for each world — home, work, the formal inter-view — to articulate its own sense of the "general" or of the "over-all." As domains of understanding, each small world might pro-duce both specific and general opinion. This would permit each question about intergenerational relations to have diverse and sun-dry answers, differentiated by small worlds, not confounded in the aggregated statistics of surveyed opinion. In this context, existing survey data concerning intergenerational relations would be opinion expressed in interview situations, not necessarily other small worlds.

Many small worlds permeate everyday life. We hear repeated references to them as people speak of how one feels "now," "here," or "when among [particular] people." The references sug-gest that communications about gaps, equity, and responsibility do not as much express situation-free, global opinion as they are re-sponses rooted in the interpersonal contexts where issues are con-sidered. For example, diverse images of what parents owe their troubled children, encountered in different therapeutic settings, provide a basis for contrasting answers to the question of intergenerational responsibility. Where one setting suggests that authority is owed, another urges that love be offered. Each setting presents its own interpretations and generalizations.

HAPPENSTANCE AND CIRCUMSTANCE

The situations that form small worlds are rooted in both happenstance and circumstance. Perceptions are formed according to when, where, and with whom, one "happens" to be associated. Understandings of intergenerational responsibility have an element of chance. At the same time, the organizational regularities of circumstance suggest that perceptions are also associated with established points of view. Accordingly, two kinds of situations particularize understandings of intergenerational responsibility: (1) *happenstance*, or chance encounters with individuals concerned with intergenerational responsibility; and (2) *circumstance*, or the engagement of questions of intergenerational responsibility in relation to established understandings.

The Small World as Happenstance

The phrase "intergenerational responsibility" rarely is heard in the two field settings studied. While various family members and service providers speak of responsibility, rights, obligations, and duties between children, parents, and grandparents, the question of responsibility is taken up in more specific terms. Even when those concerned attempt to deal with the question in the abstract or according to a principle, abstractions take on their meaning through immediately relevant particulars.

Consider how the familial experiences and personal therapeutic inclinations of individual group counselors serve as a basis for describing intergenerational responsibility in the psychiatric hospital. Focal is group therapy for families with children in the adolescent unit. The children have an average stay of six to eight weeks. They are treated for alcohol, marijuana, cocaine, and crack addiction as well as domestic misbehavior and delinquency.

Group therapy for families takes the following forms: Sundays,

beginning at noon, the families join together, without the hospitalized children, with a group counselor for an hour of Systematic
Training for Effective Parenting or STEP (Dinkmayer & McKay,
1983). A second hour is spent in open discussion of select domestic
issues, which includes the children. A third hour, with parents only,
frames the discussion of problems in terms of the Toughlove treatment philosophy (York, York, & Wachtel, 1982). Families whose
children have completed the program and been discharged meet
weekly with their discharged children and a group counselor in
what is called "aftercare," a support group facilitated by a staff
member.

STEP and Toughlove represent opposite ends of a therapeutic
continuum. The effectiveness of STEP is based on a democratic
family model, where parents and children work as equals to solve
domestic troubles. In contrast, the success of Toughlove is founded
on an autocratic family model, where firm parental authority serves
as the arbiter of misbehavior. Family members are exposed to the
full spectrum, not formally given the choice of picking among alternate treatment philosophies. As noted by the counselors, while
STEP and Toughlove contrast in their orientations to the management of intergenerational relationships, each has its merits. A common remark is, "When STEP doesn't work in dealing with inappropriate behaviors, Toughlove kicks in."

The counselors differ in their individual adherence to the treatment philosophies. Some emphasize the democratic model, others
the autocratic model. Some take an eclectic approach and combine
the two. Each counselor uses personal familial experiences in support of his or her emphasis. Parents, too, come with different sentiments about preferred parenting strategies. Some enter the program
with democratic inclinations, while others favor an autocratic approach.

To some extent, the motley collection of treatment preferences
and parenting inclinations sorts itself out in chance encounters. It is
not as if therapeutic experiences are eventually homogenized to produce a uniform sense of what parents and children are responsible
for. One important finding is that the meaning of intergenerational
responsibility depends on which counselor a parent happens to encounter in the various group therapy sessions. If a parent finds him-

or herself with a group counselor who orients to a democratic model of familial decision-making, the responsibility of parents for their children in that situation is envisioned as comprised of negotiated rules and contracts, not decisive rule enforcement.

Take proceedings led by the counselor we call Mark Pearson. Pearson regularly refers to his own, rather authoritarian father and disciplined upbringing. While Pearson teaches STEP, which stresses the democratic model, he is quick to point out that there are definite limits to intergenerational equity and rationality, repeating that the "rational consequences" for rule-infraction, written into "contracts" by children and their parents according to the STEP model, sometimes have to give way to "natural consequences," the so-called tough rules of life. Pearson describes how his father would let the law take its course when Mark got into trouble rather than taking responsibility for him. At the same time, Pearson usually adds that times have changed and what he experienced as a child probably now would be called parental irresponsibility, or perhaps child abuse.

The autocratic orientation nonetheless is repeatedly touted as the approach of last resort. Pearson habitually draws a model on the blackboard of the limits of democratic decision-making in the family, emphasizing that there is a sphere of parental affairs in all families that must remain generationally exclusive, where children have no business. This pertains to marital order and security. According to Pearson, the bounds of this sphere are nonnegotiable. An irresponsible parent permits children to define its boundary. Irresponsible children attempt to invade the space and divide the parents. To Pearson, this exclusive space sets the ultimate limits of family members' intergenerational obligations.

Another counselor, Tom Billings, is decidedly democratic in both the substance and tone of his approach. His group sessions with parents dwell on how parents and children can rationally articulate their individual rights and responsibilities. With principles of mutual respect and equal participation at the forefront, and authority and command in the background, Billings highlights co-participation in domestic decision-making. He draws examples from the many written and unwritten "contracts" he has helped to arrange, in which parents and children specify mutual responsibilities in the household. Other staff members, like Mike Pearson, also are concerned about contracts, but Billings, more than anyone, organizes his illustrations and commentary in the group sessions around the agreements and their equalitarian tenor.

The tone of Billings' sessions also contrast with Pearson's. Where Pearson forcefully makes various points about intergenerational relations and animatedly emphasizes the limits of parental responsibility, Billings talks quietly but audibly, in very measured speech, of the unlimited applications of an agreement. In voice and cadence, Billings personally exemplifies how parents and children should respond to each other. Two key phrases of his comments are "sitting down" and "talking about it" which convey calmly and rationally figuring what parents and children owe to each other. The implication is that domestic troubles are likely to persist as long as the generations communicatively engage each other in a disorderly and irrational manner.

Pearson's and Billings' approaches and emphases present parents with contrasting messages about intergenerational relationships and responsibilities. Some parents openly recognize the difference and complain about "what you hear" from one staff member as opposed to "what you hear" from another. At the same time, the differences provide wide-ranging options for the interpretation of family troubles, diversifying the understanding of intergenerational responsibility. It is evident that the meaning of ostensibly general references to matters such as good parenting, recovery, treatment, and intergenerational responsibility cannot be separated from the small worlds of understanding present in these chance encounters. While all agree that effective parenting is important and that the hospital aims to help families accomplish this, it is also evident that what effective parenting means concretely in one small world, such as Pearson's sessions, is not necessarily the same in another.

During the research period, Billings resigned from his position. This meant that newly admitted children and their parents would then "happen upon" a different range of emphases and experiences in their therapeutic encounters with staff. The small worlds' intergenerational understandings subsequently engaged parents and counselors reflected the change.

The Small World as Circumstance

Small worlds of understanding also are conditioned by the institutionalized circumstances in which families find themselves. While there is happenstance in all social settings, there also are regularities such as prevailing organization philosophies of intergenerational relationships.

The two treatment programs studied provide contrasting formal views of the meaning of intergenerational relations. We call the psychiatric hospital "Fairview" and the outpatient counseling center "Westside House." While one family counselor at Fairview, Mike Pearson, frequently stresses autocracy in managing domestic relations and another, Tom Billings, emphasizes democracy, they nonetheless work from a common definition of the basic substance of domestic relations. Like other Fairview staff members, both reference *affective* bonds as the fundamental ingredient of domestic order. Despite the broad range of treatment strategies, evident in programs like STEP, Toughlove, group support, and adolescent behavioral management, the prevailing view is that the family and intergenerational relations are a configuration of feelings. Regardless of personal inclinations, Pearson commonly asserts that what all are dealing with, in the final analysis, is love. As he reminds families, "When you really come down to it, that's what the family is all about." Likewise, even in measured and carefully modulated tones signifying rationality, Billings habitually references an affective order. What families' members basically owe one another is love and understanding.

Westside House differs in several ways. It is an outpatient facility, with treatment limited to family therapy. Families do not participate in support groups, nor are they presented diverse treatment modalities. More important, it is evident in both family therapy sessions and group supervisions where therapists discuss cases with a consultant, there is different institutional view of domestic reality and intergenerational relations. The institutional image of the family is patterned on the family process model, in which the fundamental reality of domestic life is considered to be composed of authority relations. Haley's (1976) book, *Problem-Solving Therapy*, is frequently referenced. From this perspective, small worlds of intergenerational understanding frame family troubles in terms of "dysfunctional power structures." It is familial authority, not feelings, that defines the nature of domestic relations.

Like their Fairview counterparts, Westside therapists tinker with the family's authority structure in different ways. While there are one or two who regularly explore and "work on" the feelings of select family members in therapy sessions, it is evident that these practices are tolerated, if not ignored. The idea that effective bonds are the ultimate ground of troubled domestic relations is not supported. Families who participate in the small worlds assembled at Westside House are encouraged to articulate intergenerational relations in terms of domestic authority and hierarchy, even while diverse domestic experiences, concerning both interpersonal control and feelings, are taken into account in proceedings. What family members basically owe to each other in this context is respect and the recognition of differential rights and obligations.

BROADENING THE STUDY
OF INTERGENERATIONAL RELATIONSHIPS

The concept of small worlds broadens the meaning of intergenerational relationships. Related data suggest that there is a need to examine the interpersonal sources of intergenerational relations. Just as the Fairview and Westside House data show that questions of intergenerational relations are regularly and quite contrastingly considered in these treatment settings, data gathered in diverse human service settings suggest further that intergenerational issues are the stock-in-trade of human service organizations (Gubrium & Holstein, 1990).

Rather than assuming that answers to questions of intergenerational relations and responsibility are generated out of widespread understandings or can be delineated in global generalizations, we might allow that diverse venues contain separate and distinct ways of conceiving familial relations. From the Fairview and Westside House data, it is evident that the intergenerational meaning of family trouble cannot be understood separate from local constructions. The systematic comparison of diverse venues, moreover, would make visible the manners in which responsibility is concretely interpreted, providing evidence of its social distribution. Venues, of course, vary in terms of their particular generational emphases, including settings such as residential treatment centers for emotionally disturbed children and nursing homes. Their comparison would provide a basis for contrasting understandings of intergenerational responsibility across age-groupings.

Still it is important not to overdetermine the part localized formal understandings play in defining the character of intergenerational relationships. While Fairview and Westside House offer participants different institutional images of family life, this does not eliminate the interpretive effects of interpersonal happenstance. Individual participants use what they bring with them in relation to whom they happen to encounter as they deal with intergenerational issues. As such, there is a need to be tolerant of chance, contradiction, and diversity in related affairs.

This paper has focused on the formal organization as a venue for defining the nature and character of intergenerational relationships. There are other settings to consider, such as the household and/or the neighborhood. In the varied images and encounters provided, settings can instruct us that intergenerational relationships are more complex than global states of affairs between children, parents, and grandparents. Settings situate small worlds that complicate the meaning of our relations as family members, to reveal a mosaic of intergenerational particulars.

REFERENCES

Bengtson, V. (1971). Inter-age perceptions and the generation gap, *The Gerontologist, 11*, 85-89.

Bengtson, V., Furlong, M., & Laufer, R. (1974). Time, aging, and continuity of social structure: Themes and issues in generational analyses. *Journal of Social Issues, 30*, 1-30.

Brody, E. (1985). Parent care as a normative family stress. *The Gerontologist, 25*, 19-29.

Dinkmeyer, D. & McKay, G. (1983). *STEP/teen: Systematic training for effective parenting of teens*. Circle Pines, MN: American Guidance Service.

Eisenstadt, S.N. (1956). *From generation to generation: Age groups and social structure*. New York: Free Press.

Gubrium, J.F. & Holstein, J.A. (1990). *What is family?* Mountain View, CA: Mayfield.

Haley, J. (1976). *Problem-solving therapy*. New York: Harper & Row.

Hill, R. (1970). *Family development in three generations*. Cambridge, MA: Schenkman.

Kingson, E. (1988). Generational equity: An unexpected opportunity to broaden the politics of aging. *The Gerontologist, 28*, 765-772.

Kingson, E.R., Hirshorn, B.A., & Cornman, J.M. (1986). *Ties that bond: The interdependence of generations*. Cabin John, MD: Seven Locks Press.

Mannheim, K. (1952). The problem of generations. In K. Mannheim (Ed.), *Essays on the sociology of knowledge*. London: Routledge & Kegan Paul.

National Council on the Aging. (1975). *The myth and reality of aging in America*. Washington, DC: National Council on the Aging.

National Council on the Aging. (1981). *Aging in the eighties: America in transition*. Washington, DC: National Council on the Aging.

Neugarten, B.A. & Neugarten, D.A. (1986). Changing meanings of age in the aging society. In A. Pifer & L. Bronte (Eds.), *Our aging society*. New York: Norton.

Pifer, A. (1986). The public policy response. In A. Pifer & L. Bronte (Eds.), *Our aging society*. New York: Norton.

Pratt, H.J. (1976). *The gray lobby*. Chicago: University of Chicago Press.

Pratt, H.J. (1982). The 'gray lobby' revisited, *The National Forum, 11*, 31-33.

Riley, M.W. & Foner, A. (1968). *Aging and society*, Volume 1. New York: Russell Sage.

Shanas, E. (1979). Social myth as hypothesis: The case of the family relations of old people. *The Gerontologist, 19*, 1-9.

Thomas, L.E. (1974). Generational discontinuity in beliefs: An exploration of the generation gap. *Journal of Social Issues, 30*, 1-22.

York, P., York, D., & Wachtel, T. (1982). *Toughlove*. New York: Doubleday.

Convoys of Social Support: Generational Issues

Toni C. Antonucci

Hiroko Akiyama

Theoretical issues in the field of family and intergenerational relations have focused on similarities and differences across the generations; the changing social context of intergenerational bonds; intergenerational relationships as a major agent of social change; and the nature of intergenerational ties (Bengtson, Cutler, Mangen & Marshall, 1985; Bengtson, Rosenthal & Burton, 1990; Hagestad, 1981; Troll, 1971; Troll, Miller, & Atchley, 1979). These perspectives have contributed to the understanding of intergenerational relationships. In this paper, we extend the concept of convoys of social support, both theoretically and empirically, to include intergenerational relations. We propose, through theoretical extension and empirical investigation, that intergenerational relationships be viewed within the context of convoys of social support over the life course. We believe that such a perspective provides unique input and understanding to each of the intergenerational issues outlined below.

Toni C. Antonucci is Research Scientist, and Hiroko Akiyama, is Assistant Research Scientist, Institute for Social Research, The University of Michigan, P.O. Box 1248, Ann Arbor, MI 48106.

This article was written while Toni C. Antonucci held a Research Career Development Award from the National Institute on Aging.

The data computation upon which this paper is based employed the OSIRIS IV computer software package, which was developed by the Institute for Social Research, The University of Michigan, using funds from the Survey Research Center, Inter-University Consortium for Political Research, National Science Foundation, and other sources.

ISSUES IN INTERGENERATIONAL RELATIONS

Hagestad (1981; 1990) notes that each individual progresses through time and interacts with other family and generation members differently. These differences are based on individual life time, family life time, and cohort or historical time. The value of a life-span developmental view for understanding individual development has been increasingly recognized (Baltes, Reese, & Lipsitt, 1980). The individual continually develops from birth to death. One can document, for example, the social, cognitive or physical development that an individual experiences from infancy through old age. Similarly, the individual develops as a family member. Although the family is a relatively stable entity, it too has a tendency to change and develop as does the individual's role in that family. Thus, the individual enters the family as its youngest member in infancy and lives through roles of childhood, parent and elder. And finally, regardless of age and role, each individual is a member of a particular historical cohort which significantly characterizes their life experience. Children of the Great Depression forever had a feeling of financial uncertainty and insecurity, people who were involved in the Civil Rights Movement in this country had a lasting impression of the change that could be brought about by massive collaborative efforts, whereas those who were involved in the Vietnam War remember well the feeling of fighting a war on foreign soil which was widely criticized at home. It has been suggested that the only way to gain a true understanding of adult development is to consider each, i.e., individual, family, cohort, of these parallel developmental experiences (Antonucci, 1989; Baltes et al., 1980). We propose that the same separate influences that effect individual development are important to an understanding of intergenerational relations.

One focus of inquiry in the field of intergenerational relations is the degree to which there are similarities and differences between the generations. Bengtson and Cutler (1976) discuss intergenerational solidarity, in terms of the degree to which families are similar across generations. Bengtson and Kuypers (1971) introduce the concept of developmental or generational stake, that is, the degree to which each generation is invested in intergenerational similarity or solidarity. They propose that the older generations have a greater stake in perceiving similarities across generations than younger generations. Older generations want to believe that they have contributed to younger generations in various ways, that they have socialized, transmitted, or in some other way provided the next generations with important characteristics, attitudes, or assets. On the other hand, the younger generations are more interested in making their own, separate and different contribution. Younger generations are more invested in perceiving dissimilarities across generations in order to maximize their own contribution to the family, community and society separately from past generations. These notions of solidarity and developmental stake have been studied in a variety of areas including the experience or exchange of resources and affection (Bengtson et al., 1985; Rosenthal, 1987; Marshall, Troll et al., 1979).

Many changes have been occurring within the broader societal and familial context that influence the nature of intergenerational ties. Recent demographic trends point to the acceleration in generational turnover, the increase in age homogeneity within and between generation, the increased number of multi-generation families, the emergence of long-term intergenerational bonds between adults, decreased societal or normative regulation of family and generations, and a basic increase in the number of family intergenerational relationships caused by changing family structures such as increased divorces and remarriages (Bengtson et al., 1990).

Families and intergenerational relationships have been viewed as major agents of socialization. Traditionally it was assumed that older generations socialized younger ones. Currently it is more accurate to speak of the bi-directionality of the socialization process. This bi-directionality is present in superficial characteristics such as hair and clothing styles and also in more fundamental issues such as child and parents' exchanges or expectations. Bi-directional exchanges may serve an important function of continual involvement of each generation with the other and thus provide one vehicle for maintaining intergenerational ties. These bi-directional exchanges exist over time and are part of a life-time of support relations which the individual maintains as part of his or her convoy of social support.

CONVOYS OF SOCIAL SUPPORT

The term convoy was first used by David Plath to describe the group of people with whom an individual interacts on a relatively steady basis, the group with whom one moves through life (Plath, 1975). Kahn and Antonucci (1980) expanded the use of this term to encompass attachment, roles and social support. Recently, Antonucci and Jackson (1987) explicated the concept further. The basic idea is to view social relations and social support as a life-time, ongoing set of relations that develop and change over time. These relations generally serve to enrich, fortify and reassure people but can sometimes place individuals at risk or make them more vulnerable as they move through life from birth to death.

As people grow and mature so do members of their convoy. Relationships among convoy members are likely to remain the same on some dimensions over time but to change in others over time. Indeed, the membership of the convoy may change over time. The concept social support convoy is unique because it is responsive to the change and development in the individual and, at the same time, provides an important element of stability and continuity over time. Discussions of the convoy model and empirical evidence concerning specific aspects of the model are available elsewhere (Antonucci, 1985; 1990; Antonucci and Akiyama, 1987a and b; Antonucci and Jackson, 1987). This chapter will focus on the role of the social support convoy in understanding intergenerational relations.

INTERGENERATIONAL RELATIONS
AND CONVOYS OF SOCIAL SUPPORT

The study of intergenerational relations can benefit from a life-span, continuous, hierarchical view of social relations offered by the convoy framework. Since social relations are viewed as interactional and hierarchical, it is possible to incorporate the multilevel aspects of intergenerational relations. As people grow and mature, they may attain different levels of intimacy. The nature and frequency of their interactions may change, increase, or decrease. An infant has an "intimate" relationship with her mother but that is very different from the "intimate" relationship she has with her mother when she is an adult and parent herself. Similarly, intergenerational relations between grandparent and grandchild might be frequent and loving when the child is a young preschooler but might change considerably when the cute preschooler becomes a purple spiked-haired teenager.

In the following analyses the underlying framework of the convoy model of social support is used to examine intergenerational relationships. Data from a national study of the social relationships of mature adults are used to examine intra-family intergenerational relationships. The specific issues addressed in this paper are: (1) intergenerational similarities in structure and function of support network, and (2) effects of intergenerational relationships, what we call family intactness, on support function and well-being of older persons.

FINDINGS FROM AN EMPIRICAL STUDY

Empirical findings reported here are based on the analysis of a national study of social support among older adults (Kahn & Antonucci, 1984). The purpose of this study was to provide the first in-depth national study of the social support of mature adults. The principal respondents are a national probability sample of 718 men and women ranging in age from 50 to 95 (298 men and 420 women). Respondents were asked to identify up to 20 people whom they considered part of their social networks. They were presented with a set of 3 concentric circles with a smaller circle in the center in which the word "you" was indicated. They were then asked to name the people who were "close and important" to them in each of three levels as depicted by the three concentric circles. Respondents were also asked to designate who in their social network provided for them each of six support functions and for whom they provided the same six functions. The six support functions are outlined below. Each principal respondent over 70 was requested to identify up to three network members to whom they felt psychologically most close and who lived within a 50 mile radius. In addition, if one child and one grandchild were not included among the initial three network members chosen but were in the network and lived within 50 miles, they were also added to this pool. These network members were asked the same support structure and function questions. One hundred eighty-two (182) children and sixty (60) grandchildren were interviewed.

Trained interviewers administered in-home, structured interviews which were approximately one hour in length for the principal respondents and approximately one-half hour for the network respondents. Both interviews included detailed information about social support and well-being.

1. Intercorrelations Among Structure and Function of Support Network Across Generations

Empirical investigations of social support have focused on the assessment of two types of data: support structure and support function. The former refers to the structural characteristic of the support network. These include such characteristics as the size, gender, age, and frequency of contact among network members. Support function, on the other hand, refers to what network members provide to each other. In this study, six functions were examined: confiding, reassurance, respect, sick care, talk when upset, and talk about health. In order to explore intergenerational similarities and differences in network structure and function a series of correlations were performed between principal respondents' and their children's network structure and function characteristics. Parallel correlations were also conducted examining the relationship between principal respondents' and grandchildren's structure and function variables. Results are presented in Tables 1 and 2. It should be noted that the number of principal/child pairs is considerably larger than the number of principal/grandchild pairs. This is important since it directly affects the relative proportion of significant correlations. As indicated in Table 1, fifteen of the nineteen network structure variables are significantly correlated between parents and children. With the exception of siblings in the network, all correlations were positive. Parallel correlations, examining the relationship between network structure reported by principals and grandchildren, indicate only four significant correlations among the nineteen comparisons.

Table 2 provides the correlations between the number of support

TABLE 1. Correlations between principal and network child and grandchild respondents' structural characteristics

	Child r	(N)	Grandchild r	(N)
Total Number in Network	.29**	(180)	-.10	(60)
Total Number in Inner Circle	.31**	(182)	-.07	(60)
Network Size Changed	.17*	(182)	-.09	(60)
Network Knows Community	.16*	(170)	.27*	(55)
Network Know Each Other	.19**	(182)	.08	(58)
Contact Initiative	.09	(169)	.03	(60)
Number of Males in Network	.37**	(180)	.25*	(60)
Number of Females in Network	.36**	(180)	.14	(60)
Spouse in Network	.06	(172)	-.19	(55)
Number of Children in Network	.03	(172)	.21	(55)
Number of Siblings in Network	-.18*	(172)	-.01	(55)
Number of Other Family in Network	.17*	(172)	.14	(55)
Number of Friends in Network	.23**	(172)	.02	(55)
Average Age of Network	.35**	(161)	.22	(53)
Average Years Known Network	.35**	(154)	.27*	(52)
Frequency of Contact	.34**	(159)	.08	(53)
Proximity	.44**	(163)	.37**	(53)
Personal Doctor	.09	(182)	.02	(60)
Personal Minister	.23**	(182)	-.01	(60)

*p<.05
**p<.01

TABLE 2. Correlations between principal and network child and grandchild respondents' support functions

	Child		Grandchild	
	r	(N)	r	(N)
RECEIVING				
Confiding	.04	(179)	.06	(60)
Reassurance	.16*	(176)	.24	(60)
Respect	.33**	(173)	.13	(59)
Care When Ill	.19**	(175)	.11	(60)
Talk When Upset	.10	(173)	.11	(59)
Talk About Health	.02	(179)	-.14	(60)
Total Receiving	.30**	(163)	.14	(58)
GIVING				
Confiding	.21**	(174)	.00	(58)
Reassurance	.24**	(179)	.01	(59)
Respect	.20**	(160)	.11	(56)
Care When Ill	.11	(179)	.19	(60)
Talk When Upset	.16*	(179)	.07	(60)
Talk About Health	.31**	(179)	.01	(59)
Total Giving	.26**	(161)	.13	(52)

*p<.05
**p<.01

functions reported by principal respondents and by their children or grandchildren. Again, the number of significant correlations between principal and child is greater than the number of significant correlations between principal and grandchild. These correlations were based on responses concerning the first ten people mentioned as members of the individual's network. Correlations are reported for each of the six functions received plus a total of all functions received and for the parallel six plus total functions provided. For four of the receiving and six of the providing support functions, the responses of principal respondents and their children were significantly correlated. Examination of the principal/grandchild pairs indicates no significant correlations.

In general, comparisons of principal/child and principal/grandchild in network structure and support functions suggest fairly consistent patterns. There are more significant relationships between principals and their children than between principals and their grandchildren. However, this finding may be an artifact of the smaller sample size of the latter group.

Other patterns are also evident. Generational similarities between principals and their children are conspicuous in terms of network structure. The pattern for support functions is less pronounced. Network structure for parent/child are similar for total size, number in inner circle, change in network size, network members knowing their community, knowing each other, number of males and females in network, number of siblings, other family, friends in network, average age of network members, years known, frequency of contact, proximity, and having a personal minister in their network.

There are some similarities between principals and children in support functions received, and more similarities in the number of support functions provided. Similarities between parent and child in function received are evident in reassurance, respect, care when ill, and total. Similarities between parent and child in functions provided to others are in their areas of confiding, reassurance, respect, talk when upset, talk about health, and total. People in most situations have a tendency to report that they give more than they receive and this seems to be consistent among intergeneration family members.

2. Family Intactness

In order to further explore the relationship between intergenerational characteristics and social network, a variable called family intactness was created. This variable represents the number of generations the principal respondents included when naming his/her first ten network members. Three levels of inclusion were identified: (1) neither a child nor grandchild named; (2) at least one child or grandchild named; and, (3) both a child and grandchild named as part of the first ten network members. The effect of family intactness on the structure and function of the principal's support network and well-being was examined. These analyses utilize data only from principal respondents (N = 718). Three-way analyses of variance were conducted using Family Intactness (3 levels: R only, child or grandchild, child and grandchild), Age (3 levels: 50-64, 65-74, 75-95) and Gender (male, female) as independent variables.

Network Structure

Table 3 presents analyses of variance (ANOVA) results using network size (total number of persons in network) as the dependent variable. Significant main effects of Family Intactness and Gender are evident as well as an interaction of Intactness by Gender. The main effect of Family Intactness is due to a linear increase in the total number of people in the principal's network with family intactness. Respondents reporting neither a child nor a grandchild in their networks have the smallest networks. The largest networks are reported by people who include both a child and grandchild in their networks. The main effect of Gender is a result of the fact that women have more people in their networks. The Gender by Intactness interaction reflects the fact that, although there is a consistent discrepancy in the total number of people in the principal's network (with women having more people in their network than men), this discrepancy is greatest among respondents who report neither children nor grandchildren in their networks.

The next set of analyses explored Age, Gender, and Family Intactness differences by closeness. The results are shown in Table 4. Network membership in the inner circle represents those people nominated by the respondent as so close and important that it is hard to imagine life without them. Examination of the effect of Family Intactness on the number of people in the inner circle of the network indicates that individuals with a child or grandchild in their network have more people in their inner circle than respondents who report neither child nor grandchild in their network. Principals who report

TABLE 3. Mean distribution of total number in networks (Total N = 694)

Family Intactness

	R Only		Child or Grandchild		Child and Grandchild		Total	
	Men	Women	Men	Women	Men	Women	Men	Women
	$\bar{x}$ (N)	$\bar{x}$ (N)	$\bar{x}$ (N)	$\bar{x}$ (N)	$\bar{x}$ (N)	$\bar{x}$ (N)	$\bar{x}$ (N)	$\bar{x}$ (N)
Ages								
(50–64)	5.79(29)	9.24(29)	9.15(117)	9.84(139)	9.50(2)	14.78(9)	8.50(148)	9.99(177)
(65–74)	5.80(20)	9.88(25)	6.98(57)	9.04(70)	9.75(12)	10.06(35)	7.09(89)	9.48(130)
(75–95)	4.89(9)	6.88(16)	7.91(23)	7.53(32)	9.65(20)	10.72(50)	8.06(52)	9.05(98)
Total by Sex	5.66(58)	8.93(70)	8.38(197)	9.30(241)	9.68(34)	10.86(94)	8.06(52)	
Total	7.45(128)		8.89(438)		10.55(128)			

Family Intactness Effect	$F_{(2,676)} = 13.92**$
Age Effect	$F_{(2,676)} = 2.47$
Sex Effect	$F_{(1,676)} = 17.45**$
Intactness x Age	$F_{(4,676)} = 1.55$
Intactness x Sex	$F_{(2,676)} = 3.01$
Age x Sex	$F_{(2,676)} = .77$
Intactness x Age x Sex	$F_{(4,676)} = .70$

* $p<.05$
** $p<.01$

both a child and grandchild in their network also report the highest number of people in their inner circle. The inclusion of children and grandchildren as network members apparently indicates a more general involvement in intimate relationships.

Family Intactness is significantly related to the number of friends and siblings a principal respondent included among the first ten network members. As indicated in Table 5, examination of the number of friends in the network reveals a different pattern. This suggests a compensatory process. Respondents who have neither a child nor grandchild in their network have the most friends in their network, whereas respondents who have both children and grandchildren in their network have the least number of friends in their network. Although not shown in a table, examination of the number

TABLE 4. Mean distribution of total number in inner circle (Total N = 695)

	Family Intactness							
	R Only		Child or Grandchild		Child and Grandchild		Total	
	Men	Women	Men	Women	Men	Women	Men	Women
	$\bar{X}$ (N)	$\bar{X}$ (N)	$\bar{X}$ (N)	$\bar{X}$ (N)	$\bar{X}$ (N)	$\bar{X}$ (N)	$\bar{X}$ (N)	$\bar{X}$ (N)
Ages								
(50-64)	2.21(29)	4.14(29)	3.33(117)	3.84(140)	4.50(2)	4.89(9)	3.12(148)	3.94(178)
(65-74)	2.50(20)	2.96(25)	3.14(57)	3.96(70)	2.58(12)	4.31(35)	2.92(89)	3.86(130)
(75-95)	1.78(9)	2.69(16)	2.87(23)	3.28(32)	2.90(20)	4.78(50)	2.69(52)	3.95(98)
Total by sex	2.24(58)	3.39(70)	3.22(197)	3.80(242)	2.88(34)	4.62(94)		
Total	2.87(128)		3.54(439)		4.16(128)			

Family Intactness Effect	$F_{(2, 677)} = 6.87**$
Age Effect	$F_{(2, 677)} = .25$
Sex Effect	$F_{(1, 677)} = 21.16**$
Intactness x Age	$F_{(4, 677)} = .77$
Intactness x Sex	$F_{(2, 677)} = 1.87$
Age x Sex	$F_{(2, 677)} = .27$
Intactness x Age x Sex	$F_{(4, 677)} = .70$

*p <.05
**p <.01

TABLE 5. Mean distribution of number of friends among first ten network members (Total N = 695)

	Family Intactness							
	R Only		Child or Grandchild		Child or Grandchild		Total	
	Men	Women	Men	Women	Men	Women	Men	Women
	$\bar{x}$ (N)	$\bar{x}$ (N)	$\bar{x}$ (N)	$\bar{x}$ (N)	$\bar{x}$ (N)	$\bar{x}$ (N)	$\bar{x}$ (N)	$\bar{x}$ (N)
Ages								
(50–64)	1.69(29)	2.35(29)	1.18(117)	1.29(140)	.00(2)	.33(9)	1.26(148)	1.41(178)
(65–74)	1.35(20)	4.16(25)	.91(57)	1.60(70)	.50(12)	.91(35)	.96(89)	1.91(130)
(75–95)	2.11(9)	2.31(16)	1.65(23)	1.38(32)	.30(20)	1.08(50)	1.21(52)	1.38(98)
Total by Sex	1.64(58)	2.99(70)	1.16(197)	1.39(242)	.35(34)	.95(94)		
Total	2.38(128)		1.28(439)		.79(128)			

Family Intactness Effect	$F(2,677) = 29.19**$
Age Effect	$F(2,677) = .79$
Sex Effect	$F(1,677) = 8.26**$
Intactness x Age	$F(4,677) = 1.35$
Intactness x Sex	$F(2,677) = 4.09*$
Age x Sex	$F(2,677) = 4.04*$
Intactness x Age x Sex	$F(4,677) = 1.97$

* p<.05
** p<.01

of siblings in the network revealed a similar pattern. There is also a significant interaction of Family Intactness with Gender on the number of friends which reveals a somewhat complicated pattern of results. At all three levels of Family Intactness, women are more likely than men to report friends in their network. However, the largest discrepancy between men and women in number of friends occurs among respondents who have neither a child nor a grandchild in their network; and this discrepancy is smallest among respondents who have either a child or a grandchild in their network.

In sum, network structure is significantly related to Family Intactness in several predictable ways. Respondents with neither a child nor grandchild in their network have networks which are smaller and have fewer people in the inner circle. On the other hand, in comparison with those who have children and grandchildren in their network, these respondents also are likely to report more friends and siblings in their network.

Support Functions

As in the analyses of network structure, three-way analyses of variance (Family Intactness × Age × Gender) were performed for support functions. Family Intactness is significantly related to the number of people from whom respondents report receiving both instrumental and emotional support. Table 6 indicates that people with no child or grandchild in their network report the fewest number of people who would care for them when sick. Those with either or both children and grandchildren report about the same number of people.

The number of network members who respondents report talking to when they are upset is also related to Family Intactness. As indicated in Table 7, people with neither a child nor grandchild in their network report the least number of people talking with them when they are upset. Respondents with either a child or grandchild in their support network have the largest number of people to talk to when they are upset. Those with both a child and grandchild in the network report an intermediate number.

Well-Being

Analyses indicate that the relationship between Family Intactness and Well-being is not as strong as between Family Intactness and support variables. None of the three measures of well-being, the one item life satisfaction question, the one item happiness question and the two item support adequacy index is significantly related to Family Intactness. However, as indicated in Table 8, satisfaction with Interpersonal Relationships is significantly affected by Family Intactness. Respondents with neither a child nor a grandchild in their network report the lowest level of satisfaction with Interpersonal Relationships. Respondents with either or both a child and grandchild in their network report somewhat higher levels of satisfaction with their Interpersonal Relationships.

And finally, overall Physical Well-being is also affected by an

TABLE 6. Mean distribution of number who care for respondent when sick (Total N = 686)

	R only		Child or Grandchild		Child and Grandchild		Total	
Family Intactness	Men	Women	Men	Women	Men	Women	Men	Women
	$\bar{x}$ (N)	$\bar{x}$ (N)	$\bar{x}$ (N)	$\bar{x}$ (N)	$\bar{x}$ (N)	$\bar{x}$ (N)	$\bar{x}$ (N)	$\bar{x}$ (N)
Ages (50-64)	2.83(29)	3.59(29)	3.95(117)	4.07(138)	7.50(2)	4.33(9)	3.78(148)	4.01(176)
(65-74)	2.60(20)	3.50(24)	3.88(56)	4.00(69)	3.58(12)	3.71(35)	3.55(88)	3.83(128)
(75-95)	2.44(9)	2.81(16)	3.44(23)	3.21(29)	4.11(19)	3.76(50)	3.51(51)	3.43(95)
Total by Sex	2.69(58)	3.38(69)	3.87(196)	3.94(236)	4.12(33)	3.80(94)		
Total	3.06(127)		3.91(432)		3.88(127)			

Family Intactness Effect $F_{(2, 668)} = 5.16**$

Age Effect $F_{(2, 668)} = 1.50$

Sex Effect $F_{(1, 668)} = .54$

Intactness x Age $F_{(4, 668)} = .61$

Intactness x Sex $F_{(2, 668)} = 1.06$

Age x Sex $F_{(2, 668)} = .19$

Intactness x Age x Sex $F_{(4, 668)} = .52$

* $p < .05$
** $p < .01$

TABLE 7. Mean distribution of number who respondent talks to when upset (Total N = 689)

	Family Intactness							
	R Only		Child or Grandchild		Child and Grandchild		Total	
	Men	Women	Men	Women	Men	Women	Men	Women
	$\bar{X}$ (N)	$\bar{X}$ (N)	$\bar{X}$ (N)	$\bar{X}$ (N)	$\bar{X}$ (N)	$\bar{X}$ (N)	$\bar{X}$ (N)	$\bar{X}$ (N)
Ages (50-64)	2.07(29)	2.72(29)	3.50(117)	3.73(138)	5.50(2)	2.33(9)	3.25(148)	3.49(176)
(65-74)	1.50(20)	2.40(25)	2.78(56)	2.81(69)	3.75(12)	2.97(35)	2.64(88)	2.78(129)
(75-95)	2.78(9)	1.87(15)	2.17(23)	1.97(32)	3.11(19)	2.42(50)	2.63(51)	2.19(97)
Total by Sex	1.98(58)	2.42(69)	3.15(196)	3.23(239)	3.48(33)	2.62(94)		
Total	2.22(127)		3.19(435)		2.84(127)			

Family Intactness Effect	$F_{(2, 671)}$ = 6.83**
Age Effect	$F_{(2, 671)}$ = 10.30**
Sex Effect	$F_{(1, 671)}$ = .00
Intactness x Age	$F_{(4, 671)}$ = 1.22
Intactness x Sex	$F_{(2, 671)}$ = 1.70
Age x Sex	$F_{(2, 671)}$ = .93
Intactness x Age x Sex	$F_{(4, 671)}$ = .85

* $p < .05$
** $p < .01$

TABLE 8. Mean distribution of satisfaction with interpersonal relationships (N = 671)

	R only		Child or Grandchild		Child and Grandchild		Total	
	Men $\bar{x}$ (N)	Women $\bar{x}$ (N)	Men $\bar{x}$ (N)	Women $\bar{x}$ (N)	Men $\bar{x}$ (N)	Women $\bar{x}$ (N)	Men $\bar{x}$ (N)	Women $\bar{x}$ (N)
Ages (50-64)	2.38(29)	2.43(28)	2.87(117)	2.48(136)	4.00(2)	3.11(9)	2.79(148)	2.50(173)
(65-74)	2.05(19)	2.16(19)	2.86(55)	2.52(67)	2.33(12)	2.59(32)	2.60(86)	2.48(118)
(75-95)	2.78(9)	2.40(15)	3.04(23)	2.55(31)	3.00(20)	2.54(48)	2.96(52)	2.52(94)
Total by Sex	2.33(57)	2.34(62)	2.89(195)	2.50(234)	2.82(34)	2.62(89)		
Total	2.34(119)		2.68(429)		2.67(123)			

Family Intactness Effect $F_{(2,653)} = 4.93**$

Age Effect $F_{(2,653)} = .99$

Sex Effect $F_{(1,653)} = 9.40**$

Intactness x Age $F_{(4,653)} = 1.36$

Intactness x Sex $F_{(2,653)} = 1.75$

Age x Sex

119

interaction of Family Intactness by Gender. Among respondents who have neither a child nor a grandchild in their network, men report considerably higher levels of overall Physical Well-being than women. However, women with a child and/or a grandchild in their network report slightly higher levels of overall Physical Well-being than men in these groups (see Table 9).

SUMMARY AND CONCLUSIONS

A series of cross-generational comparative analyses indicates a substantial number of similarities in network structure and support functions among principal respondents and their children. This relationship pattern is considerably less strong for the principal/grandchild dyad. An additional set of analyses examined the effect of family intactness on network structure, support functions, and well-being of the principal respondent. Results indicate a significant effect of family intactness on both structure, support function variables and to a more limited degree well-being. These data also suggest that having a convoy of social support which includes multi-generation family members may serve the important function of minimizing the gender differences that appear more prominent among respondents who do not have a child or grandchild in their network. These findings suggest that family memberships serve an even greater protective function for men than women.

At the theoretical level our findings provide some support for the convoy model of intergenerational relations. Older people with adult children do seem to have a mutual effect on each other. Parents and their adult children's support relationships are structured in a very similar fashion. This is much less true of grandchildren. Similarly, parents are very much like their adult children, but not particularly like their grandchildren, in the types of support they receive and provide. In addition, the family intactness variable was significantly related to structure, function and well-being variables, suggesting that intergenerational family convoys of social support have intergenerational family members who are similar to each other. The cross-sectional nature of these data do not permit an explication of the causal direction of these relationships but it is likely that such influences are bi-directional, that is, that while

TABLE 9. Mean distribution of overall physical well-being (Total N = 692)

	Family Intactness							
	P Only		Child or Grandchild		Child and Grandchild		Total	
	Men	Women	Men	Women	Men	Women	Men	Women
	$\bar{X}$ (N)	$\bar{X}$ (N)	$\bar{X}$ (N)	$\bar{X}$ (N)	$\bar{X}$ (N)	$\bar{X}$ (N)	$\bar{X}$ (N)	$\bar{X}$ (N)
Ages								
(50-64)	3.76(29)	2.98(29)	3.48(117)	3.59(140)	3.92(2)	2.76(9)	3.54(148)	3.45(178)
(65-74)	3.75(20)	3.14(24)	3.54(56)	3.53(70)	3.16(11)	3.38(35)	3.54(87)	3.41(129)
(75-95)	3.69(9)	3.37(16)	3.08(23)	3.13(32)	3.22(20)	3.27(50)	3.24(52)	3.24(98)
Total by Sex	3.74(58)	3.13(69)	3.45(196)	3.51(242)	3.24(33)	3.26(94)		
Total	3.41(127)		3.48(438)		3.26(127)			

Family Intactness Effect	$F_{(2,674)} = .81$
Age Effect	$F_{(2,674)} = 3.37*$
Sex Effect	$F_{(1,674)} = 1.76$
Intactness x Age	$F_{(4,674)} = 1.97$
Intactness x Sex	$F_{(2,674)} = 5.92**$
Age x Sex	$F_{(2,674)} = .22$
Intactness x Age x Sex	$F_{(4,674)} = .98$

* p<.05
** p<.01

older family members influence younger ones, the opposite is also true.

Our empirical findings provide confirmation of our view that the life-course model of convoys of social support can usefully be extended to improve our understanding of intergenerational relations. The similarities in support relations, at least among parents and their adult children, suggests the importance and influence of intergenerational socialization concerning the very nature of support relationships. However, the lack of a consistent association between well-being and family intactness or intergenerational relations does suggest caution concerning the over interpretation of the positive influences of intergenerational relationships. Our analyses tested for linear relationships only, i.e., that greater family intactness is associated linearly with either positive or negative well-being. No association was found for life satisfaction or happiness but was found for physical well-being and satisfaction with interpersonal relationships. We feel these findings suggest a note of caution in the interpretation of intergeneration family influences as always positive. It seems likely that while family intactness positively influences the structure and function of social relations as a matter of socialization, the effect of family intactness may not always be positive. Families which are intact, that is, wherein intergenerational membership is evident, may have a strong influence on the membership but that influence need not always be positive. Thus, it is important to note that the convoy of social support provides an explanatory vehicle for understanding how intergenerational family members influence each other but that influence can be positive as in the case of warm, loving family relationships, or can be negative as might be the case in a demanding or overprotecting family.

REFERENCES

Antonucci, T.C. (1990). Social support and social relationships. In R.H. Binstock & L.K. George (Eds.), *Handbook of Aging and the Social Sciences, 3rd Edition*, (pp. 205-226). San Diego, CA: Academic Press, Inc.

Antonucci, T.C. (1989). Understanding adult social relationships. In K. Kreppner & R.L. Lerner (Eds.), *Family Systems and Life-Span Development*, (pp. 303-317). Hillsdale, NJ: Erlbaum.

Antonucci, T.C. (1985). Personal characteristics, social support, and social behavior. In R.H. Binstock & E. Shanas (Eds.), *Handbook of Aging and the Social Sciences* 2nd Edition (pp. 94-128). New York: Van Nostrand Reinhold.

Antonucci, T.C. & Akiyama, H. (1987a). Social networks in adult life and a preliminary examination of the convoy model. *Journal of Gerontology 42*(5), 519-527.

Antonucci, T.C. & Akiyama, H. (1987b). An examination of sex differences in social support among older men and women. *Sex Roles*, *17*(11/12), 737-749.

Antonucci, T.C. & Jackson, J.S. (1987). Social support, interpersonal efficacy, and health. In L. Carstensen & B.A. Edelstein, (Eds.), *Handbook of Clinical Gerontology* (pp. 291-311). New York: Pergamon Press.

Baltes, P.B., Reese, H. & Lipsitt, L., (1980). Life-span developmental psychology. *Annual Review of Psychology, 31:*, 65-110.

Bengtson, V.L., Rosenthal, C., & Burton, L. (1990). Families and Aging: Diversity and Heterogeneity. In R.H. Binstock & L.K. George (Eds.), *Handbook of Aging and the Social Sciences* (pp. 263-287). San Diego, CA: Academic Press.

Bengtson, V.L., Cutler, N.E., Mangen, D.J. & Marshall, V.M. (1985). Generations, cohorts, and relations between age groups. In R.H. Binstock & E. Shanas (Eds.), *Handbook of Aging and the Social Sciences* 2nd Edition (pp. 304-338) New York: Van Nostrand Reinhold.

Bengtson, V.L. & Cutler, N.E. (1976). Generations and intergenerational relations: Perspectives on age groups and social change. In R.H. Binstock & E. Shanas (Eds.), *Handbook of Aging and the Social Sciences* (pp. 130-159). New York: Van Nostrand Reinhold.

Bengtson, V.L. & Kuypers, J.A. (1971). Generational difference and the developmental stake. *Aging and Human Development*, *2*, 249-260.

Hagestad, G. (1981). Problems and promises in the social psychology of intergenerational relations. In J. March (Ed.), *Aging: Stability and Change in the Family* (pp. 11-46) New York: Academic Press.

Kahn, R.L. & Antonucci, T.C. (1980). Convoys over the life-course: Attachment, roles, and social support. In P.B. Baltes, O.G. Brim (Eds.), *Life-Span Development and Behavior* (pp. 253-286). New York: Academic Press.

Kahn, R.L. & Antonucci, T.C. (1984). Supports of the Elderly final report.

Plath, D. (1975). Aging and social support. A presentation to the Committee on Work and Personality in the Middle Years, Social Science Research Council.

Rosenthal, C.J. (1987). Aging and Intergenerational Relations in Canada. In V.W. Marshall (Ed.), *Aging in Canada* (pp. 311-342). Markham, ONT: Fitzhenry & Whiteside.

Troll, L.E., Miller, S.J., & Atchley, R.C. (1979). *Families in Later Life.* Monterey, CA: Wadsworth Publishing Co.

Intergenerational Caregivers
of the Oldest Old

Beverly Sanborn
Sally Bould

INTRODUCTION

Intergenerational family ties are a critical caregiving resource for people aged 85 and over — the oldest old. This segment of the population has the highest potential for functional disabilities and, therefore, has the greatest need for caregiver support. The oldest old are also the fastest growing segment of the population, a condition that will continue well into the next century. Since family caregivers are the bulwark against unnecessary institutionalization and more costly forms of care, there is an urgent need to bolster the strengths of existing caregivers and to entice new helpers into their ranks.

More and more, the primary responsibility for giving care to this age group is shouldered by adult children, children-in-law, nieces, nephews and grandchildren. Care of the oldest old falls to younger generations because spousal care, the first line of defense for other age groups, is minimal for the oldest old. Spouses are in short supply, and even when they exist, they are often not physically able to provide assistance with personal care — i.e., bathing, toileting, eating, grooming; mobility — i.e., walking, transferring in and out of bed and chairs; and, instrumental activities of daily living — e.g., shopping, meal preparation, transportation, managing money, cleaning, laundry. For the oldest old, living with others of their own generation does not guarantee availability of able caregivers. Sib-

Beverly Sanborn is Vice President, Alzheimer's Services, Health Care Group, San Diego, CA. Sally Bould is Associate Professor of Sociology, University of Delaware, Newark, DE 19716.

lings and friends may not be a potential caregiving resource because they, too, are likely to be members of the oldest age groups. Therefore, intergenerational caregivers offer the only reliable hope for meeting much of the care needs of the oldest old.

More information is needed about intergenerational caregivers. Most studies have focused on caregivers in a global scene, failing to examine separately the younger generations and the spouses. Yet there is clinical, as well as research, evidence that the psychological impact and challenges faced by intergenerational caregivers differs markedly from the experience of spouses (Doty, 1986, p. 51-52; Day, 1988, p. 3; Hamon, 1988, p. 8; p. 21; Miller and Montgomery, 1989; Montgomery and Borgatta, 1989; Sanborn and Bould, 1990). An important aspect of the caregiving role is the components of the caregiver-care receiver dyad.

This paper will review the available data and explore the following questions: Who are oldest old? Who are their intergenerational caregivers? What motivates these caregivers? What are their caregiver burdens? How can these caregivers be supported by public policy and service providers? The paper proposes that issues of family caregiving for the oldest old be examined using a family systems approach within the larger context of interdependence of family and community.

DEMOGRAPHICS – WHO ARE THE OLDEST OLD?

The oldest old are largely widowed (70%) and mostly women (70%) (Longino, 1988, p. 518). This age group is growing faster than any other segment of the population. Their numbers have increased 141% since 1960, currently 2.3 million individuals are estimated to be in this age group. With continued downturns in mortality from cardiovascular disease, these numbers will continue to grow, reaching 5.4 million by the year 2000 and 7.6 million by 2020 (Longino, 1988, p. 515). Since the need for caregivers increases with age, it is probable there will never be enough caregivers to maintain oldest old people in the community. Over 70% of the oldest old have an impairment in one or more activities of daily living (Longino, 1988, p. 516). Longino (1988, p. 518) estimates that 36% of community-dwelling people of advanced years need caregiver assistance with at least one of these Activities of Daily Living (ADL) limitations.

Even though 21% of this age group are married, the spouse may not be physically or cognitively able to act as caregiver. Whether an older person lives with a spouse, an adult child or alone is a major determinant in the amount of social support immediately available. For the elder living alone the move to a nursing home is often a two-step process (Kovar, 1987). Initially caregiving is likely to be provided in the elder's own home; subsequently there may be a move into a child's home. Only later, if at all, is the final move into a nursing home necessary. The oldest old, however, may not have the two-step option; one in seven who live alone have neither a sibling nor a child to provide caregiving of this intensity (Kaspar, 1988, p. 67).

The most dramatic example for the increased need for caregivers with increasing longevity among the oldest old is Alzheimer's disease. This age group has a high risk of dementia; most recent estimates indicate that almost one in two people 85 and over experience some degree of Alzheimer's (Evans et al., 1989). Unlike other chronic illnesses, dementia requires almost constant supervision, even in the early, less disabling stages.

As the numbers in the oldest age groups grow and the need for caregivers increases proportionately, it is necessary to explore attitudes and other factors which influence family support. Specifically, the following questions must be asked: Is the grandmother generation prepared to be the caregiver for the great grandmother generation? Are there weaker ties but reliable claims for support from other members of the extended family? What is the best context for families and service providers working together?

WHO ARE THE CAREGIVERS OF THE OLDEST OLD?

Caregiving has been called the "fundamental women's issue of our decade" (Sommers, 1985, p. 6; Walker, 1983; Wilkinson, 1988). Eighty-five percent of all caregivers are women. This process begins with childbearing and ends with care of elderly parents, aging spouses and other needy family members – a virtual career in caregiving (Brody, 1985). In fact, women in their 60s and 70s—the caregivers to the oldest old--were socialized to look upon this role as their only real and valued occupation. However, women in these age groups can look forward to continuing their caregiver careers. According to Brody's 1985 study, 40% of people in their late 50s; 20% of people in their late 60s and 3% of people in their 70s have at least one surviving parent (Brody, 1985, p. 20).

These aging adult-child caregivers provide a substantial amount of care to the oldest old. Soldo and Manton (1985, p. 304) estimate that 50% of all service days needed by oldest old women are handled by adult children. Daughters provide 47% of all helper days and other women, presumably daughters-in-law and granddaughters provide 30% of helper days. The strong sense of filial responsibility among three generations of women has been documented by Brody (Brody, 1981, pp. 471-480; Brody et al., 1983, pp. 597-607). The study showed a majority of the women in all generations agreed that adult children should act as primary caregivers adjusting family schedules to meet the needs of the elderly mothers and helping to pay for professional health care when needed.

Recent attention has been directed toward the caregiving role of men. It should be noted that most of these men are spouses. Adult son, grandson and nephew caregivers are still rare.[1] With an escalating demand for caregivers, it may be necessary to seek out potential intergenerational male caregivers who are willing to assume this role. Though research is scanty, there is evidence that older male caregivers are not substantially different from older female caregivers in the way they handle the role in terms of spousal care (Fitting and Rabins, 1985). More information is needed about adult son caregivers (Raveis, Siegel and Sudit, 1990). When daughters or daughters-in-law provide for hands-on assistance, the sons tend to take more facilitive roles such as home repair, hiring outside help, seeking community services, assisting in legal, social security and welfare matters, (Raveis et al., 1990). It is unknown whether adult sons will take on the traditional "women's caregiver role" when sisters and daughters-in-law are not available to help. Perhaps the recent changes in traditional roles for men and women will be reflected in more androgynous roles when today's youth become to-morrow's caregivers.

Despite their deep commitment, normally adult children do not live with an elderly parent. This form of shared housing has been in sharp decline over the last 30 years. In 1950, for example, 32% of non-institutionalized men of advanced years lived with an adult child. By 1980, that proportion decreased to 9%. A similar trend is evident for women aged 85 and over. In 1950, 47% of this group were living with an adult child, but only 18% shared the children's residence in 1980 (Rosenwaike, 1985, Table 7.4).

In earlier decades, the elderly lived with adult children largely due to economic necessity. Today, most elderly people rank living with adult children as a "last resort" — before moving into a nursing home (Day, 1988, p. 8). The improved economic status of most elderly people allows them to enjoy their most preferred option: living independently but in close proximity to their family. In Brody's study of their generations of women (Brody, 1981; Brody et al., 1983) all agreed that sharing households was not an appropriate solution to health impairments. According to Day's study of women aged 77 to 87 (Day, 1988, p. 3) a large majority viewed living in a separate household as a "norm" for people their age. This living arrangement was definitely preferred by 67% of the respondents (Day, 1988, p. 3). The oldest old like to maintain intimate contact, emotional support and live in close proximity to an adult child in case need for help arises. Almost 8 out of 10 people of advanced years, who have adult children, live near at least one child (Kaspar, 1988, p. 65). There is high frequency of contact as well. Seventy-three percent receive daily or weekly visits from the adult child (Kaspar, 1988, p. 66). Unfortunately, one in seven of the oldest old who live alone have neither an adult child nor a sibling who can provide care or companionship when it is needed (Kaspar, 1988, p. 67).

When an adult child is available the dedication to parental care can be very strong. The levels of care provided are surprisingly intense. Adult children can handle very high levels of physical care, including all aspects of home and money management, in addition to toileting, eating, walking, bathing, (Brody, 1981). This is the case even when these parents cannot be left for more than a few hours, some only a few minutes per day. In most cases this high level of care is generally provided by adult daughters.

Research indicates that when the elderly parent's physical health worsens, family members are faced with making a decision to place their parent in a nursing home (Doty, 1986, p. 47). But what constitutes "worse"? Most caregivers, who have been studied, have spent from 8 months to 5 years in their role (Doty, 1986, p. 47). In many cases, adult child caregivers have taken the elders into their own homes prior to institutionalization. What aspects of care tipped the balance, making the burden "too much to handle"? Or, why did family members wait so long before deciding to place their parent? To answer these questions, it is necessary to find out what motivates aging adult children to make this commitment to their very old parent.

MOTIVATION FOR CAREGIVING – A FAMILY SYSTEMS PERSPECTIVE

Intergenerational caregiving can be examined from a family systems perspective. Theoretical constructs about family systems focus on three dimensions: family cohesion, adaptability and communication (Olson, 1988). In his normative study of family development, Olson identified these dimensions or processes after putting together a conceptual clustering of more than 50 existing concepts:

> The first family process, or dimension, *family cohesion* had to do with the degree to which an individual was separated from or connected to his or her family system. The second dimension was *family adaptability*, which focused on the extent to which the family system was flexible and able to change. The third dimension was *family communication* between various members. (1988, p. 59)

Olson (1988) further identifies specific concepts relating to these dimensions as:

1. Family cohesion: Emotional bonding, boundaries, coalitions, time, space, friends, decision making, and interests and recreation
2. Adaptability: family power (assertiveness, control and discipline); negotiation style; role relationships; and relationship rules
3. Communication: a facilitating dimension for the other two which includes: positive communication skills (empathy, reflective listening, supportive comments) and negative communication skills (double messages, double binds, criticism) (pp. 60-61).

These family dimensions wax and wane in positive, negative, or balanced directions over the life cycle of a family. According to Falicov, (1988), "The core concept of the developmental framework is the notion that families change in form and function over the life cycle and that they do so in an ordered sequence of *developmental states*" (1988, p. 5). Stresses occur within each state, as well as within the transition between stages and dysfunctional adjustments in the not-quite-achieved new stage.

A family system approach has not been incorporated into research on caregivers, although there has been limited attention to the study of role relationship (Hamon, 1988; Brody, 1981; Brody et al., 1983). All too often caregivers are treated as isolated individuals showing symptoms of stress. The limitations of individualistic approach are becoming increasingly more evident because global generalizations fail to differentiate between the experiences of adult child vs. spousal caregivers; male vs. female caregivers; primary vs. secondary caregivers. From a practitioner point of view, the need for a family system and family-life-cycle theoretical framework is highlighted in examinations of what motivates caregivers. The commitment probably spans many generations of family life history, and is inextricably linked to bondedness with family members, feelings of reciprocity, expectations and norms, as well as each individual's sense of self. Practitioners are grappling with such issues as: What is functional vs. dysfunctional caregiving? When should caregivers be counseled to strengthen their own network vs.

using resources from the formal system? When should a family make a decision to place a health-impaired elderly parent in a facility? How does a family's system of behaviors impede or enhance decision-making?

Doty has summarized research findings by pointing to three factors contributing to caregiver motivation: (1) love and affection; (2) a feeling of gratitude for the elderly person's past love and devotion to the family; (3) a response to higher cultural or familial values — doing what is right and living up to what is expected of an adult child (1986, p. 47). Using Olson's model, these three factors represent *family cohesion* or the sense of boundedness. Studies have shown that a sense of loyalty and filial responsibility can be a sufficient motivator even when feelings of affection are not present. However, the amount of time and intensity of care are increased if the feelings of affection are high (Doty, 1986, p. 47).

There are many satisfactions in caregiving. Using the Olson model, positive experiences of cohesion has its own rewards. It is extremely important that counselors and service providers do not assume that every caregiver feels overburdened. While the literature emphasizes the burden aspect of the role, this is a one-sided view, which does not reflect the whole experience. Most research on the subject is systematically biased because samples are drawn from service provider organizations or client groups (Matthews, 1988; Raveis et al., 1990). Furthermore, an item analysis of most caregiver burden scales indicates an expectation of burden. As Raveis et al. point out "Research on help-seeking behavior has illustrated that personality, cultural, and socioeconomic characteristics are associated with the decision to seek help, the sources approached, and the conditions under which assistance is sought" (1990, p. 56).

The families who seek out services will probably harbor at least some feelings of burden. These feelings can be expressed behaviorally as denial, depression, despair, exhaustion, or the feeling can appear as resentment directed toward other family members who are "not doing their share" (cf. Brody et al., 1989). Burden feelings may occur when motivation is high, but the caregiver feels overwhelmed by the responsibility. Since caregiving involves shifts in roles, a stress is placed on the family system to make a change in the structure, the allotments of time, and the priorities of individuals. Using Olson's model, the burden issues arise when the *family adaptability* dimension is stressed. It is important to understand caregiver burden, because these feelings, more than any other factor, can lead to decisions to institutionalize a frail elderly person.

CAREGIVER BURDEN
AND THE FAMILY SYSTEM

Caregiver burden has two dimensions to be considered: the objective and the subjective (Zarit, 1985). Objective burden is essentially what the caregiver is required to *do*, and subjective burden is the caregiver's *feeling or perception about the responsibility*. Objective burden is related to the type of disabling condition, the amount of hands-on time needed and the time period for the caregiving — whether brief, intermittent, or indefinite. Objective burden includes activities required to handle personal care as well as problem behaviors.

The amount of objective burden does not dictate the amount of subjective burden. There is enormous variability in caregiver reactions to the physical tasks and family role changes. Some caregivers feel extreme stress because a parent makes embarrassing statements in public, others are not stressed even though the parent is incontinent or does not recognize family members. It is possible, for example, that the requirements of objective burden will actually pull a family closer together, thereby increasing cohesion. The family may develop new adaptive or coping styles and the net result may be very positive and fulfilling for the family members. It is also possible that the imposition of a caregiving role will so stress the existing family system that positive cohesion is jeopardized and the family's adaptability becomes dysfunctional. The following case examples illustrate:

Mrs. D, age 87, developed Alzheimer's disease very gradually. By the time she reached 85, her 92 year old husband could no longer supervise her or care for her grooming, nor was he skilled in filling in the "women's" role of grocery shopping, cooking and cleaning. The couple had enjoyed a 57 year marriage and were loath to separate. As Mrs. D's condition grew worse, her adult daughter, Donna, age 62, and son-in-law, Jim, age 65, decided to become the primary caregivers. Donna and Jim were still running their own very demanding business, thus adding time constraints to the parent care situation. Donna and Jim held a family conference with their grown children. One son decided to enter the family business, a decision he had been contemplating for several months, to free up time for Donna and Jim to help the grandparents. Donna and Jim then divided up the tasks and, by making use of community services such as adult day care for Mrs. D., were able to set up a whole new family lifestyle. This experience pulled the family closer together and gave them a new enterprise — a sort of adventure — to work on together.

The L. family had a very different experience as caregivers. Mrs. S. was 85 and suffered from many physical ailments, which she had complained about for the last 8 years. Her daughter, Mollie, had been her caregiver. Mrs. S. always ailed, complained, and demanded constant attention, but criticized all efforts to assist her. All her physical complaints, whether real or imagined, were exacerbated by age and compounded by mild dementia. Although Mollie was retired, she was torn between the demands of her ailing and aging husband and those of her mother. She envied people who could use community services but did not know how to persuade her mother or husband to cooperate. The caregiving role strained the bonds between Mollie, her husband, and her mother. Adaptations to retirement were not made smoothly or happily. Mollie reported that both she and her husband felt depressed and hopeless.

The differences between these two families is in the subjective perception or feeling evoked by the caregiving experience. The examples illustrate the way in which each family has a life cycle, a family history, and a unique style of communication, which holds together the family boundaries and facilitates adaptation or change. Family life cycles are products of changes, both predictable and unpredictable, which occur as the life cycle unfolds. To understand subjective burden, it is useful to use a model of life cycle events and to understand the special stresses and strains which relate to each stage.

The life cycle literature is almost entirely developed around issues of child-rearing. Thus, Olson's 7 stage cycle, for example, includes: (1) childless couple; (2) oldest child is a preschooler; (3) oldest child is school age; (4) oldest child is adolescent; (5) launching the children; (6) empty nest; (7) retirement (Olson, 1988, p. 58). This model, however, ignores the fact that the years of child care can cover a very broad range of ages—i.e., a preschool child combined with launching of older children from a previous marriage. Furthermore it implies that life-cycle caregiving functions are limited to children living in the household. Family members—adult children, siblings, parents—in need of care, are excluded even if they live in the household. Instead of stopping at retirement, a life cycle model needs to include a rearrangement of family roles and/or household members to incorporate the care of a parent in their late eighties or nineties.

The care of an oldest old parent is becoming a "normative" event—i.e., it occurs for many people at similar ages. Furthermore it is an "on-time event" (Neugarten, 1977). As an anticipated life stage, families can make appropriate plans. Stresses can also be mitigated by family members sharing experiences with others of their cohort. Furthermore, the older caregivers can anticipate becoming the elder of the family when the oldest old member dies. The anticipatory socialization can strengthen bonds of reciprocity between the oldest member and the adult child caregiver while at the same time providing a role model to the younger generations.

In all likelihood, the middle-aged caregiver does not receive as many benefits from the caregiving role. First, the role is often imposed upon family obligations, involving children at home, as well as career obligations (Stoller and Pugliesi, 1989). Called the "Sandwich Generation," they are caught between two competing needs—those of their young adult and teenage children and those of their aging parents. Furthermore, the middle-aged daughter thrust into the caregiving role may have previously depended upon her mother for support (Thompson and Walker, 1984; Rosenberg, 1988).

A caregiving role can be experienced as a double problem—it is both a loss and a burden. For most middle-aged people, the caregiving experience is still an "off-time event" (Neugarten, 1977). It is not normative because it is not typical for the life stage. The demands are, therefore, unanticipated stressors which appear without prior planning or expectation. Furthermore, middle-aged caregivers are less likely to see themselves as a disabled older adult. They are, therefore, less able to identify with a parent or grandparent who needs care.

The older married adult caregiver has another advantage over the younger caregiver counterpart. The empty nest stage of marital life experienced by older caregivers is markedly happier than the launching-the-children stage characteristic of middle-aged caregivers (Olson, 1988, p. 75). Since marital happiness is highly correlated with positive adaptations to stress (Olson, 1988, p. 74), the older caregiver's family system is likely to be in a stronger position than the younger counterpart.

The differences between the older and younger caregivers also points out how subjective stress relates to issues other than the caregiving. Chiriboga, Weiler and Nielson found that adult child caregivers feel more stress from work hassles, social relationship problems and work events than from the caregiving itself. "Findings also suggested that chronic problems arising from the caregiver role may provide the context for stress overload" (Chiriboga et al., 1988-89, p. 135). Stress is a product of accumulated stressors which are exacerbated by family life stage events. Given the stress differences in life stage, it can be hypothesized that middle-aged adult child caregivers have higher levels of subjective burden than older caregivers (Dwyer, Miller and Crandall, 1989; Gibson, Antonucci and Jackson, 1989).

IMPLICATIONS FOR COUNSELORS AND SERVICE PROVIDERS

By the time caregivers arrive for counseling or seek help, the family is usually in a state of high stress because seeking outside help is not normative. It is a last resort. Gallagher et al. (1989) found that caregivers who sought help were more depressed than non-help seeking caregivers. Family members do try to care for their own. However, the concept that a capable family is one that never needs or seeks help is a pervasive belief in American society

(Daniels, 1988; Glazer, 1971). Furthermore, policy makers have had a tendency to believe in the "substitution effect" — a concern that helping a family will result in a decrease in the family efforts while adding to the public expense.[2] This perspective inhibits the development of policy options which promote the interdependence of the family and the state.

There needs to be a better understanding that family systems are not autonomous units. Families are interdependent in the context of neighborhood, community and state. Families seeking help should not be conceptualized as losing an autonomy which never existed. Just as the seeking of help for the elder's medical bills through medicare is not perceived as losing autonomy, so the seeking of help for the elder's care in the case of Alzheimer's should not be so perceived. If the overall concept is interdependence, then help can be given and accepted, without negative labels.

Demographic changes have transformed many family systems which must now deal with the needs of their oldest old members. A new life stage of the family is rapidly becoming a normative, on-time event, i.e., intergenerational caregiving for the oldest old. This caregiving role produces a change in a family system inevitably accompanied by stress, even if it is on-time.[3] Such a family system will be experiencing stresses along both its cohesion and its adaptability dimensions. New roles will be created in the family of the adult child but there are also new roles vis à vis the health-impaired oldest old.

Family members prefer relying on their own internal family resources to cope with stress (Olson, 1988, p. 77), and the caregiving burden is no exception. Families are reluctant to supplement their internal resources with community or government-sponsored programs. They feel that they should be able to adapt and manage the situation themselves. Thus, the adaptability dimension is stressed. Giving up any piece of this function can dilute cohesion and may arouse feelings of failure and shame in caregivers, especially when the situation has reached crisis proportions.

In such a crisis the counselor can reassure the caregiver that seeking help is not "giving up," and is not an indication of inadequacy. Caregivers need to understand that seeking a day care setting for their parent with Alzheimer's is therapeutic for the patient and represents families working together with communities and professionals to provide the best possible overall environment for the client.

The language of blame and responsibility should be replaced with a new language of interdependence. Counselors and family should recognize that they must work together to develop a problem-solving strategy. This approach can enhance family cohesion and adaptability while enabling the family to seek and use services.

Zarit (Zarit, Orr, Zarit, 1985) has developed a six-step problem-solving process for families with Alzheimer's victims, but the process applies to other caregiving situations as well. Counselors should help families: (1) identify the problem; (2) generate alternative solutions; (3) select a solution—pros and cons; (4) cognitive rehearsal; (5) carry out the plan; (6) evaluate the outcome (Zarit et al., 1985). A critical element for this approach is the development of an interdependent team effort fully involving the family. Zarit suggests that after initial interviews with primary caregivers, it is a good idea to have a family meeting. The goal of the meeting is to involve the entire family in the problem-solving process and to expand the primary and secondary roles so that more members are included. In this way, the family cohesion is strengthened and the counselor helps the family find positive adaptations to the demands of the caregiving experience.

CONCLUSION

Caregiving for the elderly is becoming a normative event. To understand this role, especially when it is intergenerational, it is useful to analyze caregivers from the family system perspective, not the individual's experience. By using family system models and family life stage models, caregiving can be understood within a broad context encompassing past history, expectations, role relationships, as well as feelings of inadequacy and loss. A problem-solving strategy can be employed which will enhance the family functions. In addition, families should not be stereotyped as either autonomous independent vs. needing help and dependent. To need help at various stages in family life should not be viewed as a sign of inadequacy. The family as an institution is interdependent with neighborhoods, communities, and the state; it can not function alone.

The rapid growth of the oldest old population has created a normative family life stage involving intergenerational caregiving. While caregiving can add stress at any stage in family life it is likely to be least stressful when it is an on-time event as in the case with the oldest old. The extension of life into the 80s and 90s, while requiring more intergenerational caregiving, may enable families to better adapt to caregiving. A key factor is that there are likely to be fewer competing demands on the adult child caregiver due to fewer active roles (i.e., work and parenting) and responsibilities. Furthermore, the postponement of caregiving to the retirement years provides a greater opportunity for sons and sons-in-law to be integrated into caregiving responsibilities. However, the need for help from the formal system is likely to increase, in part due to the age of the caregivers themselves. As long as the help is provided in a team approach in the context of interdependency not dependency, there is little reason to fear that overall subjective burden will increase.

NOTES

1. Male relatives do act as helpers but are not likely to provide assistance with routine household chores or personal care (Stoller, 1990).

2. Green's (1983) limited study supported this substitution effect but the large 10 state study found that family caregivers did not reduce their efforts when publicly-supported services were available (Harahan and Hamm, 1987).

3. Research reviews find that all change — even desired change such as marriage or birth of a child — produces stress. The reason that stress is so important, moreover, is that it can result in vulnerability to illness (Rabkin and Struening, 1976).

REFERENCES

Bass, D., Tausig, M. and Noelker, L. (1988-89). Elder impairment, social support and caregiver strain: A framework for understanding support's effects. *The Journal of Applied Social Sciences 13*, 80-117.

Borgatta, E.F. and Montgomery, R.J.V. (1989). The effects of alternative support strategies on family caregiving. *The Gerontologist 19*, 457-464.

Bould, S., Sanborn, B. and Reif, L. (1988). *85 + : The oldest old*. Belmont, CA: Wadsworth Publishing Co.

Brody, E.M. (1985). Parent care as a normative stress. *The Gerontologist 25*, 19-29.

Brody, E.M. (1981). 'Women in the middle' and family help to older people. *The Gerontologist 25*, 471-480.

Brody, E.M., Hoffman, C., Kleban, M.H. and Schoonover, C.B. (1989). Caregiving daughters and their local siblings: Perceptions, strains and interactions. *The Gerontologist 29*, 529-538.

Brody, E.M., Johnsen, P.T., Fulcomer, M.C. and Lang, A.M. (1963). Women's changing roles and help to elderly parents: Attitudes of three generations of women. *The Journal of Gerontology 38*, 597-607.

Chiriboga, D., Wiler, P. and Nielson, K. (1988-89). The stress of caregivers. *The Journal of Applied Social Sciences 13*, 118-142.

Daniels, N. (1988). *Am I my parents' keeper*. New York: Oxford University Press.

Day, A.T. (1988, November). Household composition and living arrangements: Structural bases of informal care of the aged. Paper presented at the 41st Annual Scientific Meeting of the Gerontological Society of America, San Francisco, California.

Doty, P. (1986). Family care of the elderly: The role of public policy. *The Milbank Quarterly 64*, 34-69.

Dwyer, W., Miller, M.K. and Crandall, L.A. (1989, June). Family caregiving for the functionally impaired elderly. Paper presented at the XIV International Congress of Gerontology, Acapulco, Mexico.

Evans, D. *et al.* (1989). Prevalence of Alzheimer's disease in a community population of older persons. *Journal of the American Medical Association 262* (18); 2551-2554.

Falicov, C.J. (1988). Family sociology and family therapy contributions to the family development framework: A comparative analysis and thoughts on future trends. In C.J. Falicov (Ed.) *Family Transitions: continuity and change over the life cycle* (pp. 3-51). New York: The Guilford Press.

Fitting, M. and Rabins, R. (1985). Men and women: Do they give care differently? *Generations 10*; 19-23.

Gallagher, D., Rose, J., Rivera, P., Lovett, S. and Thompson, L.W. (1989). Prevalence of depression in family caregivers. *The Gerontologist 29*, 449-456.

Gibson, R.C., Antonucci, T.C. and Jackson, J.S. (1989, June). Caregiving: The effects of age, gender and race. Paper presented at the XIV International Congress of Gerontology, Acapulco, Mexico.

Glazer, N. (1971). The limits of social policy. *Commentary 52*, 51-58.

Greene, V.L. (1983). Substitution between formally and informally provided care for the impaired elderly in the community. *Medical Care 21*, 609-619.

Hamon, R.R. (1988, November). Filial responsibility expectations among adult child-older parent pairs. Paper presented at the 41st Annual Scientific Meeting of the Gerontological Society of America, San Francisco, California.

Harahan, M. and Hamm, L.V. (1987). National long-term care channeling demonstration program in *Proceedings of the 1987 Public Health Conference on*

Records and Statistics (pp. 89-91). Hyattsville, MD: U.S. Department of Health and Human Services.

Hasselkus, B.R. (1988). Meaning in family caregiving: Perspectives on caregiver professional relationships. *The Gerontologist 28*, 686-691.

Hinze, E. (1989, June). Conflicts in care-taking of aged parents. Paper presented at the XIV International Congress of Gerontology, Acapulco, Mexico.

Kasper, J.D. (1988). *Aging and alone: Profiles and projections*, A Report of the Commonwealth Fund Commission on Elderly People Living Alone. New York: The Commonwealth Fund.

Kovar, M.G. (1987). The longitudinal study on aging: Some estimates of change among older Americans in *Proceedings of the 1987 Public Health Conference on Records and Statistics* (pp. 397-398). Hyattsville, MD: U.S. Department of Health and Human Services.

Longino, C.F. (1988). Who are the oldest Americans? *The Gerontologist 18*, 515-523.

Manton, K.G. and Soldo, B.J. (1985). Dynamics of health changes in the oldest old: New perspectives and evidence. *Milbank Memorial Quarterly 63*, 206-285.

Matthews, S.H. (1988). The burdens of parent care: A critical assessment of findings. *Journal of Aging Studies 2*, 157-165.

Miller, B. and Montgomery, A. (1989, June). Dimensions of caregiving strain: A comparison of spouse and adult child caregivers. Paper presented at the XIV International Congress of Gerontology, Acapulco, Mexico.

Montgomery, R.J.V. and Borgatta, E.F. (1989). The effects of alternative support strategies on family caregiving. *The Gerontologist 29*, 457-464.

Neugarten, B.L. (1977). Personality and aging. In J.E. Birren and K.W. Schaie (Eds.) *Handbook of the psychology of aging* (pp. 629-649). New York: Van Nostrand Reinhold.

Olson, D.H. (1988). Family types, family stress, and family satisfaction: A family development perspective. In C.J. Falicov (Ed.) *Family transitions: Continuity and change over the life cycle* (pp. 55-79). New York: The Guilford Press.

Ory, M. (1985). The burden of care: A familial perspective. *Generations 10*, 14-17.

Rabkin, J.G. and Struening, E.L. (1976). Social change, stress and illness: A selective literature review. *Psychoanalysis and Contemporary Science 5*, 573-624.

Raveis, V., Siegel, K. and Sudit, M. (1990). Psychological impact of caregiving on the caregiver: Critical review of research methodologies. In D.E. Biegel and A. Blum (Eds.) *Aging and caregiving* (pp. 53-75). Newbury Park, CA: Sage Publications.

Rosenberg, A. (1988, November). Equity and satisfaction in the midlife woman's relationship with her mother. Paper presented at the 41st Annual Scientific Meeting of The Gerontological Society of America, San Francisco, California.

Rosenwaike, I. (1985). A demographic portrait of the oldest old. *Milbank Memorial Quarterly 63*, 181-205.

Sanborn, B. and Bould, S. (1990, July). Transition in caregiving: A new family crisis. Paper presented at the 2nd International Conference on the Future of Adult Life, The Netherlands.

Soldo, B.J. and Manton, K.G. (1985). Changes in the health status and service needs of the oldest old: Current patterns and future trends. *Milbank Memorial Quarterly 63*, 286-323.

Sommers, T. (1985). Caregiving: A women's issue. *Generations 10*, 9-13.

Stoller, E.P. (1990). Males as helpers: The role of sons, relatives, and friends. *The Gerontologist* 30; 228-235.

Suzman, R. and Riley, M.W. (1985). Introducing the oldest old. *Milbank Memorial Quarterly 63*, 177-186.

Thompson, L. and Walker, A. (1984). Mothers and daughters. *Journal of Marriage and the Family 46*, 313-322.

Walker, A. (1988). Care for elderly people: A conflict between women and the state. In J. Finch and D. Groves (Eds.) *A labour of love: Women, work and caring* (pp. 106-128). London: Routledge and Kegan Paul.

Wilkinson, D.Y. (1988). Mother-daughter bonds in the later years: Transformation of the "help pattern." In S.K. Steinmetz (Ed.) *Family and support systems across the life span* (pp. 183-195). New York: Plenum Press.

Williamson, D.S. and Bray, J.H. (1988). Family development and change across the generations: An intergenerational perspective. In C.J. Falicov (Ed.) *Family transitions: continuity and change over the life cycle*, pp. 357-384. New York: The Guilford Press.

Zarit, S.N. (1985). New directions. *Generations 10*, 4-7.

Zarit, S.N., Reever, K.E. and Bach-Peterson, J. (1980). Relatives of the impaired elderly: Correlates of feelings of burden. *The Gerontologist 20*, 649-655.

Zarit, S.H., Orr, N.K. and Zarit, J.M. (1985). *The hidden victims of Alzheimer's disease: Families under stress*. New York and London: New York University Press.

An Intergenerational
Perspective of Marriage:
Love and Trust in Cultural Context

Ned L. Gaylin

INTRODUCTION

Marriage may be defined as the public and conscious taking of a member of the opposite sex for a life partner. No other social institution is either so indigenous to us or so defining of us as a unique species. Although cross cultural comparisons reveal all manner of variations (including homosexuality) on the typical monogamous unit we have come to know, marriage remains the most basic of all human institutions. For all cultures, marriage serves the universal function of maintaining responsible intimacy and bridging generations. Marriage has thus become one of the few remaining bastions of interpersonal security—the safehouse of love and trust.

In the present period of rapid social change, there is much conjecture about the viability of the institution of marriage. But to question the viability of marriage is tantamount to questioning the viability of civilization as we know it. The real issue facing us is how the institution of marriage is being modified and employed to help us as a species adapt to our modern world. It is not that we are not marrying; we are marrying, divorcing more frequently, and remarrying. We are continuously seeking the right relationship, the eternal match. A force that impelling—the romantic quest for the ideal state between man and woman—surely speaks to who we are and where we are going.

All mammalian species mate for sexual reproduction and it be-

Ned L. Gaylin is Professor and Director of Marriage and Family Therapy Education, Department of Family and Community Development, University of Maryland, College Park, MD 20742.

labors the obvious to note that this biological imperative is requisite for species continuance. While some infrahuman species have analogues to monogamous marriage, e.g., certain species of birds tend to mate for life, there is little evidence that any have the special consciousness of the future which the bonds of matrimony imply. Thus, marriage is palpably different from any analogous mating behavior in other animals. Marriage is a conscious contract that has an explicit past as well as an implicit future. Marriage transtemporally bridges the past by recognizing ancestry, the present by joining individuals and families, and the future by anticipating and producing heirs. Marriage, because of its link with the past and its projection into the future, is in fact humankind's attempt to overcome the limitations of the life span. By marrying, one establishes a relationship with ramifications greater than either partner's individual longevity. Thus, conscious transtemporality and generativity enable marriage to bridge and connect individuals, generations, families, communities, even empires. Marriage and its inevitable sequel, the family, are the social paradigm, the keystone in the arch of civilization (Gaylin, 1985).

Discussions of the history of marriage, research on its multiple forms, and dialogues on whether it is a functional or useful institution for these modern times abound. Textbooks attempt to dissect its nature and predict its viability, but little is written on the nonrational aspects of the institution. The nonrational or affective perspective — the poetry of our development — is fundamental to an understanding of modern marriage and family.

There are two basic elements to a workable, satisfying, and lasting marriage: love and trust. How these elements articulate within a given cultural context determines the effectiveness of marriage as an institution for the people of that culture.

LOVE

The conceptualization and understanding of love have been grappled with by poets, philosophers, and scientists. Most conclude that love is the language of the arts, not the sciences (Kaufmann, 1958; Levi-Strauss, 1969). Love is a word, an abstraction and, like all words, its meaning is derived from complex memories of myriad sensations: smells, touches, sounds, images — all stored in our individual and collective histories. Thus, while there is a timeless and universal quality to our common understanding of love, there is also a mutable quality which can subtly modify our view of it both as members of groups with common histories, and as individuals with unique histories. Our collective histories are perhaps best embodied and crystallized by our artists, musicians, and poets who project on a recognizable screen before us our universal experiences and remembered feelings. Thus, for most Westerners, David's love for Bathsheba, Tristan's for Isolde, Romeo's for Juliet, all conjure up a form of common experience with personal overtones, as might also a given painting, sculpture, or concerto.

Extrapolating from ethological evidence, Morris (1967) and Wilson (1980) note salient affective features of human sexuality which are distinctively different from animal sexuality. These features include: (a) dominance of visual over olfactory arousal cues resulting in a more personal (face to face) mating; (b) prolonged courtship employing highly complex vocal/verbal cues; and (c) absence of a relatively circumscribed estrus or heat period making sexuality more or less continuous and less focused on reproduction. The coexistence of these distinctly human features lead to a lesser emphasis on instinctive bonding and a greater emphasis on conscious awareness of the loving process.

In contrast, Freud viewed the animal sexual drive as the root of all varieties of human love from coital to altruistic (1962). While Freud recognized the vast importance of the dependency period of the immature organism for later social bonding, it was the neo-Freudian theorists (Erikson, 1964; Sullivan, 1953) and empiricists, working directly with both animal (Lorenz 1952; Harlow, 1962) and human (Bowlby, 1952; Spitz, 1945) mother-child pairs who demonstrated the power, intricacies, and ramifications of the early parent-child relationship on later social bonding. The closest we can come to imputing love to lower animals is to observe those attentive, nurturant, or passionately protective behaviors exhibited by animal parents (generally mothers) for their young. Animal courtship and the copulation which follows do not even come close to eliciting human comparison. Thus, while sex may be the basis on which species survival exists, it is the parental bond on which civilization rests.

The biological imperative which is part of the initial attraction of male and female, is by its very nature fleeting and limited. Although none would deny the impelling quality of the sensual pleasure of the arousal state or the ecstasy experienced in the orgasmic moment, this momentary exultation cannot wholly account for the continuous concern, tender tactile attentiveness, nostalgic bittersweet reverie of separation, and the anticipated joyous reunion of human lovers. Neither does the biological imperative explain the conscious desire of those in love to actualize their love for each other through the creation of children. Our awareness of these differences between biological and nurturant love tends to affect all human sexuality, and particularly love in the context of marriage.

The nature of the parent-child bond is the crucial ingredient in the transcendence of love over sex. The two uniquely human qualities of transtemporal consciousness and the protracted dependency of the young, lead homo sapiens to an awareness of kinship ties well beyond the bonding period. Memories of comfort, sustenance, and caring by parents are carried with the human organism throughout life. It is the awareness of past nurturance and anticipation of future giving and receiving of pleasure which make love a far more complex phenomenon than sex (see Gaylin, 1985 regarding the development of complex love in the child).

Knowledge of the rudiments of human love would, perhaps, not be so important if it did not play so central a role in our lives. To say that its origins are either sexual or nurturant, rather than both sexual and nurturant changes our understanding and our behavior in the way we relate to one another in all our interpersonal dealings. It is this attempt at understanding that has filled our written communication since recorded time.

Greece of the fifth century B.C.E. is considered by most social scientists to be the source of our modern ideas about love. Plato, in the *Symposium*, defines love as the inspiration of virtue and designates its hierarchy: (a) common, earthly, or sensual love (both homosexual and heterosexual) which contributes to but does not constitute divine or heavenly love, and (b) spiritual love, the noblest of pursuits. Reiss (1980) and others contrast this composite love with the hedonistic, sensual pleasures depicted by Ovid in pagan Rome of the first century C.E. With the establishment of Christianity, the concept of love was revolutionized. The varieties of love which Plato portrayed as a continuum, early Christianity reinterpreted as polar opposites. On one extreme was celibacy, the only pure manifestation of spiritual love; on the other was physical desire, the sole appropriate expression of which was limited to the conjugal bed. This dichotomization of love, with sex as a necessary evil (1 Cor. 7), led the way to the establishment of love as a sacrament, with procreation in marriage its primary purpose, a view which remained unchallenged until the Reformation and continues to be the position of the Catholic church today.

The next watershed contributing to our present ideology of love is considered by many (Linton, 1936; Biegel, 1951; Lederer and Jackson, 1968; Clayton, 1975; and Reiss, 1980) to be the period of the 12th century, the age of chivalry. While the erotic element is present in the literature of this period, it remained secondary to the hero-knight's pursuit of virtue, embodied in the image of the beatific female. This period is considered a turning point because it introduced the idea of gentleness and restraint into the consciousness of the male.

It is only with the Renaissance (14th-16th centuries) that the epic quest becomes the search for a marriage partner, thereby integrating the spiritual qualities of love with the sensual. While the periods of the Reformation and Enlightenment (16th-18th centuries) showed changes in the institution of marriage, this integrated view of love endured. The glorification of this "ideal love" in the art, literature, and music of the 19th century, with its emphasis on the ecstasies of emotion, is considered the culmination of that which we have inherited as romantic love between woman and man (Clayton, 1975). The compelling and enduring presence of the romantic ideal, as well as the evolution of the dyadic relationship based on affection, suggest that love has been a major part of selecting a mate for a large part of the population in many times.

Although our intellectual conceptualization of love has undoubtedly changed somewhat over time, perhaps it has changed not as much as we may have been led to believe. As Gay (1983) has cogently observed, often what we know of the past comes from the writings of relatively few sources, generally the social critics of the time. For example, in his analysis of the "private diaries, family correspondence, medical texts, household manuals, religious tracts, and works of art," Gay gives a distinctly different picture of Victorian private lives than that portrayed by their public images. He found that in the privacy of their homes, Victorian individuals lived sensually fulfilling lives and were less dominated by conformity and repression than by guilt and anxiety.

Furthermore, one of our major sources of information regarding the customs and mores of earlier times, the Old Testament (the writing of which is assumed to have predated Plato by anywhere from three to five centuries, i.e., 950-750 B.C.E.) is nowhere mentioned by most social scientists. This omission suggests the need for further scrutiny. It is not being suggested that the development of romantic love, as previously indicated by social scientists, is inaccurate or unimportant to the understanding of our present ideas of love, nor even that the Old Testament gives an accurate accounting of love. What is important is that the stories of the Old Testament which include as many of the facets of love as have previously been discussed, undoubtedly have had as profound an impact on what we think and feel about ourselves as the works of Plato, Ovid, Paul, or Shakespeare. From the florid erotic ecstasies of the "Song of Songs" to the "courtly" love of Jacob for Rachel, the friendly love of Jonathan and David, the fraternal love of Joseph and Benjamin, the filial love of Abraham for Isaac and Naomi for Ruth, as well as the heavenly love of humankind for God—all of these, and more, are delineated therein. Because these depictions are familiar and common to the vast majority of Westerners, they are perhaps as much a part of that which comprises our ideation of love as those of the Greeks, Romans, early Christians, and Elizabethans.

Finally, it is worth noting how our present generation of young—those who are at the appropriate developmental stage for marriage — are given an understanding of modern day love in marriage. In a recent college textbook on contemporary marriage, designed for 18 and 19 year old college freshmen and sophomores, the author presents a "mature concept of love." Delineated are "Five different elements of conjugal love: romantic love, dependent love, erotic love, friendship love, and altruistic love," (Rice, 1983, p. 57). What is most impressive about this presentation is the comprehensiveness of the formulation and its ramifications. Here love truly has become all things to all persons. If we are led to believe that marriage can meet all human affiliational needs perfectly, we are placing an enormous burden on that institution. While idealism, particularly in the young, is to be lauded, the danger of overidealization or unrealistic expectations, can quickly lead to disappointment and a sense of failure. That marriage and family have become "the giant shock absorber" (Toffler, 1970) of modern American society is a much discussed phenomenon. The question is: Can it take the load? Perhaps it is best, then, to leave this discussion of love on a simpler note. The well known theorist and psychotherapist Harry Stack Sullivan (1947) defines the state of love as existing, "when the satisfaction or security of another person becomes as significant as is one's own security." Perhaps, as Kaufmann (1958) suggests, it would be better still to leave it to the poets.

TRUST

In contrast to the vast material from widely varying sources regarding love and our understanding of it, trust as an interpersonal construct has virtually escaped or eluded attempts at scrutiny or study. Yet, ironically, throughout history we are aware of loveless marriages arranged for the purposes of establishing trust between families, clans, or nations. Few have had much to say with respect to the issue of trust in marriage. Yet without trust, marriage is, at best, a fragile contract of questionable viability. Perhaps because trust is so basic to human interaction and to society in general, its necessity and existence simply have been assumed and taken for granted.

Erik Erikson is one of the few behavioral scientists to have recognized how essential trust is in intimate human interactions. He traces the roots of trust to the first feelings of a child towards its mother. For Erikson the first year of life is characterized as the period during which a sense of basic trust is established. Trust according to Erikson is fostered by "consistency, continuity, and sameness of experience," and "the quality of the maternal relationship" (1964, p. 220). Thus, if a sense of basic trust is not established in early infancy, healthy human interaction throughout life is in jeopardy. In working with monkeys, Harry Harlow (1959, 1962) confirmed Erikson's observations. Later, Ables and Brandsma (1977) drew a parallel between the early establishment of a sense of trust between infant and mother and the ability to establish a similar relationship in marriage.

The most extensive treatment of the subject of trust in marriage appears in Lederer and Jackson's book, *The Mirages of Marriage* (1968). While they recognize trust to be "one of the necessary ingredients of a workable marriage," they take issue with the Eriksonian concept of infantile trust, describing it as unilateral—the child has no choice but to trust the parent for its basic needs. They contend that trust occurs in the interaction between the marital partners only when there is equivalence or "mutual confidence" regarding the expectations and behaviors of the other person. As such, it is dependent upon continuous communication and honesty between partners.

Reliance on confidence as a synonym or even as a test for trust is dangerous. Confidence tends to be a more specific and transitory feeling, where trust is more encompassing and comprehensive. It implies a greater permanence. For example, one may have little confidence in a spouse's driving skills yet still maintain a basically trusting intimate relationship. Trust rests on the accretion of confidence-building past experiences, and projects itself into the future as faith. Thus, it falls somewhere between the concreteness of confidence and the less tangible elements of faith, and is not so much a simple feeling state. It has both a retrospective base and a projective thrust. The most dramatic breach of confidence and trust in a marriage is adultery, which strikes at the very heart of the union. For this there is even special terminology—infidelity, unfaithfulness. One may tolerate extravagance, alcoholism, neglect (often for the sake of career), differences about childrearing, or extended family relationships. These may entail insensitivities, broken promises, even lying — stretching the confidence aspects of trust — and when extreme, the marriage may eventually be strained to the point of dissolution. But there is often much wider latitude in these and other areas than in that of infidelity. What distinguishes faith from both trust and confidence is that faith does not require proof or logic — it is there and, like love, it tends to be blind.

Faith is what makes marriage the ultimate contract. Virtually no one enters into marriage today without the belief that the union is permanent. Modern marriage vows have evolved over time, but broadly speaking, the nature of the marriage contract, the assumptions of its permanence, and the necessity of having it a public affair, i.e., witnessed, seem to be roughly similar throughout history and across widely varying cultures. It is the sanctification of pledging troth publicly that gives the union life.

Correspondingly, when faith is broken, there is loss — i.e., a form of death. The ingenuous old union no longer exists, and for a new union to be formed there are necessary conditions. Blind faith must be replaced by built trust. But, even then, the totally rational process of developing confidence, to the end of establishing trust, must often be accompanied by some form of ritual burial of the old union and ceremonious birth of the new. While some feel that the therapeutic process alone helps perform these tasks, others (e.g., Haley, 1976) take the need for a ceremony more literally.

We live in trying times; the stress placed upon intimate relationships is often chronic and insidious. We have a strong belief in science and in the rational — the need to understand ourselves, others, the world. Our twentieth century society tends to reject the more nonrational aspects of our lives. Under such circumstances, faith — unabashed and naive, given without proof or logic — is a relatively rare commodity and is what Erikson refers to when he discusses the basic trust of the infant. It is there, a priori.

As we grow and experience more of the world around us, our faith in others and in ourselves tends to be shaken. Our parents' love seems to grow conditional, dependent upon our behavior and their moods. As we age we become aware that misplaced, unequivocal faith can lead to disappointment, hurt, and anguish. Yet we continually look to others as objects of that unconditional faith: first a best friend or "chum" (see Sullivan, 1953), later a prospective spouse. Through experiences which are fired by hope and anticipation, and dampened by disappointment and hurt, we gradually learn to temper blind faith with the more rational and conditional feeling of trust which is based upon the accretion of confidence-building experiences. It is this trust, referred to by Lederer and Jackson (1968) as needing constant nurturance and validation through honesty, communication, and caring, that is the essential anchor of a successful, workable marriage.

THE CULTURAL CONTEXT

No exposition of modern marriage would be comprehensible without elaboration of what has come to be perhaps its greatest source of strain, gender role delineation. While the conflict between male and female is hardly a new one (Aristophanes, 411 B.C.E.; reprint, 1964), the intensity with which the battle of the sexes is being played out in contemporary marriage demands a clearer understanding of the nature of the conflict.

Most discussions of sex or gender role delineation begin with basic biological distinctions between the sexes and then deal with the socialization process. The scientific study of these issues is probably best traced to Darwin (1859; reprint, 1952) who represented the nature side of the controversy. Sexuality and the essential tension between the sexes was introduced into psychology by Freud (1905; reprint, 1962), who juxtaposed nurture against nature. The crystallization of the concept of gender role is attributed to George Herbert Mead (1934). It was Mead who enabled our understanding of the different socialization processes that continue to exist for men and women respectively. Historically, these processes have defined consistent sets of male and female behavior, adhered to still in various contemporary societies. Today, this battle of nature versus nurture, although not dead, is rarely a heated one, with most scholars taking a combined or biosocial approach, perhaps best embodied by Wilson, 1980.

Recent advances in the biological sciences, particularly in the field of neuroendocrinology, are telling us more and more about the basic biological differences between men and women. Those which impact most significantly on gender role are those which have remained constant, namely menstruation, ovulation, gestation, and lactation which irrefutably are characteristics of the human female. While far less important now than in earlier times, the larger skeletal frame and greater body mass of striated musculature are characteristics of the human male. Thus, premodern humankind left women those tasks relating to child care and the home. Reciprocally, men were relegated the more physically strenuous and demanding tasks of maintaining the mother and child unit, via gathering, farming, and hunting. Later, with the introduction of money and industry where previously there had been only barter and agriculture, many men turned to industry and politics, while women continued their roles in the home. As has been succinctly stated by Reiss, despite the widely varying distribution of labor in various cultures throughout time to the present, "Two features of gender roles in all cultures then, are: (a) female ties to child rearing and (b) male ties to economic power" (1980, p. 62).

It is only as recently as the middle of the 19th century that most historians mark the public questioning of classic gender role distinctions. The industrial revolution had an enormous repercussive impact on work in general. With the advent and aid of machinery, greater physical strength and speed lost their gender specificity and thereby their importance. By and large, women could perform virtually any of the skills formerly reserved for men. As in the end of the Roman period when women took over many of the managerial functions of their husbands who had gone off to war, so women also took their spouses' places on the assembly lines in America during World War II. For better or for worse, the twentieth century has seen the final reduction of gender specific behavior in human beings to one — gestation.

Any change, by its nature, creates strain. The dramatic and rapid changes that have occurred in gender roles in the last two centuries have put an equivalent load on that most basic of human institutions, marriage. Heinz Hartmann (1958) has explicated how, out of necessity and for expedience, the individual places certain behaviors out of awareness. This submergence frees the individual from being overloaded with continuous decision making. A chain of decisions is organically learned and, as Hartmann terms it, *"automatized"* at a preconscious level, thus enabling the organism to perform complicated acts. So, for example, although the beginning driver finds the process overwhelming at first, the complexities once mastered become second nature, rarely to be forgotten. The result allows the driver to attend to the road, dodge obstacles, and navigate without having to attend consciously to the clutch, brake, accelerator, etc. However, during a crisis such as a skid on a slippery road, the discrete actions may be brought to conscious awareness for reevaluation. To draw from Darwin, as ontogeny recapitulates phylogeny, so too may phylogeny parallel ontogeny. What is being suggested here is that role delineations have served as automatizers for our species. In previous times men have, by and large, known what was expected of them and what they might, in turn, expect of women, and vice versa.

SOCIAL AUTOMATIZATION

Social automatization, in its specific reference here to male/female role structuring, was crucial for the development of civilization. Cerebral decision making can maximize options, but can also paralyze through overchoice. Somewhere, then, it is necessary to strike a balance between flexibility and rigidity in everyday decisions. Just as automatization is necessary for the individual's functioning, so too is some form thereof necessary for society's functioning. Social automatizers assure a degree of expectability and predictability. They reduce anxiety, increase comfort, and at the same time mitigate or even eliminate the need for continuous decision making. These automatizers (or norms) develop over time and are gradually modified to facilitate adaptation. This is a natural evolutionary process. On the other hand, norms can become entrenched and inflexible, rigidly adhered to, and anachronistic and dysfunctional. When this happens we often have revolutions. When automatizations, for good or bad reasons, are deautomatized, that is, brought into awareness, our identity is called into question. This can happen at both an individual and a cultural level. When identity is called into question, it affects our ability to care, to love. When we are so concerned about ourselves and who we are, egoism eclipses altruism (see Maslow, 1971, and Lasch, 1978).

In many respects, we are in a state of deautomatization today. We are in the process of discarding operating procedures which are centuries old and gender specific. If we are to move on, we will have to find new roles and rules to replace the old. Emile Durkheim (1951) discussed these ideas in the framework of norms, noting that when a society, for whatever reason, upsets its established norms it creates anomie. Anomie can occur at any level within a society from the interpersonal to the economic and political. In the former situation we may observe an increase in divorce; in extremes of the latter, we may see an increase in suicide. Both observations may be made of contemporary American society.

RITUALS, CEREMONIES, AND TRADITIONS

Social automatizers may also be seen as a means by which humankind has compensated for the loss of instinctual behavior—the trade off for the growth of the cerebral cortex. The development of rituals, ceremonies, and traditions may be viewed in such a manner. Here too, contemporary Western civilization, particularly in America, is relatively lacking in the use of ceremonies to smooth out the normative crises of living such as birth, coming of age, marriage, death. The age of science has put religion, once our primary source of ritual or ceremonial practice, in a secondary position. What little ritual we retain, especially to facilitate public interactions, more aptly falls under the heading of social convention (see Goffman, 1971). Conventions are more like social habits than social automatizers. While they serve many of the same purposes as automatizers, they do so at a much more superficial level and are more easily subject to change from one generation to the next. Societal conventions are less intrinsic than automatizers and lack their timeless ability to stabilize. Further, conventions bear little of the richness and aesthetic appeal of ceremonies.

All societies have ceremonies to mark passages through life, although some have more than others. It is often noted that those subcultures in our own society which have retained more ritual practice tend to demonstrate greater family cohesion, better individual adaptation, and less propensity to social deviance. Traditionally, the Chinese, Japanese, and Jewish ethnic groups are noted for their having greater family integration and correspondingly lower rates of alcoholism, delinquency, and divorce. These same subcultures tend to surround birth, marriage, and death with rich ceremony. While it might be countered that these groups have generations of religious tradition on which to draw, one of the few studies of secular traditions of nonethnic American families (Bossard and Ball, 1950, p. 203) demonstrated similar findings: "Ritual is a relatively reliable index of family integration."

One of the few ceremonies that most Americans still retain is marriage, although even this practice appears to be diminishing. Indeed, marriage seems to be the last rite of passage which we continue to ceremonialize to any real degree. It remains the one step in our biological and social development that American culture at large recognizes as focal and best marked by ritual embellishment from the prenuptial arrangements, to the exchanging of vows and rings, to the honeymoon. Few young first marrieds and their families seem inclined to dispense with the choreography involved in such rituals, and with good reason. Marriage, in our society as in most others, demarcates the leaving of childhood and the entering into the adult world. Furthermore, the public witnessing of marriage has the impact of affirming and renewing the marriages of those who witness; their vicarious participation in the vows engenders a sense of community.

By and large our society has dispensed with the ceremonializing of the premarital developmental passages common to the majority of cultures in previous times, including the biological coming of age. Ironically, the closest thing we have to such a rite of passage is the obtaining of a driver's license. Indeed, we might have more responsible drivers if we were to celebrate more richly the adolescent's initiation into independence via physical mobility, although it might contrarily be argued that marriage licenses do not guarantee success despite all of their ritual accompaniment. Thus, marriage has become a highly loaded fulcrum with few structural supports to aid it in its work of gracefully moving both the individuals and the culture through the life-span journey.

Over a half century ago, Ruth Benedict (1938) explicated an American dilemma that she called our "discontinuities in cultural conditioning." In all cultures Benedict noted discontinuities surrounding various turning points in the life span. She explained the importance of these normative crises and the need for all cultures to facilitate its members' recognition, anticipation, and preparation for the impact of these crises. She observed that those cultures which did this best demonstrated a smoother functioning, and their members experienced greater well being. Cultures with disjunctive turning points often accomplished the transitions effectively by attending them with elaborate ceremony.

In discussing American culture of the time Benedict noted three major discontinuities between childhood and adulthood: "(a) responsible—non-responsible status role, (b) dominance—submission, and (c) contrasted sexual role" (1938, p. 163). Thus we expect childhood to be a time of play and relative irresponsibility; a time of submission to adult authority; and a time, despite high heterosexual contact, of asexuality. Benedict depicted American culture as one with great discontinuities and few sources of mitigation. That is, our transitions were abrupt and painful: We had little preparation for them, and little celebration of them.

It is not suggested here that we develop a more ritualized society as the only appropriate method for dealing with our discontinuities. Indeed, ceremony and ritual could appear to be somewhat disjunctive to our scientifically oriented culture. Benedict's point was that if a society does not adopt the means with which to mollify the normative crises inherent in life transitions, especially if the society demands radical change during those transitions, enormous strains will be placed on both the individual and society. This is particularly true of the transition from child to adult status. For several decades, many have advocated family life education as a way to moderate, through preparation, the rather difficult child-to-adult passage. However, such programs by and large have received the support neither of our educational institutions nor of the public at large (Gaylin, 1981). This notwithstanding, the social indicators of our time all validate Benedict's premise. Our protraction of adolescence well beyond its biological years, and our inability to ease the transition may well account for the recent increase in rates of adolescent drug abuse, crime, suicide, and in the young adult years, other negative social barometers such as marital dissatisfaction, divorce, and family violence. With little or no role preparation, and few ceremonies with which to mollify cultural discontinuities, the burden of expectation we place on our children to become overnight successes as spouses, breadwinners, and parents may be too great for some of our fledglings to bear.

CONCLUSION

Marriage is the ultimate and paradigmatic social institution: It is the civilizing of sexuality and the keystone in the arch of civilization. Marriage is the foundation of family and the fulcrum of the human life course. It is the intergenerational bridge which links us to our past, through our ancestors; projects us into the future, through our heirs; and sustains and maintains us in the immediate present. The key to understanding the human condition lies in our understanding of the complex interaction of both the nonrational and the rational aspects of marriage within the larger social setting: love and trust in cultural context.

REFERENCES

Ables, B. S. and Brandsma, J. M. (1977). *Therapy for couples*. San Francisco: Jossey-Bass, Inc.

Aristophanes. (1964). *Lysistrata*. Translated by Parker, D. New York: New American Library.

Benedict, R. (1938). Continuities and discontinuities in cultural conditioning. *Psychiatry*, *1*, 161-167.

Biegel, H. G. (1951). Romantic love. *American Sociological Review*, *16*, 323-334.

Bossard, J. H. and Boll, E. S. (1950). *Ritual in family living: A contemporary study*. Philadelphia: University of Pennsylvania Press. Reprint edition (1976). Westport, Connecticut: Greenwood Press.

Bowlby, J. (1952). *Maternal care and mental health*. Geneva, World Health Organization, Monograph no. 2.

Clayton, R. R. (1975). *The family, marriage, and social change*. Lexington, Massachusetts: D. C. Heath and Co.

Darwin, C. (1952). *The origin of the species and the decent of man*. Chicago: Encyclopedia Britannica, Inc.

Durkheim, E. (1951). *Suicide*. Translated by J. Spaulding and G. Simpson. New York: Free Press.

Erikson, E. H. (1964). *Childhood and society*. New York: W.W. Norton and Co., Inc.

Freud, S. (1962). *Three contributions to the theory of sex*. New York: Dutton.

Gay, P. (1983). *The bourgeois experience: Victoria to Freud. Vol. I: Education of the senses*. London: Oxford Press.

Gaylin, N. (1981). Family life education: behavioral science wonderbread? *Family Relations, 30*, 511-516.

Gaylin, N. (1985). Marriage. In M. Farber (Ed.), *Human sexuality: Psychosexual effects of disease*. New York: Macmillan.

Goffman, E. (1971). *Relations in public*. New York: Harper and Row.

Haley, J. (1976). *Problem solving therapy*. San Francisco: Josey-Bass, Inc.

Harlow, H. F. (1959). Love in infant monkeys. *Scientific American, 200*, 68-74.

Harlow, H. F. (1962). The heterosexual affectional system in monkeys. *American Psychologist, 17*, 1-9.

Hartmann, H. (1958). *Ego psychology and the problem of adaptation*. Translated by D. Rapaport. New York: International Universities Press.

Kaufmann, W. (1958). *Critique of religion and philosophy*. New York: Harper and Brothers.

Lasch, C. (1978). *The culture of narcissism: American life in an age of diminishing expectations*. New York: W. W. Norton and Co.

Lederer, W. J. and Jackson, D. D. (1968). *The mirages of marriage*. New York: W. W. Norton and Co.

Levi-Strauss, C. (1969). *The raw and the cooked: Introduction to a science of mythology*. Translated by J. and D. Weightman. New York: Harper and Row.

Linton, R. R. (1936). *The study of man*. New York: Appleton-Century-Crofts.

Lorenz, K. (1952). *King Solomon's ring*. New York: Crowell.

Maslow, A. H. (1971). *The farther reaches of human nature*. New York: Viking Press.

Mead, G. H. (1934). *Mind, self, and society*. Chicago: University of Chicago Press.

Morris, D. (1967). *The naked ape*. New York: McGraw Hill.

Plato. (1952). *The dialogues of Plato*. In R. M. Hutchins (Ed.), *Great books of the western world*. Chicago: Encyclopedia Britannica.

Reiss, I. L. (1980). *Family systems in America*. New York: Holt, Rinehart and Winston.

Rice, P. F. (1983). *Contemporary marriage*. New York: Allyn and Bacon, Inc.

Spitz, R. (1945). Hospitalism: an inquiry into the genesis of psychiatric conditions in early childhood. In A. Freud (Ed.) *The Psychoanalytic study of the child, Vol. I*. New York: International Universities Press.

Sullivan, H. S. (1947). *Conceptions of modern psychiatry*. Washington, D. C.: William Alanson White Psychiatric Foundation.

Sullivan, H. S. (1953). *The interpersonal theory of psychiatry*. New York: W. W. Norton and Co.

Toffler, A. (1970). *Future shock*. New York: Random House.

Wilson, E. O. (1980). *Sociobiology*. Cambridge, Massachusetts: Harvard University Press.

An Intergenerational Perspective on Family Ethical Dilemmas

Roma S. Hanks

INTRODUCTION

Although legal and ethical codes in Western society establish the individual as agent, there exist a number of intimate relationships within which the individual extends beyond the self and the boundaries of individualism. These corporate relationships, often existing within families, can be troublesome for researchers and philosophers whose professional orientation tends to examine responsibility and obligation in terms of autonomous rationality. The problem of agency in ethical and legal responsibility, e.g., individual versus corporate unit of analysis and action, is intensified when the family relationships under scrutiny are intergenerational.

Relationships among generations of kin involve individuals who are separated in time and often in space but identify themselves corporately as a family. Temporal and spatial distance between the generations may be a basis for agents' positions on intergenerational responsibility. However, arguments in the literature about the relationship of agents to beneficiaries who are separated from them in time and space have not been applied to intergenerational family relationships. This paper seeks to establish a basis for making such an application by linking extant literature in the applied ethical analysis of issues involving future persons and distant persons to philosophical perspectives on filial obligation. Intergenerational family caregiving is used as an example. Three questions central to this application include:

Roma S. Hanks is Project Coordinator and Instructor in the Department of Individual and Family Studies, University of Delaware, Newark, DE 19716.

1. What is the unit, i.e., who are the actors or moral agents, in intergenerational family relationships?
2. What is the actor's orientation to historic, future, and distant persons?
3. What is the impact of changing spatial and temporal configuration of the family on intergenerational responsibility?

RETHINKING THE ETHICS
OF INTERGENERATIONAL RELATIONSHIPS

Individual or Corporate Agency

Actors on both sides of an ethical dilemma "can correctly marshal moral principles in support of their substantially different conclusions" (Beauchamp & Walters, 1982, p. 4). The presentation of supporting principles on both sides is referred to as *argument* in applied ethical analysis and the actors are referred to as *agents*. The question of agency, i.e., who is the moral actor, and the appropriateness of applying ethical analysis to family relationships have been the focus of some recent philosophical discussions.

Various interpretations have been presented as to why family relationships have only recently come under ethical scrutiny. To date family relationships have been perceived as being outside the moral sphere given that the agents assumed the relationships were naturally occurring (Mann, 1988; Rawls, 1971). Since Aristotle, philosophers have asserted that ethical issues can be defined only where alternative choice exists. Theoreticians have recently presented arguments that the "family realm" is a set of relationships "created by the birth process and the establishment of ties across generations" and having different ethics from non-family relationships (Beutler et al., 1989, p. 806). This position presents two issues. First, it runs counter to the Lockean proposal that when feudalism gave way to modern individualism family life became contractual and subject to the definition of ethical issues. Second, it presents a view of family that suggests corporate agency. The moral position of individual family members must be clarified.

Definitions of personhood within the family have changed in accordance with temporal and spatial orientations in Western society.

Actors have assumed specific family roles and directed transactions with external organizations. Ethical issues within the family are of interest because society has reached a level of individualism that makes it possible to observe separate agency within a family unit.

Individualism has had the effect of bringing ethical issues in family relations to public attention. Gans' (1988) interpretation of *Middle American Individualism* demonstrates that this basic American value has been internalized by the "ordinary" citizen as well as the self-serving entrepreneur. He describes middle class individualism using various illustrations of the spatial separation which is translated into social and moral distance among agents. Gans uses examples of geographic, social, emotional, and moral distance among "ordinary" individuals and between the citizenry and social institutions.

In terms of family, the boundaries of moral agency have continued to move from the corporate toward the individual. During the nineteenth century, privacy became a "major value in family life" (Hareven, 1978, p. 211). Independent spatial and temporal units were referred to as "nuclear" families. The prevalence of generations living in the same households was reduced. Work, education, and caregiving have become increasingly segregated from family life. The nuclear unit, rather than the extended family, has gained recognition as the corporate agent in dealing with other institutions. Individuals within nuclear families have emerged as the recognized moral unit in at least two arenas: the intervention of outside institutions on behalf of dependent members and the movement of women out of dependent roles to positions of direct interaction with nonfamily institutions. The divestment of gender as a basis for moral agency has been a major influence in restricting agency to the individual level.

The social enfranchisement of women has had other effects. A feminist perspective of family responsibility proposes that gender-skewed enactments of responsibility are attributable to historical gender roles (Mann, 1988). Contemporary definitions of identity and agency have challenged former assumptions that underlie moral responsibility in family relationships. Mann argues that the question of agency in family moral responsibility has changed. Before the social enfranchisement of women, agency was "a gendered category" (Mann, 1988, p. 291). Responsibilities were defined and enacted along gender lines. Men participated in the public sphere in order to provide financial support while women performed duties in the private sphere, e.g., childbearing and homemaking. Within this contract, women were denied full personhood from birth on the basis of gender. It was assumed that a woman's actions would be primarily *for others* and that acting for others would be self-fulfilling. Her identity, and moral agency, was bound to the man who acted publicly on her behalf—even to the extent that she took his name.

Emerging individualism has had the effect of separating agents both spatially and temporally within the family. Locke reasoned that coincident with developing industrialization was the contractualization of family relationships. Functional separation, geographic mobility, and transforming values resulted in the spatial and temporal separation of the generations and laid the basis for definition of ethical issues within the extended family.

The boundaries of personhood (self) define agency. The perception of agency is the basis for relationships with historic, future, and distant persons. The family's time-ordered nature (Larzelere & Klein, 1987) allows members to perceive corporate agency as existing across generations. *Corporate agency* includes historic, future, and distant persons in the personhood of the agent. Any individual member acts as an agent representing the corporate unit in all transactions. The Japanese concept of an individual as representative of the family is an example of inclusive personhood and corporate agency.

In contrast, *individual agency* emphasizes the person as agent. All interactions within and outside the family occur between separate persons. The agent represents the self in transactions with other agents; the agent does not represent corporate interests. In some families, the boundaries of personhood are extended to a very small number of "special" relationships. For example, spouses and other individuals who exist together in time and space may be part of an inclusive personhood while historic, future, and distant persons are excluded. This limited corporate agency has been recognized in legal statutes which have made spouses equally responsible for marital debts and have protected them from involuntarily testifying against each other in court.

While philosophical discussion will continue around individual versus corporate agency as it applies to family relationships, it is sufficient for the purpose of this paper to note that definitions of moral agency may vary with individual and family perceptions of personhood. The remainder of this analysis focuses on the relationship of actors to historic, future, and distant persons with whom they are involved in intergenerational relationships.

Distant Persons

In some families, geographic distance between the generations is great. In others, either emotional bonds or contractual relationships are missing. Does filial obligation exist among emotionally and geographically distant kin? Can that responsibility be reassigned to closer non-kin without moral blame?

Two kinds of welfare rights of distant persons have been discussed in applied ethics literature: (1) rights that are based on specific relationships and hold against nameable persons and (2) rights that do not require specific contractual or role relationships (Sterba, 1983). In the example of elder care, elders hold rights to have basic needs met to insure a decent life. Arguments arise around the rights of elder parents to specific kinds of care from their children based on role and contractual relationships.

Discussions often turned to motivations for family elder caregivers in sessions sponsored by the research committee on aging at the recent XIIth World Congress on Sociology in Madrid. Marvin Sussman's (1980) proposal that family members who provide care be reimbursed was among those creative options debated (Streib, 1990; Riley & Riley, 1990). The suggestion that family members need incentives to provide elder care implies the availability of choice in making caregiving decisions. In contrast, research evidence shows family caregivers are often chosen by proximity, motivated by attachment and feelings of obligation, and sustained in spite of feelings of burden and stress (Kahana & Young, 1990; Cicirelli, 1981). The issue of choice is complex. American policy recognizes economic responsibility for non-kin through taxation of the wage-earning generation and obligation for family caregiving through filial responsibility legislation. However, support is inadequate for kin who choose to forfeit participation in economically rewarding jobs in order to provide elder care and for family members who must purchase non-kin care for geographically distant relatives.

In a free society, individuals distribute resources to other individuals. Nozick (1987) proposes that these distributions are results of individual decisions and voluntary exchanges in historic and current time. Individuals in "special" relationships designate each other as giver or recipient of care and whatever resources are associated with reciprocity in the relationship. These individual arrangements are made within kin networks and non-kin networks. Although morally commendable, voluntary non-kin responsibility is not currently recognized in policy as substituting for filial responsibility. However, it is possible to argue that non-kin care is morally equivalent to kin care and can be exchanged for relief from legally binding filial obligations. Caregiving in this context is morally commendable because it results from free choice.

Relationships are between individuals; obligations, on the other hand, may be between aggregates. Individual and collective duties are distinguishable (Bayles & Henley, 1983). For example, the wage-earning generation may be obligated to share its resources with the adjacent non-earning generations, the young and the old, to assure that all co-existent persons have decent lives. However, whatever rights exist to specific exchanges exist through individual relationships. Social obligations are fulfilled as long as the numbers of wage earners or caregivers contributing to the numbers of non-earners or beneficiaries remain in balance.

Future Generations

In all families, the generations are separated by time, although the amount of time varies. Two axioms are essential to responsibility toward future generations (Green, 1983):

1. "We are bound by ties of justice to real future persons" (p. 335).
2. "The lives of future persons ought ideally to be 'better' than our own and certainly no worse" (p. 337).

Extending personal interest across generational lines requires the examination of future as well as historic persons on whom our actions have impact. The obligations of both parents and children must be clarified (Rheinstein, 1965). For example, the consumption of resources affects the quality of life of future generations. Caregiving that involves conflict between the interests of parents and children is another arena where ethical battles are fought.

A family oriented toward future generations may be more concerned with the obligation of parents toward children. The historically oriented family focuses on the obligation of children to parents. Different temporal orientations in families are reflected in different reasons for having children and may result in different views of intergenerational responsibility. It has been suggested that children owe gratitude to parents for the gift of life. If children are conceived to give pleasure to the parents, do parents become obligated to children in return for whatever pleasure they derive from them?

It is troublesome to think of parent/child relationships as contractual since they begin when the children are developmentally unable to negotiate. Thus, a wider definition of relationships which fulfill intergenerational obligations is appropriate. Adult children and non-kin have the opportunity to choose among alternatives in meeting the needs of the parental generation. Formal and informal exchanges across generational lines are well-documented (Sussman, 1962, 1965; Sussman & Burchinal, 1962; Kreps, 1965; Shanas, 1973). The emotional content of relationships between parents and children influences them to enter contractual relationships for exchanging resources. Although exchanges occur in separated families, spatial, temporal, and emotional distances result in designation of different agents to the intergenerational contract for some types of caregiving.

Arguments for familial duties such as caregiving often rest on principles of gratitude and benevolence. Parents perform acts that are beneficial to the child. Therefore, the child acts out of gratitude to perform caregiving tasks for the parent. Jecker (1989) argues that parental acts are not based on benevolence. The creation of a child does not benefit the child, but the parent. Child care, i.e., education and nurturing, become *duties* given that parenthood benefits the parents more than the child. Does the child then owe gratitude to the parent who performs her duty?

To find a more appropriate rationale for filial duties, Jecker (1989) explores the condition of loyalty. The *family* as an institution and *parents* as specific persons with whom one has a relationship can be candidates for the child's loyalty. However, loyalty can be expressed in a number of ways. Not all expressions of loyalty are demonstrated through physical care. Jecker concludes, "Although children owe parents loyalty, then, this does not suffice to show that parents are entitled to receive specific services or sacrifices" (p. 78).

Post (1988) presents arguments counter to Jecker's (1989). His discussion of filial morality is primarily Christian teaching focusing on the nature of family relationships. He discounts the contractual nature of family relations and emphasizes their naturally occurring and intimate qualities. He cites Sommers' (1986) interpretation of the "differential pull" of relationships that are intimate over those that are casual. Non-family relationships lack the emotional weight of family relationships in Post's analysis. He concludes that the "special" relationships of the family must be supported by public policy that supports family caregiving across the generations.

Wider Definitions
of Intergenerational Responsibility

Post fails to address "differential pull" in non-familial relationships that are emotionally intimate. If we accept Mann's, Locke's, and Rawls' positions that the basis of filial obligation is contractual in current Western society, then we can extend the limits of obligation by allowing a wider definition of "special" relationships. These relationships include any contractual arrangement in which the agent has extended her or his personhood to include the other agent in a corporate one.

It is not necessary for individuals to be related in order to feel special obligations. It is simply necessary for the agents to extend their self-definitions of personhood so the resulting relationships occur within an extended personhood or corporate agency. The relationship is then "special" in the sense that a natural "differential pull" develops and duties within that relationship are defined differently than those perceived to occur in the general society. This extension of Post's argument assumes that similar responsibility could follow consanguine *or* emotional ties. For example, a person could feel responsibility for an aunt or other relative who is emotionally and geographically distant or a friend who is emotionally and geographically close. Either relationship has some differential pull, although the basis of the relationships is quite different.

This argument exists in various religious interpretations of relationships between followers of the same faith. For example, Christian teaching asserts that the "household of faith" or "Church Universal" house the primary relationships within which filial duties exist. The relationships are spiritual, not physical (Post, 1988). In Apache and Navajo traditions, humanity is one with nature and special obligations exist in relationships with both human and non-human extensions of the self. The Mormon concern about the relevance of one's actions through time implies a special relationship among agents who are temporally separated (Kluckohn & Strodtbeck, 1961).

The extension of the self beyond the individualistic boundaries of duty is possible under secular contract as well. "Special" relationships can be designated and contracts for care drawn between the agent and the designee. Libertarians assert that the only truly moral action is one which is chosen freely (Nowell-Smith, 1961). Suppose we agree that persons in one generation have some responsibility for persons in the generations adjacent to their own. Designating the recipient of actions that fulfill that responsibility assures that the agent will have acted out of choice and therefore will be morally commendable for those actions. While social welfare programs that are supported by taxes are necessary, it is difficult to argue that one who pays taxes is morally commendable for choosing to be benevolent toward program beneficiaries.

Documentation exists on voluntary non-kin aid to dependent populations (Goodman, 1984; Pynoos et al., 1984) and reciprocity in friendship groups (Komarovsky, 1964; Babchuck & Bates, 1963). The evidence is that unreciprocated aid is higher among family members than among friends and neighbors (Hochschild, 1973; Troll & Smith, 1976). Redefining "special" relationships on the basis of extension of personhood requires qualitative research to explore kin and non-kin relationships in relation to inclusive personhood and corporate agency. What differential pull exists in such intergenerational ties as mentor/protégé? Are the obligations of these relationships qualitatively similar to those in parent/child relationships? It may be that some relationships defined as family are qualitatively closer to friendship or colleagueship and some non-kin relationships are closer to inclusive personhood. Current research on AIDS caregivers (Matocha, 1990) has begun to examine non-kin relationships that are qualitatively similar to family relationships.

POLICY AND RESEARCH IMPLICATIONS

Policy makers recognize the need to motivate younger people to provide aid for elders and for elders to conserve resources for the young (Riley & Riley, 1990; Callahan, 1986). Such action is critical in an aging society. Suggestions for policy directions include: developing educational curricula to strengthen the sense of obligation young people feel toward their elders with the intended outcome of making them aware of the need for reciprocity (Wynne, 1986); de-emphasizing the prolonging of life at all cost in order to achieve equitable distribution of resources among the generations (Callahan, 1986); and developing coherent national elder care policy that recognizes the changing needs of caregivers (Hooyman, 1990; Gilliland & Havir, 1990). These suggestions imply that policy will be directed toward all generations involved. Both young and old must be educated to extend their personhood across generational lines. The caregiving generation must be supported.

Return to the premise that shrinking spatial and temporal orientations of persons in this society have resulted in sharper definitive lines between agents. The resulting individualism isolates agents who are temporally and spatially separated. Family units are separated into households (spatially) and generations (temporally). Obligation is at best recognized as a component of relationships in adjacent generations (temporally adjacent) and proximate households (spatially adjacent). Obligation can be extended when the definition of personhood is extended spatially to distant persons and temporally to future and historic persons. This extension creates the "differential pull" that has been argued as the basis for moral responsibility within "special" relationships. Specifically, obligation is based on temporal and spatial connections among humans. The disconnected individualist has little basis for moral obligation or responsibility and lacks motivation to act in any way other than self interest.

It may be easier to motivate individuals in a generation to act on their responsibilities to other generations if there is some emotional or intellectual bond that is the basis for actions. From society's perspective, the central issue is whether each generation fulfills its responsibilities not that those responsibilities occur within recognized family boundaries. Intergenerational responsibility in an individualistic society is contractual. Policy must protect the interests of the generations that need care and recognize needs of the caregiving generation. Individual contracts can be negotiated in kin and non-kin relationships within policy guidelines that protect aggregate rights.

More can be learned about a culture by examining variations in the value orientations of its members and subgroups than by looking at dominant values (Kluckhohn and Strodtbeck, 1961). Questions about intergenerational responsibility and obligation may require an investigation of variations among subcultural groups and individuals along spatial and temporal orientations. This kind of research could begin to turn policy and curriculum development from the current focus on "competition for resources" and "reciprocity by guilt" to focus on building intergenerational connections.

REFERENCES

Babchuck, N. & Bates, A.P. (1963). The primary relations of middle class couples: A study of male dominance. *American Sociological Review*, *28*, 377-384.
Bayles, M.D. & Henley, K. (1983). *Right conduct: Theories and applications*. New York: Random House.

Beauchamp, T. & Walters, L. (1982). *Contemporary issues in bioethics* 2nd edition. Belmont, CA: Wadsworth.

Beutler, I.F.; Burr, W.R.; Bahr, K.S.; and Herrin, D.A. (1989). The family realm: Theoretical contributions for understanding its consequences. *Journal of Marriage and the Family, 51*(3), 805-816.

Callahan, D. (1986). Health care in the aging society: A Moral dilemma. In A. Pifer & L. Bronte (Eds.), *Our aging society: Paradox and promise* (pp. 319-340). New York: Norton.

Cicirelli, V.G. (1981). *Helping elderly parents: The role of adult children.* Boston: Auburn House.

Gans, H.J. (1988). *Middle American individualism: The Future of liberal democracy.* New York: The Free Press.

Gilliland, N. & Havir, L. (1990). Public opinion and long-term care policy. In D.E. Biegel & A. Blum (Eds.), *Aging and Caregiving: Theory, Research, and Policy* (pp. 242-253). Newbury Park: Sage.

Goodman, C.C. (1984). Natural helping among older adults. *The Gerontologist, 24,* 138-143.

Green, R.M. (1983). Intergenerational justice and environmental responsibility. In M.D. Bayles & K. Henley (Eds.), *Right conduct: Theories and applications* (pp. 334-341). New York: Random House.

Hareven, T.K. (1978). The Last stage: Historical adulthood and old age. In E.H. Erikson (Ed.), *Adulthood* (pp. 201-216). New York: Norton.

Hochschild, A. (1973). *The Unexpected Community.* Englewood Cliffs, NJ: Prentice-Hall.

Hooyan, N.R. (1990). Women as caregivers of the elderly: Implications for social welfare policy and practice. In D.E. Biegel & A. Blum (Eds.), *Aging and caregiving: Theory, research, and policy* (pp. 221-241). Newbury Park: Sage.

Jecker, N.S. (1989). Are filial duties unfounded? *American Philosophical Quarterly, 26*(1), 73-80.

Kahana, E. & Young, R. (1990). Clarifying the caregiving paradigm: Challenges for the future. In D.E. Biegel & A. Blum (Eds.), *Aging and caregiving: Theory, research, and policy* (pp. 76-97). Newbury Park: Sage.

Kluckhohn, F.R. & Strodtbeck, F.L. (1961). *Variations in value orientations.* Evanston, IL: Row, Peterson.

Komarovsky, M. (1962). *Blue collar marriage.* New York: Random House.

Kreps, J. (1965). The economics of intergenerational relationships. In E. Shanas & G. Streib (Eds.), *Social Structure and the Family: Generational Relations* (pp. 267-288). Englewood Cliffs, NJ: Prentice-Hall.

Larzelere, R.E. & Klein, D. (1987). Methodology. In M.B. Sussman & S.K. Steinmetz (Eds.), *Handbook of Marriage and the Family* (pp. 125-155). New York: Plenum Press.

Mann, P.S. (1988). Personal identity matters. *Social Theory & Practice, 14*(3), 285-316.

Matocha, L. (1989). [Unpublished doctoral dissertation]. University of Delaware.

Nowell-Smith, P.H. (1961). Ethics. In R.B. Brandt (Ed.), *Value and obligation* (pp. 405-417). New York: Harcourt, Brace, & World.

Nozick, R. (1987). Distributive justice. In P.A. French & C. Brown (Eds.), *Puzzles, paradoxes, and problems* (pp. 453-464). New York: St. Martin's.

Post, S. (1988). An Ethical perspective on caregiving in the family. *Journal of Medical Humanities and Bioethics*, 9(1), 6-16.

Pynoos, J., & Hade-Kaplan, B. (1984). Intergenerational neighborhood networks basis for aiding the frail elderly. *The Gerontologist*, 24, 233-237.

Rawls, J. (1971). *A Theory of justice*. Cambridge, MA: Belknap.

Rawls, J. (1987). Two principles of justice. In P.A. French & C. Brown (Eds.), *Puzzles, paradoxes, and problems* (pp. 465-472). New York: St. Martin's.

Rheinstein, M. (1965). Motivation of intergenerational behavior by norms of law. In E. Shanas & G. Streib (Eds.), *Social Structure and the Family: Generational Relations* (pp. 241-266). Englewood Cliffs, NJ: Prentice-Hall.

Riley, J.W. & Riley, M.W. (1990, July). *The lives of retirees and changing social roles*. Paper presented at the XIIth World Congress on Sociology, Madrid, Spain.

Shanas, E. (1979). The family as social support system in old age. *The Gerontologist*, 10, 160-174.

Sommers, C.H. (1986). Filial morality. *Journal of Philosophy*, 83(8), 439-456.

Sterba, J.P. (1983). Welfare rights and future generations. In M.D. Bayles & K. Henley (Eds.), *Right conduct: Theories and applications* (pp. 327-334). New York: Random House.

Streib, G. (1990, July). *Politics, aging, and the family context*. Paper presented at the XIIth World Congress on Sociology, Madrid, Spain.

Sussman, M.B. (1962). The isolated nuclear family: Fact or fiction? In M.B. Sussman (Ed.), *Sourcebook in Marriage and the Family* 3rd Edition (pp. 89-95). New York: Houghton Mifflin.

Sussman, M.B. (1965). Relationships of adult children with their parents in the United States. In E. Shanas & G. Streib (Eds.), *Social structure and the family: Generational relations* (pp. 62-92). Englewood Cliffs, NJ: Prentice-Hall.

Sussman, M.B. (1980). Future trends in society and social services. *Proceedings of the National Conference on Social Welfare*. Columbus, OH, New York: Columbia University Press.

Sussman, M.B. & Burchinal, L. (1962). Kin family network: Unheralded structure in current conceptualizations of family functioning. In M.B. Sussman (Ed.), *Sourcebook in Marriage and the Family* 3rd Edition (pp. 72-82). New York: Houghton Mifflin.

Troll, L. & Smith, J. (1976). Attachment through the lifespan: Some questions about dyadic relationships in later life. *Human Development*, 19, 156-171.

Wynne, E.A. (1986). Will the young support the old? In A. Pifer & L. Bronte (Eds.), *Our aging society: Paradox and promise* (pp. 243-263). New York: Norton.

Sharing or Competition:
Multiple Views
of the Intergenerational Flow
# of Society's Resources

Barbara Hirshorn

Over the last several years, there has been a growing awareness of tension between people who are at different points along the lifecourse. This tension has centered on the distribution of resources — especially those impacting public policy. While some analysts and commentators assign the attribution of "conflict," specifically, *intergenerational* conflict, to this tension, others stress sharing and even cohesiveness between the generations. Still others interpret the intergenerational distribution of resources through perceptions of the heterogeneity of human behavior and activities regarding group and individual needs. These various perspectives on the intergenerational flow of resources are prominently featured in a variety of publications — ranging from a cover page story of a weekly news magazine to a presidential address featured at an annual meeting of a social science professional organization (Preston, 1984a). Yet one is often left with a confusing jumble of arguments that frequently contradict each other — and even themselves — in either thesis, assumptions, or suggested outcomes.

This article attempts to relieve some of the confusion by classifying several of these arguments into an organizational structure; by pointing out similarities and differences among them on underlying factors related to the distribution of resources in a social context;

Barbara Hirshorn is Assistant Professor for Research, Institute of Gerontology, Wayne State University, Detroit, MI 48202.

and by describing some of the arguments themselves. While the perspectives represented are not always mutually exclusive in their component assumptions and/or conclusions, an attempt has been made here to describe an array of arguments and, in so doing, to give an indication of the breadth of data, opinion, and feeling about the subject.

IMPORTANT FACTORS TO CONSIDER REGARDING THE INTERGENERATIONAL DISTRIBUTION OF RESOURCES

Prior to considering the different viewpoints, it is important to note several factors that underpin and delimit each. These include: the concept of the "generation;" the idea of "distributive justice;" the question of whether it is relative or absolute loss/gain of resources that matters to individuals or groups; and, the perception of the resource "pie" to be distributed.

The concept of the "generation" has been used freely, frequently with multiple meanings, even in the same argument. Since ancient times, it has been used in the genealogical sense as a biological tracer to mark the descent of offspring from some progenitor. Beginning with the early nineteenth century, the word has also been used as a sociological term incorporating the concept of time, the process of aging, age groups, and social structure (Bengtson et al., 1985). In recent years the word has taken on additional meanings. Often it now denotes the effect of being in a certain birth cohort. Within this context "generation" refers to what happens to people who are seen as a group on the basis of having been born at the same point in historical time, socialized in youth at a certain time, and likely to carry common experiences with them across the life-course as they confront a variety of personal and societal issues. Lastly, the idea of the generation is associated with a group that shares a collective mentality and set of concerns (Bengtson & Cutler, 1976).

Another issue that frequently results in confusion concerns different concepts of the criterion establishing distributive justice — fairness in the manner in which resources are distributed among people.[1] For instance, shall resources be distributed in equal shares, e.g., equal shares of an estate when a parent dies, equal monthly Social Security retirement fund allocations? Shall resources be distributed according to some measure of merit for work well done, e.g., in the family, to the daughter who assumed the bulk of the caregiving responsibilities prior to the death of a parent; to those people who benefitted the community through some creative effort? Alternatively, shall resources be distributed in greater allotments to those individuals who have greater needs? For instance, in a parental bequest, more to those children who are struggling to make ends meet than to those who are financially comfortable; on the societal level, more to older people who are barely getting by than to those who have a vacation home and considerable additional assets. Lack of consensus regarding the purpose and definition of distributive justice strongly affects individual and group assessments of the fairness of the distribution of resources and whether or not there are feelings of resentment and anger over the distribution process and its outcomes.

Related to these two concerns is that of the absolute or relative context for loss or gain. This is a matter of fixing on whether the focus is on an actual, perceived, or threatened *absolute* loss, or on a *relative loss* while others appear to be gaining. For example, is the individual's or group's major concern a matter of not having enough to meet personal needs; not having enough to meet needs while others do; or not having enough to meet needs *because* others are appropriating the resources? These issues lead one to question: to what extent are some suffering while others are benefitting? Alternatively, does the individual or group envision that what others receive is, in some circumstances, also a personal gain? Or as long as one has enough to meet personal needs, what others receive is of little consequence?

This leads to the final issue — the perception of the resource pie to be divided. Is it perceived as a "fixed pie," implying a constant amount of resources that must be distributed based on existing needs? If so, then during times of resource scarcity (for which a credible argument can usually be made) there will be competition among the different interested parties for the same piece of the pie. On the other hand, with the perception of an "expandable pie," there is greater elasticity in the amount of distributable resources;

more resources may be a consequence of economic growth, additional sources of tax revenue, and eliminating wasteful expenditures. This perception provides at least the possibility of serving a wide variety of interests simultaneously.

Any description of the various arguments regarding the distribution of resources requires a consideration of these four factors. Each helps to define the conceptual framework and terms of debate within which the distribution of resources is discussed. Moreover, insofar as the *discussion* of the resource distribution process can *affect* that process, particularly in the public sector, it is important to know what delimits the discussion. It may be that much of the inter-group tension regarding resource allocation is due to variation in how these concepts are defined.

DESCRIPTIONS OF THE ARGUMENTS

Conflict-Based Arguments

Conflict-based arguments emphasize tension between identifiable subgroups of the population regarding the amount of resources at stake as well as the distribution process. Very often, these arguments are marked by emotionally charged symbols of wealth or ownership used repeatedly to illustrate inter-group inequities. Of the six conflict-based arguments discussed here, all but the last tend to: use the concept of the "generation" as basically synonymous with "cohort;" use "equal shares" as the criterion for distributive justice; emphasize relative deprivation; and perceive a "fixed pie" of resources. The position of the sixth on these issues will be described presently.

The first of the conflict-based positions regarding the intergenerational transfer of resources assumes an *inverse relationship between the welfare of the young and that of the old*. While this argument frequently is drawn in terms of young and old *age groups*, it places *birth cohorts* in clearly adversarial positions regarding the sharing of resources. From this perspective, to the extent that the well-being of older persons, i.e., "current cohorts of the elderly," is improved by the infusion of public resources, younger people suffer. Proponents of this position often cite, as justification, data indicating that older people, as a group, are better off financially than they were two or three decades ago and, moreover, that, as a group, they are currently better off than young people are. Used in support, in the past, for example, are U.S. Bureau of the Census figures indicating that in 1983, a full percentage point more of the population under age 65 (15.4 percent) was below the poverty line than was the over 65 population (14.1 percent) (Council of Economic Advisers, 1985, chap. 5).

From this perspective, older people are no longer penurious. Rather, they have begun to indulge themselves with a new-found affluence and, abetted by additional years of good health, have sought an "active life-style" that includes luxury items, travel, and, in general, the enjoyment of accumulated assets augmented by non-cash benefits such as Medicare (Longman, 1985). In contrast, the young are portrayed as *not* benefitting from public policy entitlements and actually struggling to make ends meet or else going without — as had the elderly a few decades ago.

Analysts Axinn and Stern (1985) see the roots of this situation in a historical shift in the pattern of distribution of entitlements *away* from the young and *toward* the elderly. They point out that, before the Great Depression of the 1930s, public financial assistance was available, in a very restrictive and modest form, for both the old *and* the young. Change occurred with the advent of the Social Security system in 1935 and with the restructuring, during the 1950s and 1960s, of the legal definition of "family responsibility" to dependent family members. The result was an *easing* of the responsibility of adult children for their parents yet a *retention* of the responsibility of adults for their minor offspring. Thus, Axinn and Stern state, "the aged, reaping the benefits of a vast array of public programs, improved their economic and social circumstances while children, increasingly the responsibility of their parents, reaped a bitter harvest of poverty and lost opportunities" (1985, p. 666). To alleviate the current status of children in this country and begin to address this perceived resource distribution problem, medical ethicist Daniel Callahan maintains that we, as a society, must not only rethink our resource allocations to *children* but also encourage the elderly to be concerned with the welfare of the young, more so than their own (Callahan, 1987).

Closely related to the "inverse relationship" position is one that focuses on the idea that *population aging has had and will continue to have a negative effect on current, and possibly future, cohorts of younger people*. It is clear that the population of the United States *has* aged during this century. This is evident by the facts that fewer women of childbearing age are having children, the median age of the entire population is rising, and the proportions of the population over the age of 65 and the age of 85 have increased. Advocates of this viewpoint link the increase in *social expenditures* on the elderly and the diminution of such expenditures on the young *directly* to what they maintain is an outcome of population aging—the concomitant increase in the political and economic influence of older people as they have become a greater proportion of the total population (Preston, 1984a; 1984b).

Proponents of this view are often at their gloomiest when discussing the future. Two commentators voicing this perspective warn that "future demographic trends and current benefit laws guarantee an enormous growth in resource transfers to older generations over the next 50 years." They maintain that the aging of America is not a "one-time blip that we can 'tough out'" until the Baby Boom cohort has died. Rather, they assert, because of the low fertility levels and the improvements in the survival rates of old people, the preeminence of the elderly and their needs is an "enduring reality to which our economic, political and social institutions must adapt" (Hewitt & Howe, 1988, p. 9).

A third viewpoint regarding the intergenerational transfer of resources is *the national profligacy argument*. Central to this perspective is the idea that the current combination of high federal governmental and trade deficits, low personal savings rates, and low reinvestment in the private sector and physical infrastructure will take its toll on current and future generations of young Americans. Proponents of this view maintain that the process of deferring payment on present-day borrowing to keep the federal government afloat is one of the largest "intergenerational transfers" from today's old to tomorrow's young.

Why is this "transfer" often perceived as stemming from the old, specifically, and not from adults of *all* ages? Because, advocates maintain, the most costly portions of these obligations are the pensions for public employees and the Social Security system. Unlike private sector pension funds which are usually fully funded (have sufficient assets to pay pensioners at any given time without drawing down on later contributions), the federal government's civil service and military retirement systems for states and local jurisdictions are only partially funded for the most part. Thus, proponents assert, our national debt is fueled to an estimated $1.5 trillion to support these public pensioners. As for Social Security, at least one proponent of this perspective foresees an estimated $5 trillion in unfunded liabilities, *despite* the adjustments made to the system in 1983 to make it fiscally stronger (Leonard, 1988).[2]

The problem is only compounded, according to those who hold this perspective, by the diminution of the national rate of savings, resulting in an anemic rate of reinvestment in the American business infrastructure. According to one concerned analyst:

> With personal savings providing very little industrial capital, American firms are highly dependent on retained corporate earnings and on open capital markets for funds to invest and create new jobs. What capital is left is obtained only at very high rates. A myopic fiscal regime is robbing America of the financial tools we need to grow and compete. (Moody, 1988, p. 3)

Also, deferred maintenance of the *public* infrastructure—roads, bridges, railroads, and public utilities is often mentioned. It is claimed that this reduces still further the net value of such transfers to future generations and insures that these future generations, rather than current generations of adults, will have to pay much more dearly to keep both the public and the private sector going (Leonard, 1988).

Another conflict-based argument is the *interest group perspective* which again places the personal interests of the young and the old in an adversarial position. In this case, public expenditures for health care in old age and pensions are pitted against public expenditures for educational health and nutritional programs for the young. This argument is one of the strongest levelled at older people; it places their self-interest directly in conflict with the self-interest of the most vulnerable of the younger age groups—children. Indeed, it assumes that the amount of public expenditures for these various resources are directly related to the size, wealth, and empowerment of the individuals in the age groups to which these resources go. Since children do not vote, the argument continues, the elderly win, hands down. For instance, one analyst suggests that communities composed of large proportions of old people, who tend to turn out in substantial numbers at the polls, will vote against measures that support allocations for public education and will vote for measures that support allocations for health care and pensions for the elderly (Preston, 1984a). Once again, one sees the inverse relationship between the well-being of the young and the well-being of the old. *Size* of the constituent group is not the only important factor here; the *number of voters* is also of great importance. Thus, a neighborhood with a small number of elderly and a large number of welfare mothers and children may still not result in a well-endowed school system.[3]

Others link organized interest group activity to the inability of government in this country to either protect those who are unorganized or to pursue interests that are for the long-term common good. Indeed, one writer asserts that, while we may never be able to rid ourselves of factions, we *can* penalize politicians and special interest groups that do not distinguish between serving the interests of rich and poor elderly (Longman, 1987).[4]

The fifth perspective, the *angry baby boomer argument*, focuses on the perceived relative deprivation faced by one particular cohort, those born in this country between 1946 and 1964, in contrast with the perceived more bountiful resources available to, and enjoyed by, those born during the preceding five decades. Indeed, proponents contend that, in terms of personal wealth, the "baby boom" cohort is quickly becoming the "baby bust" cohort, reflecting a growing disparity between baby boomers and older birth cohorts on *all* resources necessary for well-being. This argument focuses upon the relative diminution of resources and options facing those who are currently young adults in comparison with the resources and options available to their parents. As commentator Michael Moore has stated:

Contrary to the popular myth that the baby boomers are a privileged class of yuppies with Gold Cards and compact discs, the
truth is that our generation, unlike any generation in the history of this country, is worse off than our parents. Unlike our
parents, most of us cannot afford to buy a house. We do not
trade in for a new car every two or three years. We save less
but have to spend more. . . . The worst part of being a baby
boomer though, is the total lack of job security. No longer
does hard work or the profitability of the company have anything to do with guaranteeing that you'll be working there tomorrow. . . . (Moore, 1987, p. A9)

In its more conflictive "angry yuppie" form, this argument
echos the complaint of a 30-year old public health dentist who
wrote in the op-ed column of NEWSWEEK a few years ago regarding the perceived relative advantages enjoyed by those currently old
in comparison with the lot of those currently young:

How are older Americans faring today? Like bandits . . . A
married man whose wife did not work and who retired in 1982
at 65, got back all of his [Social Security] payroll contributions
since 1937 in 14 months. . . . Retired persons often have stabi-
lized, if not entirely rigid expenses. Almost 70 percent own
their own home; others have a sizable nest egg from its sale.
Their fixed incomes do not decrease because of a company
layoff or because of increases in FICA withholding. Medicare
covers major hospital expenses . . . Public transportation is
cheap . . . And virtually every amusement can be obtained for
a discount. Contrast this with the expenses of a 30-year-old
"Yuppie" couple. The typical monthly mortgage payment in
1983 reached $741. Total home payments are higher. There is
no rebate on your property tax, which many seniors in my city
get. Or on a bus that costs 75 cents, but serves seniors for a
dime. (Anderson, 1985, "My Turn" Column)

The *alienated near-poverty level elderly* position also assumes a
"fixed pie" of resources, uses "equal shares" as the criterion for
distributive justice, and emphasizes "relative deprivation." In this

case, however, the conception of a "generation" is not based on birth cohort masked as age but on ethnic background or on economic class. Older people who voice this argument, usually in letters to the editors of local newspapers, live precarious lives, surviving mainly on Social Security checks, unable to afford current food prices or property taxes, and frightened that they will lose what modest resources they have. They maintain that their problem is the direct result of the material enhancement of other groups in society — in this case not the young, or any other age group for that matter — but rather of greedy businessmen, people on welfare, or illegal immigrants. Thus, the adversaries for the fixed pie of *public* resources are easily identifiable individuals who are as vulnerable or even more vulnerable than are these older people who are slightly above the poverty level. Opponents for resources within the context of the *private* sector are easily identified symbols of that power structure — particularly local businessmen who are directly responsible for the diminution of personal resources when a transaction is made.

Solidarity-Based Arguments

Solidarity-based arguments stress a commonality of needs and the assumption that what is good for individuals in one group is usually good for individuals in other groups. Frequently, there is an interest and stake in the welfare of individuals not in one's own identity group. Rhetoric used in these arguments tends to include symbols of intergroup cohesion such as the "general welfare;" the "needs of society as a whole;" "working together toward a commonly-shared future."

The two particular solidarity-based arguments discussed here use multiple meanings for the concept of the "generation:" a birth cohort; generations in the family; and a collective reflecting a common set of concerns. These arguments hedge on a criterion for distributive justice by stressing the need to be aware that different distribution decision rules exist and that the context for assessing loss and gain is often an indirect or long-term one. With these perspectives, the resource pie is an expandable one.

The *common stake argument* maintains that individuals in every generation, however the word is defined, have a common stake in a variety of transfers that move across age groups and birth cohorts. Included in this common stake are transfers of personal services such as care-giving, culture, technology, biomedical advances, as well as cash and in-kind benefits (Kingson, Hirshorn, & Cornman, 1986, chap. 2). This perspective stresses the *inter*dependence of individuals and contends that, while one does not give to and receive from *particular* individuals in equal amounts, over the course of a lifetime, most of us both give to *and* receive from others in considerable portions. Thus emphasis is on a longitudinal, rather than a cross-sectional, view of the transfer of resources. Proponents of this perspective emphasize the common stake most members of U.S. society have in public transfers, such as Social Security retirement or disability payments, Aid For Families With Dependent Children (AFDC), GI Bill entitlements, that may affect *directly* one member of a family while at the same time affect *indirectly* members of different generations in a family (Kingson et al., 1986).

Nowhere is this position more vigorously proposed as it is in support of one particular public transfer—the Social Security system. From a "common stake" perspective, there are costs and benefits to Social Security that flow *directly* to Americans as family members and members of society (e.g., in the form of financial support in retirement, maintenance in the event of a disability, or in the event of the loss of a family breadwinner). These costs and benefits also reach Americans *indirectly* as family members and members of society who would, otherwise, have to devote considerable amounts of alternative resources to support individuals in these life circumstances. Such transfers can be viewed both cross-sectionally, at one particular point in historical time, and longitudinally— over decades. Indeed, it is when one takes a longitudinal view of both the direct and indirect flow of Social Security as a resource transfer that the "common stake" in it is most obvious (Kingson et al., 1986, chap. 4).

This argument has received support recently from unexpected quarters. Some conservative groups, notably the Eagle Forum, assert that Social Security's spouse and widow benefits are pro-family and, thus, deserve support (Carlson, 1987). After years of contending that Social Security ought to be phased out, conservative economist John Mueller now concludes that "privatizing Social Security would subject the baby boom to a whopping tax increase, and materially hurt the family" (Mueller, 1987, p. 46). Moreover, he maintains that, if one assumes that the family is the basic unit of society, then "basing everyone's pension solely on cash earnings means forcing mothers willy-nilly out of the home." Consequently, it is worthwhile to continue to make Social Security workable (Mueller, 1987, p. 47).

Another perspective, *the stake of the no longer young on the well-being of children*, is based on several factors. Couched specifically in terms of the stake that the *elderly*, in particular, have in the well-being of children and youth, it contends that those who are no longer young must weigh both moral and practical concerns when considering inter-age group resource allocations. Regarding moral considerations, one source points out that: (1) our societal value system dictates that children have the right to a decent standard of living and to some means with which to try to fulfill their potential and (2) the society-wide belief system in the United States includes the idea that adults assist those who will inherit the civilization (Kingson et al., 1986, chap. 7).

Justification for this argument involves several points. One is the notion that many individuals who are no longer young have a practical interest in the *future* productivity of today's children. This concern, advocates maintain, rests on an understanding that sufficient support must be transferred to individuals when they are children to insure that they will be equipped as adults to engage in productive activity as workers, designers of public policy, community leaders, and parents. Furthermore, today's worker will be turning to individuals who are today's young children for both public and family-based support during the retirement years. This argument proposes that an ill-equipped child will not be in a position to provide that support as an adult (Kingson et al., 1986, chap. 7; Vobejda, 1987). To help insure that today's children are equipped to be tomorrow's producers, one analyst suggests that, as a society, Americans provide free medical care for all children, the human resources of the future, from the time of conception until the age of 12 (J. Morgan, personal communication, January 25, 1989).

Secondly, for some there is a concern for the safety net function of public policies directed at the family. Those adhering to this perspective point out that substantial proportions of *both* the old and the young are poor and/or not in good health and would be in even worse circumstances without Medicaid, Supplemental Security Income, public housing, etc. (Kingson et al., 1986, chap. 7).

Finally, those holding this perspective often voice the idea that there is a potentially unifying effect for young and old in the response, through public policy, to so-called "family issues," e.g., government supported child and adult day care. This resurgence of interest has led one analyst to note: ". . . a shift toward family policy will automatically produce intergenerational policy proposals that will require the aged to not only share lobbying time with other age groups but resources as well" (Wisensale, 1988, p. 777).

Heterogeneity-Based Arguments

These are arguments that stress the diversity among individuals and groups without necessarily assuming that tension exists over the distribution of resources as a result of that diversity. The case is made for channeling resources to certain individuals or groups. In contrast with conflict-based arguments over the distribution of resources, in which age frequently is used as a proxy for birth cohort, the justification for that channeling is based on differentiating characteristics that tend to either cross-cut the age distribution of the population or consider age irrelevant. With this perspective, the emphasis upon heterogeneity precludes a concern with the concept of generation—except, perhaps, in the loosest sense of "differences in social structure." The criterion for distributive justice is a redressing of need, regardless of whether or not additional allocation criteria are also used. The context for loss or gain is one of absolute need, and the perception of the resource pie is usually an expandable one (or a fixed pie for those who mix a conflict-based perspective with the "needs-based" argument described below).

The *diversity of the elderly perspective* takes as its credo a state-ment written by Boston College economist Joseph Quinn:

> . . . never begin a sentence with 'The elderly are . . .' or 'The elderly do.' No matter what you are discussing, some are, and some are not; some do, and some do not. The most important characteristic about the aged is their diversity. (Quinn, 1987, p. 64)

It is the *economic* heterogeneity of the elderly that proponents of this perspective contend is paramount in maintaining the flow of society's resources, particularly old age entitlements such as Social Security retirement funding and Medicare. The concern is that a failure to recognize the economic diversity of older Americans will result in the disregard of the substantial pockets of poverty still existing among older people. For instance, approximately 31 per-cent of elderly blacks, 23 percent of elderly Hispanics, 27 percent of all elderly women not living with family, and 60 percent of el-derly black women not living with family were below the poverty threshold in 1986 (U.S. Bureau of the Census, 1987).

The *needs-based perspective* is rooted in the criterion for distrib-utive justice that maintains that resources should be distributed to each according to the exigencies of his/her own material circum-stance. Many of those who argue that the elderly are consuming too great a proportion of society's resources, especially those who maintain that young people are suffering as a consequence, also support this position. However, the perspective stands on its own as a possible alternative to those with age-based distribution criteria, or to other bases for meting out society's resources. This position requires the identification of individuals who, irrespective of any other characteristic, "share a problem or a life condition that calls for intervention by a public or private agency" (Neugarten & Neugarten, 1986, p. 45). Often tagged "age-neutral" policies, needs-based policies attempt "to provide services on the basis of demonstrated or assessed need, rather than on the basis of member-ship in a group defined by an arbitrary chronological age" (Austin & Loeb, 1982, p. 276).

Regarding the elderly specifically, Bernice Neugarten, a proponent of this viewpoint, urges a closer examination of the blanket use of "chronological age" as the basis for policy design. She acknowledges that, since a large proportion of the elderly in the 1950's and 1960's *were* poor and without health insurance, many of the age-based programs created during that period as a consequence *did* provide crucial assistance to those who were also in great need. However, she points out, chronological age is a poor predictor of physical, intellectual, or social status during the second half of life. Thus, Neugarten maintains, it is, by itself, a weak criterion upon which to peg the development of social policy (Neugarten, 1982).

Analysts such as the Neugartens, who have given considerable thought to the validity of an age-based versus a needs-based distribution system for society's resources, suggest that it may not be easy to determine the circumstances in which one or the other of these approaches is the wisest. They maintain that these issues "do not usually take the form of simple either/or decisions, but involve complicated combinations of age and need" (Neugarten & Neugarten, 1986, p. 47). Thus, by stressing the "both/and" rather than the "either/or" nature of heterogeneous populations, the Neugartens acknowledge how challenging it is to decide upon just criteria for the distribution of society's resources and to design policies that will satisfactorily implement those criteria.

CONCLUSION

This article has discussed perspectives that have gained wide currency in recent years regarding the intergenerational transfer of resources. In doing so, it has described the importance of several factors that underpin and delimit the way in which these perspectives are framed. These are issues that are likely to be topical well into the next century. Therefore, it is important that, as members of a global community, citizens of this country, community members, and family members, we are aware that a broad range of perspectives regarding the flow of resources across "generations"/age groups/the lifecourse exists. Each perspective entails certain assumptions about the resource distribution process. With this awareness, we are in a better position to avoid the acrimony that often imbues discussion of these issues while maintaining an awareness of the inevitability of multiple perspectives.

NOTES

1. The most influential work on distributive justice in the last 50 years is John Rawls' *A Theory of Justice*, which describes a two-pronged theory of "justice as fairness": (1) each individual in a society has an equal right to various basic freedoms; however (2) insofar as there are inequalities in the distribution of resources, those resources must be focused upon enhancing the well-being of society's most disadvantaged. Others who have dealt extensively with the subject are Nicholas Rescher (1966); Hugo Bedau (1971); and, at the other end of the philosophical spectrum, the libertarian orientation of Robert Nozick (1974). There also have been, especially during the last two decades, a spate of works focusing specifically upon the equity of the criteria through which health-related resources are distributed — viz. especially the writings of Dan E. Beauchamp, James Childress, Gene Outka, Charles Fried, Daniel Callahan, and Norman Daniels.

2. Critiques of this perspective abound. For instance Minkler asserts that, as part of what later evolved into a "victim-blaming process," the elderly were the objects of a humanitarian federal action program during the economically good times of the 1960s and early 1970s which then resulted in the labelling of the elderly the major cause of the subsequent fiscal crisis (Minkler, 1983). Estes maintains that the assignation of the elderly as "a problem to society," fueled by the images of a graying budget, graying society, and aging population, has solidified the symbolic linkage of economic crisis with old age (Estes, 1983a; also Estes, 1983b for a discussion of the way in which the elderly are portrayed as the source of "the problem" with the Social Security system). A related critique is offered by Binstock who contends that the elderly in the United States are scapegoated for a range of current political and economic ills. He finds the roots of this scapegoating in "compassionate ageism," prevalent until the late 1970s, which characterized the elderly as poor, frail, and politically impotent and which has been turned on its head in the present era of economic uncertainty (Binstock, 1983). Binstock also focuses this critique on the context in which those over the age of 85 are often considered in the controversy over health care cost containment (Binstock 1985).

3. While investigations during the 1960's and early 1970s appeared to support the contention that older people are apt to vote against school bond issues (e.g., Piele & Hall, 1973; Hamilton & Cohen, 1974) recent studies provide considerable countervailing evidence. For example, Chomitz looked at three survey-based studies of public education expenditures (Rubinfeld, 1976; Bergstrom, Rubinfeld, & Shapiro, 1982; and Lankford, 1985) and at four community-based studies of per pupil educational expenditures explained by such factors as the median income in the community (Feldstein, 1975; Inman, 1978; Ladd, 1975; and Lovell, 1978). As it turns out, Chomitz found that there is *no* significant effect on voters'

per pupil educational expenditures that could be attributed to the age or to the cohort of the voters. Moreover, wealthier, higher-income, and more educated voters supported *greater* educational expenditures (Chomitz, 1987). This conclusion is seconded in a recent analysis of the voting patterns on school bond referenda of the elderly in Florida which determined that, at least in the last several years, the presence of politically organized, educated, and relatively affluent older people tends to lead to *increased* support for local education (Button and Rosenbaum, 1989).

4. Again, it is worthwhile noting Minkler's analysis. She maintains that it was the instrumentation of a social welfare federal action program, instituted through the use of a block grant system in the 1960s, that set up a dynamic whereby the advocates of the young and the old were placed in adversarial positions which have been felt most acutely during the subsequent era of fiscal austerity (Minkler, 1983).

REFERENCES

Anderson, T. A. (1985, January 7). The best years of their lives. *Newsweek*. "My Turn" Column.

Austin, C. D. & Loeb, M. B. (1982). Why age is relevant in social policy and practice. In B. L. Neugarten (Ed.), *Age or need? Public policies for older people* (pp. 263-288). Beverly Hills, CA: Sage Publications.

Axinn, J. & Stern, M. J. (1985). Age and dependency: Children and the aged in American social policy. *Milbank Memorial Fund Quarterly/Health and Society*, *63*(4), 648-668.

Bedau, H. (1971). *Justice and equality*. Englewood Cliffs, NJ: Prentice-Hall.

Bengtson, V. L. & Cutler, N. E. (1976). Generations and intergenerational relations: Perspectives on age groups and social change. In R.H. Binstock and E. Shanas (Eds.), *Handbook of Aging and the Social Sciences*, 1st Edition (pp. 130-159). New York: Van Nostrand Reinhold.

Bengtson, V. L., Cutler, N. E., Mangen, D. J., & Marshall, V. W. (1985). In R. H. Binstock and E. Shanas (Eds.), *Handbook of Aging and the Social Sciences* 2nd Edition (pp. 304-338). New York: Van Nostrand Reinhold.

Bergstrom, T. C., Rubinfeld, D. L., & Shapiro, P. (1982). Micro-based estimates of demand functions for local school expenditures. *Econometrica*, *50*(5), 1183-1205.

Binstock, R. H. (1983). The aged as scapegoat. *The Gerontologist*, *23*(2), 136-143.

Binstock, R. H. (1985). The oldest old: A fresh perspective or compassionate ageism revisited? *Milbank Memorial Fund Quarterly*, *63*(2), 420-451.

Button, J. & Rosenbaum, W. (1989). Seeing gray: School bond issues and the aging in Florida. *Research on Aging*, *11*(2) 158-173.

Callahan, D. (1987). *Setting limits, medical goals in an aging society*. New York: Simon & Schuster.

Carlson, A. C. (1987, Fall). Is social security pro-family? A response to John Mueller. *Policy Review*, p. 49.

Chiriboga, D. (1988). Review of *Born To Pay. Generations*. 79-80.

Chomitz, K. M. (1987). Demographic influences on local public education expenditures: A review of econometric evidence. *Demographic Change and the Well-Being of Children and the Elderly (National Research Council)* (45-53). Washington, DC: National Academy Press.

Council of Economic Advisers. (1985). Economic status of the elderly. *Economic Report of the President*. Washington, DC: U.S. Government Printing Office.

Estes, C. L. (1983a). Fiscal austerity and aging. In C. L. Estes and R. J. Newcomer (Eds.), *Fiscal austerity and aging, shifting government responsibility for the elderly* (pp. 1, 17-40). Beverly Hills, CA: Sage Publications.

Estes, C. L. (1983b). Social security: The social construction of a crisis. *Milbank Memorial Fund Quarterly, Health and Society, 61*(3), 445-461.

Feldstein, M. S. (1975). Wealth neutrality and local choice in public education. *The American Economic Review, 65*(1), 75-89.

Hamilton, H. D. & Cohen, S. H. (1974). *Policy making by plebiscite: School referenda*. Lexington, MA: D.C. Heath.

Hewitt, P. S. & Howe, N. (1988). Generational equity & the future of generational politics. *The Generational Journal, 1*(1), 8-9.

Inman, R. P. (1978). Testing political economy's "as if" proposition: Is the median income voter really decisive? *Public Choice, 33*, 45-65.

Kingson, E. R., Hirshorn, B. A., & Cornman, J. M. (1986). *Ties that bind, the interdependence of generations*. Washington, DC: Seven Locks Press.

Ladd, H. F. (1975). Local education expenditures, fiscal capacity, and the composition of the property tax base. *National Tax Journal, 28*(2), 145-158.

Lankford, R. H. (1985). Preferences of citizens for public expenditures on elementary and secondary education. *Journal of Econometrics, 27*, 1-20.

Leonard, H. B. (1988). Shadows in time: The perils of intergenerational transfers. *The Generational Journal, 1*(1), 1-2.

Longman, P. (1985, June). Justice between generations. *The Atlantic Monthly*, pp. 73-81.

Longman, P. (1987). *Born to pay, the new politics of aging in America*. Boston: Houghton Mifflin.

Lovell, M. C. (1978). Spending for education: The exercise of public choice. *The Review of Economics and Statistics, 60*(4), 487-495.

Minkler, M. (1983). Blaming the aged victim: The politics of scapegoating in times of fiscal conservatism. *International Journal of Health Services, 13*(1), 155-167.

Moody, J. (1988). Dollars & debt: Can America pay the price of liberty. *The Generational Journal, 1*(1), 3-4.

Moore, M. (1987, February 11). Not having it all. *The Ann Arbor News*, p. A9. (Written for *Newsday*, distributed by the *Los Angeles Times-Washington Post News Service*.)

Mueller, J. (1987, Fall). A subsidy for motherhood: Why I now support social security. *Policy Review*, p. 46.

Neugarten, B. L. (1982). Policy for the 1980s: Age or need entitlement? In B. L. Neugarten (Ed.), *Age or need? Public policies for older people* (pp. 19-32). Beverly Hills: Sage Publications.

Neugarten, B. L. & Neugarten, D. A. (1986). Changing meanings of age in the aging society. In A. Pifer & L. Bronte (Eds.), *Our aging society, paradox and promise* (pp. 33-52). New York: W. W. Norton.

Nozick, R. (1974). *Anarchy, state, and utopia*. New York: Basic Books.

Piele, P. K. & Hall, J. S. (1973). *Budgets, bonds, and ballots: Voting behavior in school financial elections*. Lexington, MA: D.C. Heath.

Preston, S. H. (1984a). Children and the elderly: Divergent paths for America's dependents. *Demography*, 435-457.

Preston, S. H. (1984b). Children and the elderly. *Scientific American*, *251*, 44-49.

Quinn, J. F. (1987). The economic status of the elderly: Beware of the mean. *The review of income and wealth*, Series 33, No. 1, 63-71.

Rawls, J. (1971). *A theory of justice*. Cambridge, MA: Harvard University Press.

Rescher, N. (1966). *Distributive justice*. Indianapolis: Bobbs-Merril.

Rubinfeld, D. L. (1976). Voting in a local school election: A micro analysis. *The Review of Economics and Statistics*, *59*, 30-42.

United States Bureau of the Census. "Money Income and Poverty Status of Families and Pension in the United States: 1986." (1987, July). *Current Population Reports*, Series P-60, No. 157. Unpublished data from the March 1987 Current Population Survey.

Vobejda, B. (1987, October 11). Fewer students may make the grade: Poverty, language, home life raise barriers to graduation. *The Washington Post*, pp. A1, 22.

Wisensale, S. K. (1988). Generational equity and intergenerational policies. *The Gerontologist*, *28*(6), 773-778.

Ancestor Worship
as an Intergenerational Linkage
in Perpetuity

Kris Jeter

When a father stoops to help his son, they both laugh.
When a son stoops to help his father, they both cry.

— Yiddish saying

She looked at me with wise
bluebell eyes
and told me Grimm
had it all wrong
for it was grandmother
who gobbled up the bad wolf
and not the other way round.

He had it all wrong,
for grandmothers you see
are very strong.

— Ada Aharoni
Grandmother and the Wolf

In this era when the individual is recognized as a viable entity, the family is defined by theorists as any group of persons who want to consider themselves to be a family. Indeed, a family may be a horizontal age group of adults without the vertical strata of elders and youngsters. In this highly mobile society, the family becomes a place where individuals of like concerns meet and exchange talents, and, hopefully, nurture, love, and care for each other.

Kris Jeter is a Principal in Beacon Associates LTD Inc., a social research and consultation firm, 800 Paper Mill Rd, Newark, DE 19711-3316.

The illusion of the individual, "able to take care of myself"—to live in a secured care-free condo, purchase home delivered deli meals, buy any service, conduct work on the personal computer, and find distraction at the home entertainment center—leads to the rupture of generations. The illusion of the family, an intergenerational connection of empathy and intimacy, is seen beneath its veil by some individuals. As "memories light the corners of the mind," the intergenerational family homestead becomes crystallized into the heart.

The 1989 San Franciso earthquake alerted Californians to the importance of the generation as a measure of time important to the human memory. One scientist announced that even though the "big one" was not predicted to occur for ninety years, it was important for each generation to endure an earthquake. Experience alone would promote sufficient respect for the splitting and shaking of the ground and lead to proper preparation for this natural phenomenon. Because of lack of experience within a generation, Californians had grown blasé about the potential destructive force. The telling of stories by survivors would ignite changes in social policy and individual action. Architectural structures and transportation ways could be made to withstand earthquakes. Each home, work site, and vehicle could store emergency water, first aid kit, flashlight, and food.

The generation is a valuable measure of time. In the *Hebrew Bible*, *Mahabarata*, the *Edda*, and other ancient texts, we read litanies of generations. In fact, some translators believe the Icelandic word, *edda*, actually means grandmother and that these stories were told by generations of grandmothers. The Brothers Jacob and Wilhelm Grimm were so convinced of the relationship between grandmothers and future generations that they made it their life mission to collect German stories. There is a wisdom behind the ancient definition of the family that relies on a vertical line of generations. Had there been no intergenerational connection, the actual presence and the viable wisdom of the grandparents, the hominids would never have survived.

Ancestor worship is a cross-cultural phenomenon which connects generations of a family and a people. Average life spans have only rather recently in the history of the hominid allowed children to learn from grandparents and great grandparents. Thus, ancestor worship with its accompanying recitation of stories has connected generations over time. Intergenerational connections provide the key to remembrance and forgetfulness.

Traditionally, the human is born into and dies within a family. However, with sufficient ancestor worship, a human lives forever in the bosom of the family. Paradoxically, the family provides not only birth, but immortality in perpetuity for its members.

Today in the West, age-old norms of family behavior have lost their usefulness. For instance, ancient custom deemed it necessary that Wilma Mauler, my maternal grandmother in the Alps, the eldest of three daughters, marry first. Only then, could the other daughters marry. Wilma was 30 and sturdy, and Friedel, the next younger daughter, was physically beautiful and the recipient of many marriage proposals. Thus, my grandmother obeyed the custom by answering an advertisement for a German bride, sending to American a picture of the beautiful sister signed "Wilma"!

In the past, trust in tradition and the fates was considered the key to a good life. Now, with increased autonomy, few Westerners feel a bond to moral obligations of cultural mores. However, if we cannot trust the age old customs, can we trust the actions of our recent ancestors, who did the best they could in a vacuum of directions and a circus of options?

Traditional ancestor worship has given way to contemporary doubt and mistrust of ancestors which requires psychoanalysis to repair the psychic damage. Therapist Harold H. Bloomfield teaches in a book and on an audio-tape, *Making Peace with Your Parents: The Key to Enriching Your Life and All Your Relationships* (1983). Author Nancy Friday tells of her finding her inner self when she investigated *My Mother My Self* (1977). Jungian analyst, Linda Schierse Leonard works with *The Wounded Woman: Healing the Father-Daughter Relationship* (1983). Other professionals speak of re-birthing and re-parenting.

This schism between generations is furthered by rapid-paced modernity. In China, sixty percent of the population is under the age of thirty. The 4 June 1989 massacre of students at Tiananmen Square in China has been explained by some to be a conflict of youth, knowledgeable, many personally, of the liberty of the West, and elders, who recollected their own power when rebelling as youth against their elders. An ironic joke on intergenerations told at the time in China was, "The 80-year-olds are calling meetings of 70-year-olds to decide which 60-year-olds should retire" (Birnbaum and Chua-Eoan, 1990).

Meanwhile, Westerners live in horizontal families, cutting rain forests, drilling and spilling oil. Many die to become ancestors whom the living should doubt, mistrust, and even enter into therapy in order to create within their memories better ancestors for themselves and hopefully to transfer this information to make themselves into better ancestors for their children.

In this analytic essay, I describe psychological and social implications of three cultures of ancestor worship: Early Chinese objects plus later Chinese domestic deities; the Mexican Day of the Dead; and the Maring *kaiko*. I shall then summarize patterns of ancestor worship representative of different cultures and ages and propose that much of the practice of twentieth century psychology is actually an attempt through intergenerational connection to recreate ancestor worship in contemporary dress. The time-honored practices actually speak to the current adage, "You think your parents ran your life when they were alive, wait till they are dead!" Moreover, they speak to the connections from generation to generation over centuries and even millennia of time. I conclude this article with a case study illustrating how the ritual of ancestor worship contributed to the ultimate demolition of the Berlin Wall.

CHINESE ANCESTOR WORSHIP

Archaeologists have found burials from 3000 B.C.E. China. Tremalite (jade) from the hills of Shanghai was fashioned very laboriously with wooden and bamboo tools. The completed jade pieces were then placed in every body cavity with the purpose, it is thought, of keeping the soul within the body.

Around 2000 B.C.E., China's climate became dryer, the vista stark and dusty, the northern area a treeless wasteland. During this time period, the appearance of bronze is one evidence of the emergence of the state bureaucracy. The working of bronze requires a high level of labor organization, management, and authority to mine ore, create models, and rapidly pour melted ore into large molds.

Among the objects in existence today are *ding* or 250-pound tripod vessels inscribed with tributes to ancestors, such as "Shou made this precious vessel for Father Geng." These vessels were used for the serving of sacrificed flesh carved from the carcasses of humans captured in war specifically for ancestral offering. During rituals, the dead and living were gathered together around the vessel for communion. With each dip into the deep cauldron, the eldest would not only serve food but, through ritual, nurture all of the generations of the family, living and dead, and thereby the state. Ancestor worship was important for the elite. They alone had the resources to display wealth of jade and bronze plus human sacrifices.

Bone divinations have been excavated dating from 1700 B.C.E. A question was written on the bone which was then slightly burned and cracked. The answer was then divined and often written on the bone fragment.

In approximately 700 B.C.E., the middle class emerged. Jade and bronze could be buried only in graves of the upper class. Coins, ivory, mirrors, and malichite were buried in graves of the middle class. The ceremonial vessels used for ritual communion between the dead and the living were made of pottery for the middle class. Thus, we find that burials with jade became burials with glass and eventually today have become burial with paper ("Symbols of the Ancestors: The Power of Chinese Bronze and Jade", 1990).

Wooden statues started to appear in the fifth century B.C.E. Archaeological excavations in the Ch'u area, south of the Yangtze River, have yielded *Chang-mu-sho*, wooden statues which protect the burial site (Ecke, 1977).

Before me sits a collection of one brass and seven wooden Chinese ancestral figures. They are transportable statues carved of camphor, cypress, and other aromatic woods. The fragrance has repelled insects and preserved the statues. The statues were originally coated with plaster so that features could be formed with ease, smoothly, and expressively. They were then painted in gold and red ochre, and in later times, painted in a variety of colors.

The ancestor figures are gentle looking, especially the female figures; they reflect how the people beheld themselves — beneficent and kindhearted. Upon the death of a respected relative, the family would commission the creation of a statue to reside with others on a home altar. Relatives were neglected if they did not earn remembrance. In bad times, the statues would be exchanged for food; in good times, they would be retrieved and once again worshipped.

The oldest of the statues in this collection are the Scholar and the Scholar's Wife, or as I prefer to call them, the Dual Career Scholars. Their well-carved robustness and simplicity suggest that they are as early as the late Ming period from Shalong, Sichuan, the Three Minor Gorges. They smile benevolently and gently. With each hand enveloped in large sleeves, they hold their skirts upward. The male has large ears, a long beard, and furrowed brow. He has earned wisdom through careful listening, advanced years, and hard life. The female is crowned with sculptured hair, high cheekbones, and expressive eyes. She has earned wisdom through patient perseverance, positive attitude, and keen observation.

This family had other notables. The Official, who carries a tablet of the law in his left hand, is a desirable relative to have for survival within the bureaucracy. The Heavenly Ministry rides a white tiger, a cat's face in his left hand, and a driving stick in his right hand. He wears a stylish golden robe with green trim and a burnished helmet. He is in charge of wealth and is favored by tradespeople. The Mistress of the White Crane sits in elegant red and golden robes with blue leggins atop a white crane with a long green beak. She provides comfort to all those in need (Ecke, 1977).

Three deities complete the collection. Buddha, with traces of original red paint, sits in meditation. With his right hand placed palm down over the right folded knee, he touches the earth and vanquishes every spirit and force. The left hand lying upon the lap of his legs crossed in lotus position receives the divinity. There are holes inside of the statue of Buddha, where apparently later family members must have searched for papers and valuables which might have been hidden in him (Jung, 1990).

There are two statues of Kuan Yin. A moss green colored brass head of Kuan Yin has large eyes and ears. She sees and hears all, and because of this input is compassionate and empathetic. Curls fall gracefully on each side. Her neck is creased which is considered to be an attribute of wisdom. The bun of hair which crowns her head is polished to a patina, individuals having rubbed her head requesting mercy. Pre-Buddhist stories tell that Kuan Yin lived before the world began, creating the element of water. She poured water out of a vase to fill the rivers that flowed into the oceans.

A wooden statue of Kuan Yin portrays her sitting in a modified posture of royal relaxation, her head slightly reclined, her right arm supported by the raised right knee, her left foot tucked under her, and her left hand holding a boy child. As a madonna, she receives prayers from women wanting sons. As in the tradition of the Chinese family, it is only when these boys marry, that the woman will attain the status of mother-in-law and be able to rule over someone.

Later Buddhist stories associate Kuan Yin with a human woman. In the more popular versions, Kuan Yin's father disowns her because of her devotion to Buddha. In one version, she sacrifices an eye, and in a second version, she cuts flesh from her arms to restore the health of her father. Imagine an archetype, important to generations of women, who was abandoned by her father and then bears sons so that after their marriages, she can finally have power over someone in the family! This historical Goddess of Mercy manifests acts of patient forbearance for the offenders and provides blessings of divine compassion to the distressed. Kuan Yin is an archetype who deserves more research.

Ancestor worship was the source of the concept of filial piety. Confucius taught filial piety, the worshipers submitting while alive to the wishes of parents, burying them with honor, and sacrificing to them regularly. Defiling the ancestors of another is considered the most abusive form of dishonor.

THE MARING KAIKO

Marvin Harris (1974) has investigated the Maring, a horticultural tribe who live in villages located in the Bismarck Mountains of New Guinea. Family members are both pig and human, living and dead. The *kaiko* is a ritual held by each generation to bring living humans, pigs, and ancestors into harmony with each other and the environment.

The Maring man prepares gardening plots in the thick tropical forest. Torrential rains leach nitrogen and other nutrients from the soil, making a plot viable for only two or three consecutive years. The man clears and burns a portion of land which as time goes on becomes more and more distant from the home and the village.

The Maring woman grows sweet potatoes, taro, and yams; prepares meals; constructs clothing; weaves baggage for transporting goods; and rears children. The infant human and infant pig are carried by the woman on her back to the work sites and often during each task. Upon weaning, the pig is taught to follow the woman. The four-or five-month-old pig scavenges each day for food in the forest and then returns home when called and is fed low-grade produce. The pig is embraced, petted, and spoken to by name with endearment. The pig sleeps and eats with the family—just like a human relative. An adult pig might easily weigh 150 pounds. The Maring family may have six pig members.

About once or twice a generation, the intensity of the intra-family and inter-family conflict escalates to an intolerable pitch. The pig population has multiplied to a number which threatens the food supply as well as the health status of both the human and the pig population and so disturbs the social ecosystem. Women grumble about the responsibility of caring for large families of pigs. They object to carrying increased amounts of produce from plots cleared further and further in distance away from home to feed the family. Pigs trespass on the neighbor's property; families quarrel over the territory encroachment. The clan mourns the loss of security felt when all families lived and farmed in close proximity to each other. The men, in time, decide that the number of pigs is sufficient to hold a *kaiko* and so uproot the rumbin tree, symbol of peace, from its sacred ground.

The *kaiko* is a year-long festival involving extensive preparation, ritualistic sacrifice, and the slaughtering of nearly all the pigs. The family attends to the departed ancestor's yearning for pork. Each family is to club down a loved pig family member on the burial place of a human ancestor. The dead pig is then roasted in an oven constructed over the grave. The family patriarch feeds his brother-in-law cool saline stomach fat with the intention of obtaining devotion from the extended kin. "The climax of pig love is the incorporation of the pig as flesh into the flesh of the human host and of the pig as spirit into the spirit of the ancestors" (Harris, M., 1974, p. 39).

The clan through the *kaiko* can restore communal ties and insure triumph in war. Clan members, kin, and guests devote much time and energy into painting and wearing the appropriate image, which is then displayed during ceremonial dancing. Single men and women survey each other in search of a potential marital partner. Possible allies are persuaded to participate in a war. It is not unusual for each person to eat twelve pounds of pork in five days! Gluttony becomes the basis for reuniting communal ties and preparing for conquest.

Within the three months of the last convening of the *kaiko*, the warriors, strengthened by nutritious protein and fat along with the spirit of the pig and human family members, conduct a war against a neighboring enemy. Land, of course, is either gained or lost in this struggle.

A ceremony is then held to proclaim the end of the war. Each adult male touches the sapling rumbin tree with his hands as it is planted on holy ground. The war magician expresses gratitude to the ancestral and living clan for the safe return of the warriors and the low number of surviving pigs. It is now the intention of the clan to increase the number of pig and human members of each family. War will not resume until sufficient pigs can be sacrificed to satisfy again the yearning of the human ancestors for pig meat and pig spirit.

THE MEXICAN DAY OF THE DEAD

An example of ancestor worship that carries the intentions of the ancients is found in the Mexican celebration of the Day of the Dead, All Saints' Day and All Souls' Day, 1 and 2 November. Each family gathered in reunion constructs an altar in the home and each community builds an altar in the cemetery so that the dead can be remembered and honored. On these altars are placed bread baked in the shape of a skeleton and the favorite items of each dead relative, such as a preferred type of sweet or a brand of tobacco. The spirit of the object is ingested by the dead, and the substance is given to friends outside the family. The brilliant yellow marigold, the pre-

Columbian blossom of the dead, decorates the altars, homes, and streets.

The celebration of the Day of the Dead allows a myriad of activities, carried out in the protection of costume, often sexually provocative and adorned with extraordinarily large phallic symbols. Some may keep vigils of prayer. Others may walk from house to house singing ancient songs. In the cemeteries where bands provide music for dancers and listeners, many will often be under the influence of alcohol, engaging in sexual flirtation and play.

The symbol of the skeleton is found everywhere. Skeletons constructed of pleated lace paper swing in the breeze. Adults give skeleton toys to children. Lovers exchange skulls of sugar candy on which their beloved's name is carved. Families light the firecracker embodied within a papier-mâché skeleton. In store windows, mannequins are replaced by skeletons dressed in seasonal finery. No one of importance escapes portrayal as a skeleton — business owners, movie stars, police, politicians, religious dignitaries, and soldiers.

Thus, in this hallowed time and place, the participant communes with death, expresses feeling to the dead, discharges personal guilt, becomes comfortable with the ultimate life event, and sees her or himself as a link in the continuity of the community. The fertility of the individual and the prosperity of the community are dependent upon this ritualistic celebration of the Day of the Dead incorporating a mixture of Incan, Mayan, Mexican, Roman Catholic, and Spanish metaphors. Ultimately, Octavio Paz (1961) witnessed and wrote, this ritual allows for the embrace of the reality of death.

The word death is not pronounced in New York, in Paris, in London, because it burns the lips. The Mexican, in contrast, is familiar with death, jokes about it, caresses it, sleeps with it, celebrates it. It is one of [her or] his favorite toys and . . . most steadfast love. True, there is perhaps as much fear in his attitude as in that of others, but at least death is not hidden away: [she or] he looks at it face to face, with impatience, disdain or irony.

ANCESTOR WORSHIP

. . . behold before ye
Humanity's poor sum and story;
Life — Death — and all that is of Glory.

— Barry Cornwall
"History of a Life"

Eighteenth century social thinkers observed the prevalence of ancestor worship throughout the world and began to postulate theories. Philosopher Herbert Spencer (1877-1896) proposed that ancestor worship was the very source of each religion. The respect that a people have for remarkable ancestors who created arts and invented skills became a belief formalized into a theology. By contrast, anthropologist Andrew Lang (1887) in his research of mythology and religion determined that a creator of the world was at the basis of each cosmology. Only after human beings came into existence was the inevitability of human death recognized and followed by the practice of ancestor worship.

There are eight patterns of ancestor worship representative of different cultures and ages.

1. Ancestors are perceived as friends. Bodies of the dead are often buried in the home, under a sleeping platform or near the fire. Relics are saved. Banquets are held and the guests of honor are the dead ancestors. Ancestors can serve the living as advocates and allies.
2. Ancestors are perceived as enemies and must be appeased. The whole spectrum of emotions is possible with the dead, just as with the living.
3. Ancestors provide information. Hellenic Greeks believed that ancestors emerged from caverns in the earth and could be divined as oracles.
4. Ancestors are the source of disease. Today, epidemiologists studying the inheritance of genes by progeny agree.
5. Ancestors are believed to come to earth again as animals. For instance, Sumatrans revere tigers as their ancestors.
6. Images are created of ancestors, especially in Africa, the

Americas, Asia, and the Pacific Islands. Since the art of photography is only one hundred and fifty years old, statues are the time-honored way to preserve the physical appearance of ancestors within the memory of their progeny.

7. Humans want to bear a child who will fullfill the rituals that will sustain them as ancestors in good stead. The Western custom of placing wreaths on graves each holiday is becoming more difficult for the progeny who have relocated away from home.

8. Ancestor worship is essentially a family cult that may expand into the political realm. For instance, the worship by royalty of their ancestors can become a state religion, as in Japan.

RITUALS

"That's not a mere plank-bridge, Benjamin—our ancestors in heaven have interceded to save us!"

— Mendele Mocher Seforim *"The Ancestors Intercede"*
The Travels and Adventures of Benjamin the Third

We have a yearning for visible signs, for rituals that sustain intergenerational connections. The off-off-Broadway play, *Tony n' Tina's Wedding*, has been playing for over a year in Greenich Village and has recently opened in Philadelphia and Los Angeles. Play-goers pay $75 to attend a traditional Italian-American wedding ceremony and reception, complete with cake-cutting, dancing, and family fights!

Family rituals are rites of passage that serve to create and maintain family ties. Through ritual, family members are nourished with the significance of their place in society and history. Research on family relations has largely neglected the study of ritual. The literatures of anthropology and religion have provided the most comprehensive information on ritual in the family. Contemporary women's magazines have been publishing articles on the conducting of family rituals.

In most parts of the world, possibly no family members so utterly exemplify the rites of passage of families and kin networks as do the ancestors. Several texts from second millennium B.C.E. tell of

Gilgamesh, a ruler of the Sumerian city-state Uruk, known as Erech in the *Hebrew Bible*. These texts preserved a story and ritual dating six hundred and fifty years before. We learn that Gilgamesh endeavors to evade death by calling upon his ancestor Sitnapishtim, the Babylonian Noah, who had successfully avoided death. This ancient story tells us that ancestors were considered to be powerful family members to whom one could plead for intercession. Also, these state texts which have survived indicate that honor and devotion were given by a city-state to its dead leaders or "fathers."

Ancestor worship became a familial ritual of the home and a political ritual of the state. Epic poetry tells that the king is the son of a goddess. For instance, Japanese emperors were said to be the son of Amaterasu Omikami, the sun goddess.

Through ritual and worship, ancestors in Chinese, Indian, Japanese, and Roman kinships became the most important members of families. Ancestors in unison repress and restrain distinctive individuality, a trait especially prevalent in contemporary Western society. Furthermore, the embodied family as a corporate organism strives to conserve and preserve the family through encouraging normative behavior. To be abandoned without kin support meant sure death in the ancient world. Thus, the power of the ancestors, dead intergenerational family members, persisted.

Anthropologist Jack Rankine Goody (1962), in his study of inheritance systems in Africa, has addressed the psychological stresses of intergenerational transfer. He defines inheritance as the generational authorized transfer from holder to heir of exclusive rights, such as restricted property, sexual roles, and office rights.

Although inheritance is perpetuated by serial reciprocity, the transmission of exclusive rights does carry emotional overtones. The heir may experience anticipatory tension. Inheritance issues can create anxiety as even parity propels up from below and odd parity shoves down from above. The transfer of property can often divide possible heirs into the haves and have nots. Where divisions do not occur strain is placed on the inheritor who may then have responsibilities for the non-inheritors. Conflict is endemic to such an outcome.

The death of a family member may indicate the destruction of a portion of the family heritage which can lead to a social projection of guilt experienced by heirs. Thus, inheritance may cause solidarity because of the felt need to continue familial ties. It not only affects the descent groups after death, it actuates and renews kin relationships. Funeral rituals and ancestor worship act to cement intergenerational linkage in perpetuity.

PSYCHOLOGY

Joke: "I found a girl just like my mother, she dresses like her, kavetches like her, looks like her, cooks like her. — My father doesn't like her!"

Joke: Three mothers are talking on the Miami boardwalk. The first mother says, "My son loves me best because he has given me a ballerina-length silver fox coat and a Mercedes automobile." The second mother says, "My son loves me best because he has given me a floor-length mink coat and a house on the beach." The third mother says, "My son loves me the best of all. Each day he goes to a psychologist and pays $150 an hour to talk about me!"

Sigmund Freud and Carl G. Jung wove their psychological theories hearing clients tell stories of their personal and family life while seated amidst large cross-cultural collections of archaeological artifacts, including ancestor statues. Freud listened carefully to his clients recount their memories and fantasies about sexual experiences with parents; thus, came his theories of the Oedipal and Electra complexes. Jung found archetypes, forces of innate energy, living in the personal and collective unconscious. Images of ancestors, natural forces, and paradigms rise in dreams to assist individuals in understanding themselves. Jung urged his clients to work with symbols in their own familial, cultural, and religious backgrounds.

Other more recent psychological theories speak of ancestors. In Transactional Analysis, persons are perceived to communicate with others, replaying messages of parents and children responding to parents, as well as creating messages as adults. Other theories recommend that individuals enter swimming pools and hot tubs to be massaged and lullabied into a rebirth.

Political activist of the 1960s, Jerry Rubin in *Growing (Up) at 37* (1976) details his internal quest in the 1970s during which he engaged in popular-psychology movements ranging from Arica to *est* to Gestalt to yoga. During an exercise in which he wrote lists of his grandparents' traits, he had an astonishing insight. "Those two ancient people — my grandmother and grandfather — I was just like them! Not only did I discover that I *am* my grandmother and grandfather, but I began to see that in my blood are the values and beliefs of nineteenth-century Russia! Here I am — a modern, hip, radical yippie. But if you look close, what I really am is a nineteenth-century Russian orthodox religious Jew. That is my programming."

INTERGENERATIONAL WORSHIP

Remember, then, what when a boy I've heard my Grandma tell,
"BE WARNED IN TIME BY OTHERS' HARM, AND YOU SHALL DO FULL WELL!"
Don't link yourself with vulgar folks, who've got no fixed abode,
Tell lies, use naughty words, and say they "wish they may be blowed!"

Don't take too much of double X! — and don't at night go out
To fetch your beer yourself, but make the pot-boy bring your stout!
And when you go to Margate next, just stop, and ring the bell,
Give my respects to Mrs. Jones, and say I'm pretty well!

— Richard Harris Barham (Thomas Ingoldsby, Esquire)
"Misadventures at Margate"

In 1981, my mother, Lee Klinger Jeter, who died at the young age of 56, was an accomplished artist in varied media from photography to opera to radio production to writing. She was able to visualize the picture, the song, the show, the story compose itself and then stop that moment from ever going away by recording it with a camera or a rendition.

Upon my mother's death, a number of friends gave me empathy and counsel. One, Judith Morley (1981), spoke from her experience saying that our parents, even though they might have died, are still with us. We can talk with them, tell them of our lives, hear their responses, feel the intergenerational connection. In this communication, respect is acknowledged, worth is honored, worship is carried out. On the humorous side, there is even one advantage. Ma Bell will not be making monetary profits from our conversations!

I wonder what would occur if not only would I talk with my mother, but my grandparents and relatives before them. I would talk to my paternal grandparents, East Texas farmers, whom I never actually knew because they died before I was born. I would talk, without the need of a translator, with my maternal foreparents from the Bodensee on the German-Swiss frontier. In a sense, this communication would be the remembrance of their worth on this earth, a form of worship.

I am reminded of psychologist-philosopher Jean Houston's exercise of harvesting the wisdom of the ancestors, of physically walking backwards and recollecting our past, and then walking forward, enlightened with this enhanced knowledge. This exercise is certainly a personal intergenerational connection.

Talking with the past, our ancestors, is not enough. We must speak to the future, our progeny. This is a difficult job. Psychologist Robert D. Strom (1988-1989) has taught a course for 200 individuals on how to be a better grandparent. The grandparent needs to live in the 1990's, and be aware that family members are using computers and laser disks, may rear children born from ethnic synthesization and even test tubes, and may even die before their grandparents from a decade-old disease such as AIDS. Imagine talking to the unborn of an unknown world of the future. Empathy for the unknown world of each generation is required.

Sociologist Richard Hessler (1989) has recently reported on his 24-year research involving the interviewing of 1,700 elders from 64 culturally distinct communities in Missouri. Hessler has isolated four predictors to survival: age, formal social networks, health, and sex. Involvement in networks is the most important predictor. No matter how physically well a person is, those who in 1966 were active in formal social networks have been most liable to continue to live.

Ancients across the ages and cultures have emphasized involvement in networks—living and dead. Abandonment, desertion, and exile were the worst curses a society could place upon another. Perhaps it is time once again to embrace life fully, to bestow worth upon — to literally worship — friends and kin through our formal social networks and communication with our ancestors and progeny.

MARTIN'S DAY AND THE BERLIN WALL

Once upon a time in the hills of Lebanon, two sages encountered each other under a large cedar tree. One sage said, "What is your destination?" The second sage replied, "I am looking for the fountain of youth. What is your destination?" The first sage said, "I am looking for the secret of death." They then began to debate the metaphysical rigor of their missions.

The nearby hamlet's dullard happened by and overheard their debate. "My esteemed sages. You use dissimilar phrases to describe a similar mission. You both have the same destination." The sages smiled and agreed to travel together in search of their mission.

> — Kahil Gibran
> *The Quest*

"Ich geh' mit meiner Laterne." ("I go with my lantern.")

> — Martin's Day expression

On 10 November 1989, the Berlin Wall came tumbling down. Politicians point to factors such as economics, the *perestroika* policy of Soviet President Mikhail Gorbachev, and the flight of East Germans to the West. I propose that there are additional factors that rise from the deep memory of Germans for human ancestors, an over-sixteen-hundred-year reverence for St. Martin and an over-four-hundred-year reverence for Martin Luther.

St. Martin of Tours

In 314 C.E., Martin of Tours was born into a Roman military family in what we know as Hungary today. He was reared in Pavia, Italy and adopted his father's profession. One frigid day upon seeing a beggar on the road, Martin cut his cloak in half and presented a portion to the alms seeker. That night in a dream it was revealed to him that the beggar was Jesus. Martin was baptized and requested to be discharged from the army as a conscientious objector, offering to stand without arms between two firing lines to prove his bravery.

As a civilian, Martin lived on the Adriatic coast. In 360, he established the first monastery in Gaul. Ten years later, he was ordained a Bishop. Martin was an aggressive missionary, destroying non-Christian sanctuaries and converting pagans. He was accused of being a magician and condemned to death by Emperor Maximus of Spain. However, his metaphysical mastery so incited wonder in believers from the Mediterranean to the Black Sea to the North Seas that he was victorious over the Emperor's brutality and rage. Martin died on 11 November 397 C.E. A most prominent fact is that St. Martin is one of the first holy people to be canonized as a saint without having been persecuted as a martyr.

Martin Luther

Martin Luther was born 10 November 1483 in Eisleben, the son of a family prominent in the copper industry. His father was inflexible and ironhanded. Luther received a Master's degree in liberal arts from the University of Erfurt and set out to study law in accordance with his father's demands. However, within two months, during a formidable and ominous tempest, Luther encountered a resounding fireball which led him to promise Saint Anne, the grandmother of Jesus, to leave law school and become a monk.

Luther became associated with the rigorous and mystical Monastery of the Eremites of Saint Augustine in Erfurt, and two years later in 1507, was ordained into the priesthood. His initial observance of the Mass was a peak spiritual experience. Luther felt integrated with himself and the universe, fully functioning, and master of his fate. He then began his formal instruction in religion. In 1509, Luther earned his Bachelor's degree and three years later his Doctorate degree in Bible studies. He became a professor as well as parish preacher and vicar of his order.

Luther's study of the Bible and, some would say, his relationship to his father caused him to question authority. On 31 October 1517, Luther is said to have nailed the Ninety-five Theses on the door of the Wittenberg Castle Church. He became an immediate hero because the Ninety-five Theses contained prevailing political, economic, and religious themes. Public dialogue resulted and the Reformation was born.

In 1521, after his lighting of a highly visible fire of church papers calling him a heretic, he was excommunicated. Four years later, Luther and Katharina von Bora, a former nun, entered the state of marriage, or, as they described it, an institution for the building of constitution. The remainder of his life was conducted as a writer, reformer, and protester. In 1537 he died, uncomfortable till the end with church and nation politics.

Luther challenged people to live in accordance with their spirit and the grace of God rather than theological dogma. His belief in the "priesthood of all believers" has reshaped the practice of Western religion. Protestantism was concerned with essence instead of structure, veracity instead of standardization, autonomy instead of procedure. Reformationists discarded Latin and utilized the vernacular languages. They rejected formal legal briefs and employed such varied media as brochures, cartoons, discussions, parody, and theatre.

Both St. Martin and Martin Luther were spiritual mystics who lived with integrity and followers were inspired by their willingness to act upon their strong beliefs. St. Martin used the sword of distinction and Martin Luther used the pen of distinction to accentuate their positions. St. Martin cut his cloak to warm a beggar which led to his missionary work converting heathens to Catholicism. Martin Luther penned and posted his words to protest an economic/political bureaucracy and to reform spritual practice.

Annual November Rituals

Germany has drab, foggy, hazy drizzly weather in November. The crops have been gathered and the landscape is stark. The November holidays ask people to face the barreness with rituals of remembrance. On 1 November, *Allerheiligen*, Catholics acknowledge saints who do not have individual feast days. On the next day, *Allerseelen*, all dead are honored. Protestants contemplate their behavior of the past year on *Bussund Bettag*, the second to the last

Wednesday before the first Advent. On the following Sunday, *Totensonntag*, they pay respect to dead family and friends.

Then, on 10 November, the Germans nurtured by their recent acknowledgement of all saints and ancestors, celebrate the life of Martin. Catholics commemorate the brilliance of St. Martin; Protestants, Martin Luther who by synchronicity was born on this day and named Martin; and the pagans, the moon-light and star-shine. Children cut colored transparent paper into lanterns and place them on lengthy rods. During the evening, the children promenade around the community and are presented apples, sweets, and nuts.

The next day, *Sankt Martinstag*, everyone feasts. In the Bodensee, my grandmother, a Lutheran, Wilma Mauler Klinger, would bake *Bettelmannpudding*, a Catholic celebratory "Beggars Pudding," alternating layers of rye bread crumbs, currants, apples, butter, sugar, and cinnamon. Hogs and geese were considered fattened for the season and the slaughtering would start. Cattle were led to their barn stalls where they would reside for the winter. The herders and other workers were rehired or fired (Gilgenast, 1982).

It is no surprise to me that the Berlin Wall would open during this holiday season. Even though the actual practice of holidays changes with time, the deep memory is excited with the symbology of the season, ignited by the gathered crops, barren landscape, and dreary weather.

The deep memory recollects St. Martin's presentation of half of his cloak to the beggar. The deep memory recalls St. Martin's triumph over brutality through spiritual practice and his attainment of Church Office without suffering martyrdom. The deep memory reminisced about Martin Luther and his successful protest for religious autonomy. The deep memory retained the wisdom of all of the saints and the dead, and upon reflection of the past months and years, sought to further the cause of freedom and unity. The deep memory charged the Germans "to go with their lanterns" — their lamps of freedom like those led by the sweet, strong symbol of the Statue of Liberty in the New York Harbor. Their recent memory was still scorched with the images of Chinese students, who, just months before, followed the Goddess of Liberty to their death in Tiananmen Square.

Linguist Alfred Wedel (1990), after listening to my proposal, told me of the saying popular in Spain, "To every pig comes St. Martin's Day." There are those who would transpose the saying into, "To every 'Communist pig' comes St. Martin's Day!" Moreover, on this St. Martin's Day, there would be no annual automatic renewal of employment for Communist leaders; now, there would be democratic elections in which the best person, of any party, could be elected.

The Berlin Wall, which has separated families and a people for over a generation of time, has through the harvesting and application of ancestral wisdom, fallen. East Germans visited West Germany, each receiving $50 welcome funds and a bouquet from florists in the Netherlands. Families and friends have become reacquainted. The mood has been festive; people have danced all night on and near the wall. Large hoses have sprayed water into the air. The symbology of cleansing water and joyous celebration portends a rebirth of a united culture, intent upon cooperative pursuit and maintenance of freedom in a world increasingly aware of the delicate balance of its nature.

The challenge of unification is for East and West Germany to successfully go past its history in which, as the saying goes, "every step on German soil is a step on bloodshed." Unification is needed to satisfy deep psychic as well as political requirements; each land, each people has strengths of value to the other. The vivid class distinctions need to be viewed as inverted strengths to avoid further bloodshed. With mindful communication, the German family—ancestors and progeny, East and West—can again be a functioning kinship unit.

The demolition of the Berlin Wall is a testimony to the power of ancestor worship. In the linking of generations—living and dead—there is comfort and wisdom available to individuals, families, and cultures.

The intergenerational connection is pervasive in all time and space. The linkage exists for cohorts as well as individuals. For instance, the Apache have long recognized the importance of the vertical strata of elders and youngsters in families and communities; indeed, they use the same word to denote grandfather and grandson. Moreover, the continuity between ancestors, elders, youth, and descendents is emphasized, as indicated in the saying, "We do not simply inherit the land from our ancestors; we lease the land from our children.''

The presence of departed ancestors is expressed in the ideas, ideologies, and values we remember as well as genetic codings which have their origins in the beginnings of the hominid. Through intergenerational ancestor worship, we are what we have interwoven from the past to procreate into the future.

> *. . . So the multitude comes, even those we behold,*
> *To repeat every tale that has often been told.*
>
> *For we are the same our fathers have been;*
> *We see the same sights our fathers have seen, —*
> *We drink the same stream and view the same sun,*
> *And run the same course our fathers have run.*

—William Knox
"O, Why Should the Spirit of Mortal be Proud?"

REFERENCES

Attwater, D. *Dictionary of Saints*. Second Edition revised and updated by Catherine Rachel John. New York, NY: Viking Penguin Inc., 1983.

Birnbaum, J. and H.G. Chua-Eoan. "Despair and Death in a Beijing Square." *Time* 133: 24 (12 June 1990) 27.

Bloomfield, H.H. *Making Peace with Your Parents: The Key to Enriching Your Life and All Your Relationships*. New York, NY: Random House, Inc., 1983.

Ecke, T. Yu-Ho. *Chinese Folk Art in American Collections, Early Fifteenth Century to Early Twentieth Century*. Honolulu, HA: University of Press of Hawaii, 1977.

Fischer, L.R. *Linked Lives: Adult Daughters and their Mothers*. New York, NY: Harper and Row, 1986.

Friday, N. *My Mother My Self: The Daughter's Search for Identity*. New York, NY: Dell Publishing Company, 1977.

Gilgenast, T. *Das Mehl Ist Anders*. Dover, DE: North Light Studio, 1982.

Goody, J.R. *Death, Property and the Ancestors*. Stanford, CA: Stanford University Press, 1962.

"Grandparents: Keep up to Date." *Modern Maturity* 33:1 (February-March 1990) 96.

Harris, M. *Cows, Pigs, Wars and Witches: The Riddles of Culture*. New York, NY: Vintage Books, 1974. Page 39.

Hessler, R.M.; J. Guinn; D. Huesgen; and L. Wolter. "Research Entry: A

Twenty-Year Longitudinal Study of the Rural Elderly." *Qualitative Sociology* 12:3 (Fall 1989) 261-277.

Hessler, R.M.; S.H. Pazaki; R.W. Madsen; and R.L. Blake. "Predicting Mortality among Independently Living Rural Elderly: A Twenty-Year Longitudinal Study." Columbia, MO: University of Missouri-Columbia, November 1989.

"Ting: The Cauldron." *The I Ching or Book of Changes*. The Richard Wilhelm Translation rendered into English by Carry F. Baynes. Third Edition. Princeton, NJ: Princeton University Press, 1967.

Jeter, K. "A Historical, Interdisciplinary Analysis of the Animal and Human Social Ecosystem." *Pets and the Family: Marriage and Family Review* 8: 3/4 (Summer 1985) 223-238.

Jeter, K. "Jack Goody and Inheritance." *Family Systems and Inheritance: Marriage and Family Review* 5:3 (Fall 1982) 105-112.

Jeter, K. "Metaphor: Building a Bridge, the Road to Community." *Voices: The Art and Science of Psychotherapy* 24:2 (Summer 1988) 62-72.

Jung, L. Personal Communication. Wilmington DE. 10 January 1990.

Leonard, L.S. *The Wounded Woman: Healing the Father-Daughter Relationship*. Boulder, CO: Shambhala, 1983.

Lang, A. *Myth, Ritual, and Religion*. New York, NY: A.M.F. Press, 1968. Originally published in 1887.

Morley, J. Personal Communication. 30 November 1981.

Neilson, W.A., (Ed.) "Worship." *Webster's New International Dictionary of the English Language*. Second Edition. Unabridged. Springfield, MA: G. and C. Merriam Company, Publishers, 1955. Page 2955.

Paz, O. *The Labyrinth of Solitude*. Lysander Kemp, Translator. New York, NY: Grove Press, 1961. Pages 57-58.

Rubin, J. *Growing (Up) at 37*. New York, NY: Warner Books Edition, 1976. Pages 158-159.

Spencer, H. *The Principles of Sociology*. Three Volumes. London, England: William and Norgate, 1877-1896.

Staiger, J. Personal Communication. Newark, DE. 14 March 1990.

Strom, R.D. "Becoming a Better Grandparent: An Educational Program for Grandparents to Help Strengthen Families." Tempe, AZ: College of Education, 1988-1989.

"Symbols of the Ancestors: The Power of Chinese Bronze and Jade." University Museum of Pennsylvania. Philadelphia, PA. February 1990.

Tony n' Tina's Wedding. Conception by Nancy Cassaro. Original production in New York by Joseph Corcoran and Daniel Corcoran. Created by Artificial Intelligence.

Wedel, A. Personal Communication. Newark, DE. 21 February 1990.

GENERATIONAL AND INTERGENERATIONAL CONNECTIONS WITHIN THE FAMILY AND THE COMMUNITY

Studying Adult Children
and Their Parents

Jetse Sprey

The intention of this paper is to present an analytical position toward the explanation of multi-generational families. Empirical information is cited only for illustrative purposes. Its value is heuristic, intended to improve the quality of our questioning.

A discussant of a theoretical presentation on "parent-child solidarity in aging families" (Bengtson and Roberts, 1988) offered the following comment:

> What amazes me in the practice of family theory building is the analogue to the laboratory experiment, its unwholesome artificiality, done without regard to contextual realities, done without concern to the circumstances of everyday life and the cauldron of forces which impinge and shape dyadic interaction. (Sussman, 1988, p. 5)

This astute observation provides a useful starting point to the position presented below. Laboratory experiments in the natural sciences do not violate the intrinsic nature of the phenomena under study. Their settings are, ontologically speaking, as "natural" as real life ones. Attempts among social scientists, however, to emulate controlled reality—through statistical manipulation, simulation, or "causal" modeling, produces an artificiality that may border on the "unwholesome." Explanatory models, regardless of the

Jetse Sprey is Professor of Sociology, Case Western Reserve University, Cleveland, OH 44106.

The author wishes to acknowledge the support of a grant from the National Institute on Aging (AG-03484). All case materials quoted throughout this paper are derived from the study funded by this grant (cf. Matthews and Sprey, 1987).

"theoretical" loadings of their composite variables, remain static constructs and are only capable of prediction under relatively familiar and stable conditions. Where the future is characterized by the presence of risk or uncertainty the quality of their forecasts seems no better than simple common sense. Here, then, Sussman's references to contextuality and, especially, the continuously changing contingencies that characterize *normal* family life are quite to the point. The difficulty of capturing such contingencies is illustrated in a respondent's answer to a question about how he and his two brothers meet their parents' needs:

> There's nothing really set up. They would call whoever is available. We also use our wives to assist. They have taken Mom to places and things like that . . . nobody organizes anything. Just as it occurs, we decide who's gonna do it . . . Rides to the doctor, take care of the lawn, the car, the home, plumbing, things like that. We don't take him [father] shopping usually; he'll go on his own. George is not mechanically inclined, so he doesn't work on their car. He's a salesman — if something has to be resolved over the phone, he'll take care of it. Matter of fact, this last incident with the doctor, he handled that. He's good with people. I kind of shy away from that; maybe I lose my temper. Ben really doesn't do anything from Chicago. He has come in from Chicago, only for a day or two at a time. If there's a crisis, he'll fly in. He flew in this last incident [mother's hip dislocated].

How far can we remove ourselves from the above reality without losing touch? At what level of abstraction do our neatly specified models become mere castles in the sky, elegantly designed but relevant only to a reified conceptual scheme?

There is, of course, no perfect way out of this dilemma. To deal with it, however, requires that our first decisions be conceptual rather than research-technical. It is often overlooked that an indication of the logical-positivistic imprint on mainstream family scholarship is its focus on the individual as the unit of analysis. Most of us still adhere to what the philosopher McMullin calls "an ontology of individuals linked by similarities instead of by common natures" and follow "an induction that takes the form of generalization from resemblances and issues in probable knowledge only" (1988, p. 30). This way of thinking makes it difficult, if not impossible, to contemplate the explanatory power of *any* social entity larger than a single individual. It means, for example, that for the case cited above, our analysis will be directed towards and limited to an investigation of how each individual brother feels about his parents. It is clear, however, that much of their actual behavior reflects how they feel about, perceive, and interact with one another.

The perspective proposed here, then, challenges any conceptualization which sees individual states of mind and/or intentions as sufficient explanations of social interaction patterns between siblings, spouses, or parents and offspring. It is not proposed that attributes of individuals are irrelevant, nor that quantitative research strategies are, categorically, unsuited to the study of intergenerational family ties. That would be one-sided and merely create a "straw" issue. However, conceptual decisions, because they precede a choice of research strategies, do influence techniques of data collection and/ or analysis.

The analytic position presented below is based on the review of some recently published research that is theoretically oriented. It is augmented by the use of illustrations derived from an ongoing study about how adult siblings share responsibility for their elderly parents (Matthews and Sprey, 1987). I see conceptualization, that is, the formulation of a coherent analytical vocabulary, as a first move toward further theoretical thought. Data observed in this context do not pretend to prove anything in particular but serve as a reminder of the phenomena to be explained.

THE QUEST FOR INNER FORCES:
FAMILY SOLIDARITY

The individual-centered approach to the explanation of inter- and intra-generational family relationships is a search for "inner forces." It directs the analysis toward individual states of mind so that phenomena like love, indifference, and attraction, are hypothesized as basic causal variables in the explanation of behavior like mutual aid, visitation, and other forms of cooperation. This is, of course, not categorically wrong as long as the presumed causal linkage between personal feelings and actual behavior remains hypothetical until empirically verified. But this is not always the case. If, for example, "attachment" is defined as the "propensity or tendency for psychological closeness and contact," as an attribute of adults, and "attachment *behavior*" as "a class of behaviors including the interaction of communication over distance to maintain psychological closeness and contact" (Cicirelli, 1983b, p. 816) it becomes quite difficult — if not impossible — to think about *any* form of non-random contact between adult children and their parents as not "explained" by feelings of attachment.

Some recently published work within this individual-oriented tradition represents an attempt to inductively formulate a "theory of solidarity" in aging families (cf. Bengtson, Olander, and Haddad, 1976; Bengtson and Roberts, 1988; McChesney and Bengtson, 1988; Atkinson, Kivett and Campbell, 1986). The idea of family solidarity is seen to provide theoretical access to the phenomenon of parent-child bonding throughout the life span in that it "opens examination of issues of warmth, affection, attraction to and interaction with one another, [and] providing assistance when needed" (Bengtson and Roberts, 1988, p. 3). Implied is the premise that personal feelings, like warmth and affection, may well lead to and maintain cohesion of the system. Such a "steady state," in turn, accounts for behavior like mutual support. This is logical, but it should be noted that in this explanatory context "systemness" per se, is not an explanatory variable. Instead, it appears to be only an environmental condition which is understood as an outcome of joint individual activities. *Why*, and *how* individual attributes conjointly may lead to a more, or less, stable familial process remains unexplored and unexplained in this analytical context. The possibility, for example, that certain family members may truly like one another but may also, for some reason, neglect a sibling or parent simply does not fit into an explanatory framework in which mental states are linked to specific types of behavior. Such conduct may be included only by defining it as either "erroneous" or "deviant." The same holds for the possible association of mutual indifference and helping behavior among family members. For example, a respondent who is one of three sisters said:

My sister's work schedule gives her freer hours in the day-
time. She feels very responsible . . . Everyone does her fair
share, but she does a lot. My out-of-town sister says maybe
she has taken on too much.

The "overly responsible" sister was not their mother's favorite but
she did contribute, not always happily, disproportionately to the
collective caring effort.

The disjunction between what daughters feel towards and actually do for their elderly mother, is relevant to the findings of Bengtson's and Roberts' extensive research which did not support their
original assumption that "solidarity among older family members
could be conceptualized as a linear additive composite of the members' degree of affection, association, and ideological agreement"
(1988, p. 18). An independent test by Atkinson and her coworkers
also failed to support such a "theory of family solidarity" (1986,
p. 415). Further manipulation of the data by Bengtson and Roberts
did lead to the conclusion that

the child's affect for the parent did not directly predict levels
of association, but exerted an indirect influence through its
positive effect on levels of parental affect. (1988, p. 19)

Pertinent also to my argument is the authors' contention that:

In essence, the empirical tests demonstrated that the theory
may have been too abstract too soon. That is, the proper foundation had not been established for the interpretation of higher-
order characteristics of families. (1988, p. 18)

This is a revealing comment. What *is* the precise meaning of "too
abstract"? Is it equivalent to "too artificial" in the sense Sussman
used the term? And what "theory" exactly? The authors seem to
vacillate between proposing a general theory of small-group solidarity and one about the usefulness of a carefully constructed *concept* labelled "family solidarity." Finally, what *are* those elusive
"higher-order" family characteristics?

Families, as living systems, consist of relationships between concrete human beings. Where, then, do we find the complexity re-

ferred to in the above? I doubt that the lack of predictability implies a higher order levels of structuring.

Herbert Simon's comment on the complexity of the individual human psyche is illuminating:

> A man, viewed as a behaving system, is quite simple. The apparent complexity of his behavior over time is largely a reflection of the complexity of the environment in which he finds himself. (1981, p. 65)

Analytically, the systemic nature of family process can be viewed as analogous to that of an individual's behavioral system. This helps clarify its seeming complexity and "higher-order" characteristics. Furthermore, it directs the attention to the many ways in which families manage to handle the contingencies of everyday life.

There is a tendency among researchers to jump from the individual to the collective level of family analysis by means of simple addition. This remains, however, a leap of faith since small group process is not just a summation of its contributing parts. Families especially are made up of people who, by virtue of their common membership and shared fate, are special to each other. Simple addition cannot capture this and may produce more "noise" than relevant information.

The usage of "generation" as a relatively homogeneous category within family systems is such an example:

> The extent to which the familial link between generations is female-based strongly predicts the amount of help received and given, and, it is more important for the child than for the parent to be female. Women do indeed appear to be the keepers of kin. (Atkinson et al., 1986, p. 415)

This observation contains an element of empirical truth, but its explanatory value is limited by the very real possibility that contemporary family members often may not deal with one another as representatives of different generations. Instead, they interact, or bond, as "mother and only daughter," "father and youngest son," or "mother and her least favorite daughter," to mention a few ties that constitute actual families. Such "relational" realities are not additive, nor can they be reduced to confrontations or collaborations between generations or age cohorts. Statements like the one made by Atkinson et al., do not provide answers to such issues as to whether aging parents without daughters will be neglected; or that we may expect competition for the role of kin keeper or principal caregiver in all-daughter families. At best, one may assume that this claim will hold for families that contain brothers and sisters. But, if that would be the case, what *are* we looking at: bonding between the "generations" or between siblings? Or both? Frankly, I doubt whether it makes theoretical sense to look at intergenerational linkages *within* family systems.

An approach, which, focuses on individuals, only allows for addition and subtraction. Consequently, its explanations reflect what occurs inside family members rather among or between them. One other example of such a person-oriented stance, expressing the relationships between adult children and their elderly parents, is quite close to that of this paper. The author, Professor Cicirelli, is well aware that such bonds "should not be considered in isolation, since they constitute only one subsystem of a larger subsystem in which the relationships within any one subsystem affect and are affected by the ongoing relationships within the other family subsystems" (1983a, p. 31). Once having stated this position, however, he continues:

> While it is recognized that interactions with other subsystems of the larger family system may influence the relationship between an adult child and the elderly parent, this chapter will focus on the parent-child relationship itself. The influence of other family subsystems on this relationship will be discussed only when particularly relevant. (1983a, p. 31)

Parent-child bonding is then placed within a "perspective of life-span attachment theory" (Cicirelli, 1988, p. 31), and the impact of "other family subsystems" is treated as an "intervening" variable, only to be included when "particularly relevant." One question for the researcher to study is *the* parent-child relationship in families with several children. In such cases, do we compute an average or select a modal bond; or do we choose the most convenient and/or accessible parent-child dyad to represent all others? When and why does one pay attention to the impact of other family subsystems? Illustrations furnished by a brother/son respondent set may clarify these points:

> Now we communicate almost every day because of our parents. We didn't always see eye to eye, but we always worked it out.

Or, as a different brother/son explained:

> In the past I would say most of the conversations I had with my brother were about anything that intimately involved any of us. Now that's changing—the discussion I have had with Bill and undoubtedly am going to have, will be more pointed about the family. I think that will affect the relationship. And I think John's moving to Tucson will change things. When both of them lived in the area (of parents), they were too close by to share the emotional or practical burdens; to be called on. I didn't feel too concerned then. Now with John moved I feel a greater share of the responsibility. Probably also a sense of guilt—not to them (parents), but to Bill because he is the only one on the spot.

Such comments illustrate that phenomena like "closeness" seem to vary as a function of the perceived well-being of the parents, geographic proximity, and the array of contingencies that constitute "normal" living in aging families. Multi-generational family relationships, thus, must be seen as a more or less bounded process of structuring. Not necessarily as a complex one, but rather a continuously adapting, negotiated state of affairs.

Analytically, there is no reason why one cannot focus on specific subsystems or relationships, such as mother-daughter dyads. The overall system, however, must remain the ultimate explanatory context. Knowing someone to be one of four brothers, or the only sister of two brothers, for example, not only defines that person's position in his or her family but also is a necessary condition for explaining interaction and its consequences for the family and its members.

AGING FAMILIES
IN A STRUCTURAL PERSPECTIVE

This paper does not advocate the elimination of "inner states" from attempts to explain the dynamics of family process. It proposes that personal feelings and attitudes at best may account for necessary conditions of family coherence and solidarity. It does not make sense to attach any explanatory power to individual intentions or motivations separate from a structure which is to be considered *sui generis*.

Structural thinking about family process directs attention to the implications of patterned *relationships* between its members (cf. Wellman, 1988, p. 16; Broderick and Smith, 1979). Systemness implies "a set of different things or parts . . . that meet two requirements: first, these parts are directly or indirectly related to one another in a network of reciprocal causal effects; and second, each component part is related to one or more of the other parts of the set in a reasonably stable way during any particular period of time (Kantor and Lehr, 1976, p. 10). The ideas of system and structure obviously are closely related. Without exploring the many facets of their interdependence, it suffices here to say that the former directs attention to boundary related phenomena, while the latter accentuates the patterned relationships between constituent parts.

Reflected in the foregoing is the premise that people pass through life as members of groups but also as partakers in bonds with special others. These two forms of social participation are not mutually exclusive (cf. Breiger, 1988, p. 86). Family systems in particular, because of their culturally ascribed and socially recognized status, *implicate* or entangle their members in a form of involuntary membership. They also, however, give rise to a wide range of interpersonal bonds of varying degrees of specialness and intensity. This "latent" quality remains an essential aspect of contemporary family structures (cf. Riley, 1983). It implies that individuals, because of their joint membership, and regardless of their personal feelings, may be expected to engage in supportive behavior when such is deemed necessary. Refusal to participate will be seen as a violation of both familial *and* social obligations. Obviously, in this context "solidarity" — in contrast to feelings of personal loyalty — is an attribute of family systems and has become institutionalized, that is, culturally defined and socially sanctioned. This is not a new idea and can be traced to Durkheim who wrote

> if the division of labor produces solidarity . . . it is because it creates among men an entire system of rights and duties which link them together in a durable way. (Durkheim, 1933, p. 406)

Talcott Parsons, among others, continued this theme:

> Loyalty is, as it were, the uninstitutionalized precursor of solidarity, it is the 'spilling over' of motivation to conform with the interests or expectations of alter beyond the boundaries of any institutionalized or agreed obligation. Collectivity-orientation on the other hand converts this 'propensity' into an institutionalized obligation of the role-expectation. Then whether the actor 'feels like it' or not, he is obligated to act in certain ways. . . . (Parsons, 1951, p. 98)

Both of these theorists make a clear conceptual distinction between the feelings individual family members may harbour toward one another and those obligations that involve *all* by virtue of their common membership.

This point is not new to the study of aging families. Rosow, for example, stressed the importance of a clear distinction "between formal responsibility for old parents and the emotional tie between generations" (1967, p. 25). The analysis of family process must come to terms with individual behavior that cannot be understood as merely individualistic. Most current research on familial bonding fails to take this into account.

Let us return briefly to a point touched on earlier, namely Bengtson and Roberts' comment on the presumed "higher-order characteristics" of families, and their conclusion that their theory appeared "too abstract too soon" to successfully interpret the functioning of family solidarity. I feel, however, that their problem reflects the combined effects of inadequate conceptualization and a highly abstract measurement model. This combination creates a level of "artificiality" which hinders our understanding of *any* aspect of family living, let alone its perpetual need to deal with uncertainty and contingency.

The presumed complexity of family life must be grasped conceptually before it can be studied rationally. For example: simple arithmetic tells us that within families consisting of three individuals three different dyadic "subsystems" are logically possible. For a size of four this number increases to 10, namely 6 dyads and 4 triads. Five-member families allow for 24 different combinations and/or potential alliances among its members, to wit: 10 dyads, 9 triads, and 5 quartets. Complexity, then, even in relatively small families, is a function of its organizational potential. Its resulting relationships can be of short or long duration, competitive or cooperative, exploitative or altruistic. Clearly, this reservoir of possible bonds and/or alliances is finite for each individual family and not difficult to identify. I do not see it as a higher order characteristic. On the other hand, the structuring potential of aging family systems must be part of the causal explanation of their process. Focussing only on individuals in families, or on dyads which are lifted from their actual setting, will provide some knowledge but not enough.

AN IMAGE OF PROCESS IN AGING FAMILIES

Thinking theoretically about any social phenomenon requires an "image" or "model" of what is to be explained. This means a speculative point of departure which allows for the choice of a conceptual vocabulary, a relevant line of questioning, and an appropriate research design (cf. Sprey, 1988, p. 882). Such models exist not only in the research literature but also in our culture. Scholars are not always in complete agreement, so that it is up to the skill of theoreticians to identify the most useful one.

About our subject, for instance, Blau, writes:

Children have an enduring sense of diffuse obligation as long as their parents live; but enduring solidarity, if solidarity means close bonds of affection and intimacy, will probably not last long . . . Adult children, as a rule, fulfill their material obligations and dutifully maintain some contact with aging parents, but their separate existence, interests, and daily experiences lessen intimacy between the generations, and estrangement, carefully hidden on both sides, begins. (1981, pp. 51-52)

She sees, then, "a mutual interest among parents and children. . . . to preserve the fiction that parents are 'insiders' and not 'outsiders'" (1981, p. 54).

Cicirelli, on the other hand, disputes this picture of the aging family:

> Based on the research we have reviewed and presented, we conclude that most adult children and their elderly parents do maintain a relationship that is based on the affectional bond between them. While the relationship is not one of day-to-day contact or close personal intimacy, neither is it one of mere obligation, pseudo-intimacy, and estrangement, as Blau (1981) suggests. (1983, p. 45)

Which of these is the most appropriate image? I see both models as not totally contradictory because they accentuate different aspects of family process. Information so far gleaned from our ongoing study on the division of filial responsibility among adult children supports this. In 49 "daughterless" families, for example, not surprisingly, "brotherhood" varied in the extent that adult brothers saw themselves as "close" to one another and to their family. However, the differing degrees of "affiliation" of such brother systems did not seem to affect their expressed loyalty to and actual support for their aging parents (Matthews, Delaney, and Adamek, 1989). In other words, solidarity, as a "social fact," indeed does seem to operate on a different "level" than that of the individual. The inevitable estrangement between parents and their grown, often absent, offspring, as emphasized by Blau does not necessarily threaten the contact with and care for the parents. Nor does it negate strong individual, and or dyadic, attachments between *specific* children and parents.

This point is echoed in the findings of an exploratory investigation of the impact of divorce on grandparenthood (Matthews and Sprey, 1984). It was found that parents not (yet) touched by the divorce of an adult child considered marital dissolution quite unlikely, and, should it happen, expected to know in advance. In contrast, the large majority of those *with* a divorced child did not anticipate it and were not consulted or told in advance. This suggests that,

> most of these grandparents were not aware of what really went on in their children's marriages. They were very much part of their extended family systems but, at the same time marginal to it. Some were more involved than others, of course, depending at least in part on geographic proximity and age. The participation of most of them, however, did not seem to penetrate deeply behind the closed doors of their children's married lives. (Matthews and Sprey, 1984, p. 43)

What happens in such extended families, therefore, is *not* that people stop caring for one another, but rather that individual members, depending on the circumstances, become less aware and part of the deeper content of each other's daily lives. This seems true for the relationships between parents and their adult offspring, but also for those between and among adult siblings. By the same token, under normal conditions solidarity and cohesion become more latent.

So we ask, why, and how such latent systems become "activated" when the need arises? What role do personal feelings play when familial crises do arise? And, finally, how does the resulting interaction feed back into the continuing reciprocity among adult siblings? These are systems-oriented questions, ones that imply feedback, adjustment, and readjustment processes that operate within a context of systemic rather than linear causality.

CONCLUSION

Family systems did change during the past two and a half decades, especially demographically. The life expectancy of individuals increased, while the average family size has grown smaller. This doubtlessly affected the scope of current family life, and may have influenced its quality. There seems no reason, however, to question the following observation:

> There exists in modern urban societies, particularly in American society, an extended kin family system, highly integrated within a network of social relationships and mutual assistance, that operates along bilateral kin lines and vertically over several generations. (Sussman, 1965, p. 63)

The main thrust of this paper, then, has been to propose the *causal* relevance of such systems for the explanation of what happens in aging families.

The position presented in this brief article has been conceptual. It took issue with a psychologistic approach towards the study of process in older family systems and suggested a more systemic view. The rationale is simple: like all living systems families age; adult children leave home and, as a rule, become part of other family structures. The latter remain, however, *implicated* within their own families of origin, regardless of their age or that of their parents.

It was illustrated that even relatively small families possess a large organizational potential. Consequently, problems of definition and measurement abound. Despite this I see most of the "surface" unpredictability that characterizes family process as a reflection of an uncertain, varied, and perpetually changing environment. The analytical path one follows to unravel the complex interaction between aging families and environmental contingency can incorporate individual attributes only within a systemic explanatory context. Its resulting theory need not be highly abstract as long as it allows us, to come to terms with, to paraphrase Sussman's comment, the circumstances of everyday life in aging family systems and the cauldron of forces which structure its process.

REFERENCES

Atkinson, M.P., Kivett, V.R. & Campbell, R. (1986). Intergenerational solidarity: An examination of a theoretical model. *Journal of Gerontology, 41,* 408-416.

Bengtson, V.L., Olander, E.B., & Haddad, A.A. (1976). The 'generation gap' and aging family members: Toward a conceptual model. In J.F. Gubrium (Ed.), *Time, Roles, and Self in Old Age* (pp. 237-263). New York: Human Sciences Press.

Bengtson, V.L. & Roberts, R.E.L. (1988). Parent-child solidarity in aging families: An exercise in theory construction. Paper read at the Theory Construction

Jetse Sprey 235

and Methodology Workshop of the National Council on Family Relations, Philadelphia, PA, November, 1988.
Blau, Z.S. (1981). *Aging in a changing society*. New York: Franklin Watts.
Breiger, R.L. (1988). The duality of persons and groups. In B. Wellman & S.D. Berkowitz (Eds.), *Social structures: A network approach*. New York: Cambridge University Press.
Broderick, C. & Smith, J. (1979). The general systems approach to the family. In W. R. Burr, R. Hill, F.I. Nye, & I.L. Reiss (Eds.), *Contemporary theories about the family*, Vol. 2. New York: Free Press.
Cicirelli, V.G. (1983a). Adult children and their elderly parents. In T.H. Brubaker (Ed.), *Family relationships in later life*. Beverly Hills: Sage Publications.
Cicirelli, V.G. (1983b). Adult children's attachment and helping behavior to elderly parents: A path model. *Journal of Marriage and the Family, 45*, 815-827.
Durkheim, E. (1933). *The division of labor in society*. Illinois, Glencoe: The Free Press.
Kantor, D. & Lehr, W. (1976). *Inside the family*. Washington: Jossey-Bass.
Matthews, S.H. & Sprey, J. (1984). The impact of divorce on grandparenthood: An exploratory study. *The Gerontologist, 24*, 41-47.
Matthews, S.H. & Sprey, J. (1987). *Dividing filial responsibility in adult sibling groups*. Proposal funded by the Department of Health and Human Services. Public Health Service.
Matthews, S.H., Delaney, P.J. & Adamek, M.E. (1989). Male kinship ties: Bonds between brothers. Unpublished Paper.
McChesney, K.Y. & Bengtson, V.L. (1988). Solidarity, integration, and cohesion in families. In D.J. Mangeb, V.L. Bengtson, and P.H. Landry, Jr. (Eds.), *Measurement of Intergenerational Relations*. Beverly Hills: Sage Publications.
McMullin, E. (1988). The shaping of scientific rationality. In E. McMullin (Ed.), *Construction and constraint*. Notre Dame, Indiana: Notre Dame University Press.
Parsons, T. (1951). *The social system*. Illinois: The Free Press.
Riley, M.W. (1983). The family in an aging society: A matrix of latent relationships. *Journal of Family Issues, 4*, 439-454.
Rosow, I. (1967). *Social integration of the aged*. New York: Free Press.
Simon, H.A. (1981). *The Sciences of the artificial*. Cambridge, MA: MIT Press.
Sprey, J. (1988). Current theorizing on the family: An appraisal. *Journal of Marriage and the Family, 50*, 875-890.
Sussman, M.B. (1965). Relationships of adult children with their parents in the United States. In E. Shanas & G.F. Streib, (Eds.), *Social structure and the family*. Englewood Cliffs, NJ: Prentice-Hall.
Sussman, M.B. (1988). Commentary on V.L. Bengtson & R.E.L. Roberts, Parent-child solidarity in aging families: An exercise in theory construction. Theory Construction and Methodology Workshop of N.C.F.R., Philadelphia, PA, November, 1988.
Wellman, B. & Berkowitz, S.D. (1988). *Social structures: A network approach*. New York: Cambridge University Press.

Between Mothers and Daughters

Lucy Rose Fischer

How different are daughters' lives today from their mothers' lives? Between some generations, there seems to be very little similarity at all. For example, women who reached adulthood in the 1950s and early 1960s were taught to "save" sexuality for marriage. They, in fact, may have engaged in premarital sex; but they understood that it was not socially acceptable. Most married at a young age and expected to stay married until "death do us part." They tended to leave the paid labor force when they had children and to view marriage and motherhood as central to their lives. In contrast, women reaching adulthood in the 1970s and 1980s — the daughters of these women — often shun patterns that were accepted as normal by their mothers' generation. The most recent cohorts of young women cohabit in increasing numbers before they marry and they marry at later ages. They not only anticipate working after marriage and motherhood but their wage-earner role has become increasingly essential to maintain their standard of living. They are having fewer children, and they are divorcing in record numbers (see Cherlin, 1981; Glick, 1984). With all these changes, is there still a "mother-link" — a special bond between mothers and daughters?

Sociologists, anthropologists and psychologists have described a special closeness between mothers and daughters over all stages of the life course, from the infancy of the daughters to the old age of the mothers. (For a review of recent research on the mother-daughter relationship, see Boyd, 1989; see also Baruch and Barnett,

Lucy Rose Fischer is Senior Research Scientist at Wilder Research Center, Amherst H. Wilder Foundation, 1295 Bandana Boulevard, Suite 210, St. Paul, MN 55108.

237

1983; Fischer, 1986; Hagestad, 1981; Hammer, 1976; Walker and Thompson, 1983.) Mothers are said to identify with daughters more than with sons; daughters are more likely than sons to be caregivers for their elderly mothers. Potentially, however, recent changes in women's roles undermine the special mother-daughter bond. These trends may widen the "generation gap" so that mothers' experiences may have little relevance to their daughters' actual futures. More specifically, the fact that an increasing proportion of women remain childless, along with the salience of professional careers in the lives of many women, means that the mothering role often is *not* passed down from mother to daughter.

LINKED LIVES

It has been over ten years since I did the research for my book, *Linked Lives: Adult Daughters and Their Mothers*. For that project, I conducted in-depth interviews with about 40 young adult daughters and their mothers. The daughters in my sample were born between 1948 and 1958; thus their mothers were part of the 1950s "mothering cohort," the decade marked by the highest rates of marriage and fertility in this century. The daughters were entering adulthood in the mid to late 1970s, a time of decline in both marriage and fertility, along with rising rates of divorce and female labor force participation. In demographic terms, the contrast between these two mothering cohorts is striking.

In my sample, only a few of the women in the mother generation pursued careers for most of their lives. Those few who had successful careers still tended to espouse the "traditional" ideology of motherhood—that is, the principle that mothering is woman's central role and that it is preferable for women not to work when they have small children. Most of the women in the mothers' generation, however, had dreams of pursuing other careers. Almost two thirds of these women described *unfulfilled* career aspirations. Several of them commented that education was not available to daughters in their families.

Many of the mothers and daughters insisted that the daughters' lives were better, in both economic and personal terms. Their daughters had purchased homes earlier in their lives and, in many ways, seem to have more material goods and to enjoy a higher standard of living. Some of the mothers also described the daughters as "freer," more "independent" and having more "open" relationships with their husbands. The daughters' husbands were said to spend more time with their wives and children than their fathers (Fischer, 1986, p. 105).

The daughters in my sample seemed to be trapped between two ideologies — "traditional mother" and "modern woman." They wanted to be both, but they often expressed frustration about how to reconcile these ideologies. One daughter, for example, spoke of her commitment to working as a registered nurse, but then also noted: "I feel I miss a lot with Joanie. I went back to work when she was five weeks only. The first word or whatever — she always did it with a babysitter" (Fischer, 1986, p.113).

In the conclusion of *Linked Lives*, I argued that the mothering role, conceived broadly, provides the framework for the mother-daughter bond.

> The family roles of women provide a meeting ground for the interweaving of generations. The caring orientation of adult daughters and their mothers — the centrality of mothering in both of their lives — means that their lives are linked from generation to generation. (Fischer, 1986, p. 201)

If I were to begin this research now — as we approach the last decade of the twentieth century — I wonder if I would draw the same conclusion. In the last decade, there has been a sharp rise in the labor force participation of mothers of *infants*. Also, increasingly, young mothers today are the daughters of working mothers — a factor which has been shown to affect women's attitudes toward work and careers (see Macke and Morgan, 1978; Pearson, 1983; Rollins and White, 1982). A number of theorists have argued that there is a continuity in women's roles — as wives and mothers — in contrast to the disjunction between fathers and sons whose lives tend to be focused around their work and who rarely (in this country) share the same work roles. To the extent that daughters enter the work world, the role disparity between mother and daughter should begin to be as wide as that between father and son.

THE MOTHER-LINK

Various classical studies have reported that the mother-daughter bond is the closest link between kin. Images of close mother-daughter bonds are especially vivid in portrayals of working class families. For example, Willmott and Young, in *Family and Class in a London Suburb*, based on observations of family life in London in the late 1950s, commented on the "striking" interdependence of mothers and daughters. They noted that if the mother is sick, it is the daughter who comes to help. They also said that daughters see their mothers more often than sons do, and maternal grandparents see their grandchildren more than paternal grandparents (Willmott and Young, 1960). Similarly, Peter Townsend, another anthropologist who was studying British family life around the same time, described family relationships as dominated by women—with the mother-daughter bond as the linchpin of family interactions (Peter Townsend, 1957). In her study of American working class families, Komarovsky reported that wives often use their mothers as confidantes and that a "wife's emotional investment in her mother remains strong" (1962, pp. 208, 246).

A number of studies of middle class families also have found greater closeness between mothers and daughters than between other intergenerational pairs. Adult children in white collar families are more likely to live at a distance from their parents than the sons and daughters of blue collar families. But daughters appear to be "kin-keepers" (that is, maintain contact) more than sons with both geographically near and distant relatives (see, for example, Adams, 1968; Fischer, 1983, 1986; Sussman, 1953).

The special bond between mothers and daughters emerges from the social construction of gender. Chodorow (1978, p. 39) has proposed that the ability to mother is "reproduced" from mother to daughter and that the structure of family relationships is a crucial factor in creating a psychological basis for mothering.

> Women's capacities for mothering and abilities to get gratification from it are strongly internalized and psychologically enforced, and are built developmentally into feminine psychic structure. Women are prepared psychologically for mothering

through the developmental situtation in which they grow up, and in which women have mothered them. (Chodorow, 1978, p. 39)

Freud reported that his female clients who had children often felt a revived identification with their mothers (Freud, 1933, p. 33). I reported a similar finding from my own research. One young mother, for example, stated: "Now that I had children I realized what she had been through. Before that . . . it just didn't dawn on me what kind of responsibility she had." Moreover, their shared role is not simply the generic mother-role but, as I have found in my study, adult daughters tend to replicate their mothers' mothering in specific and idiosyncratic ways (Fischer, 1986, pp. 74, 87).

This mother-link, however, can be viewed negatively. Both Chodorow and Dinnerstein have pointed to the problematic nature of women's position as mothers. Dinnerstein wrote:

So long as the first parent is a woman, then woman will inevitably be pressed into the dual role of indispensable quasi-human supporter and deadly quasi-human enemy of the human self. She will be seen as naturally fit to nurture other people's individuality; as the born audience in whose awareness other people's subjective existence can be mirrored; as the being so peculiarly needed to confirm other people's worth, power, and significance that if she fails to render them this service she is a monster, anomalous and useless. And at the same time she will also be seen as the one who will not let other people be, the one who beckons her loved ones back from selfhood, who wants to engulf, dissolve, drown, suffocate them as autonomous persons. (Dinnerstein, 1976, pp. 111-12)

The daughters in my study often viewed their bond of identity with their mothers in negative terms. Either they saw resemblances to their mothers as a tainted inheritance (characteristics that they did *not* want) and/or they insisted that their lives were or would be very different from their mothers' lives. One daughter, for example, told me that she was determined never to learn to play bridge and join bridge clubs because that was what her mother had done and she felt that bridge clubs just "kill time." This daughter—as a non-bridge player—had defined part of her identity through negation of her mother's identity, a theme that I found particularly common for educated daughters.

Between mothers and daughters, there is a liability of mutual rejection. In a review of recent literature on mothers and daughters, Werlock writes:

> The intense anomaly of the mother-daughter bond is clearly voiced through a comparison of statements by both Friday and Arcana: whereas Friday affirms that if a mother tells her daughter motherhood is inglorious, she in effect says "I shouldn't have had you," Arcana points out that if daughters fail to imitate mothers "then we are rejecting what they have accepted; we are rejecting them." (Werlock, 1989, p. 7)

I noted, above, that nearly two-thirds of the mothers in my sample reported aspirations which they were not able to accomplish in their lives. Most of these women also said, however, that they had "no regrets" about how their lives turned out. Perhaps for these mothers, regret over life choices could only imply a rejection of their own husbands and children.

FEMINIST PERSPECTIVES ON THE MOTHER-DAUGHTER BOND

There has always been some confusion, in feminist writings, between two very different sources of power for women: the power of motherhood and the power beyond motherhood. These power bases emerge from two types of perspectives on women's rights: the "women-are-different" and the "women-are-equal" perspectives. These different sources of power have divergent implications for relationships between adult daughters and their mothers.

Women-Are-Different. Motherhood has been a traditional source of power for women. As Oakley points out, children "are the inalienable property of women, who are otherwise placed by society in a propertyless condition" (Oakley, 1981, p. 228). In this sense, the mother-daughter bond is something like a trade-union—"a source of help in troubled times, a financial protection in the event of marital breakdown and, perhaps most importantly, a common basis for self-esteem'' (Oakley, 1981, p. 272).

Those feminists who emphasize how women are different from men have attempted to transform and expand this traditional basis of women's power. Thus, for example, daycare becomes a specifically women's issue — under the implicit or explicit recognition that women are the primary ones to care for children.

This is not a simple issue. On the one hand, this perspective lets men off the hook — with little expectation of equal participation in parenting. On the other hand, if men are *assumed* to be equal and to carry equal parenting responsibilities, there is considerable risk to women. Women may lose traditional resources; and their supposed equality with men may offer little in the way of concrete compensation. A striking example is the change, in virtually all states, from fault-based to no-fault divorce. Part of the rationale for no-fault divorce was that women today are capable of being earners and therefore should not need lifetime support from ex-husbands. The flaw in this argument, of course, is that women still earn considerably less than men and their earning ability is diminished by their investment in motherhood. The trend toward no-fault divorce has been responsible, in part, for the "feminization of poverty" (see Weitzman, 1985).

From the women-are-different perspective, women are special because their lives are oriented toward "mothering" — i.e., caring for others. The mother-daughter bond represents both the training ground for caring and the most enduring woman-to-woman relationship. One of the hallmarks of the mother-daughter bond is mutual nurturance. Just as daughters learn from their mothers how to mother their children, they also provide emotional and physical support to their mothers in later life.

The feminist women-are-different perspective emphasizes the power of sisterhood. From this perspective, mothers and daughters are potential allies in a sisterhood of women. My research and other studies in the 1970s (see, for example, Hagestad and Snow, 1977) found daughters socializing their mothers in terms of feminist consciousness. A number of daughters in my study, in their attempt to differentiate themselves from their mothers, also tried to change their mothers. Some daughters, for example, counselled their mothers with marital problems; several daughters pressed their mothers to divorce an abusive spouse. Komarovsky, in *Blue Collar Marriage*, also depicted a form of sisterhood between mothers and daughters in working class families, but the political tone is quite different. In her sample, mothers and daughters provided sympathy to one another at the same time that they supported the status quo. Their mutual sympathy was based on a shared understanding of their fate as women, because, in effect, "boys will be boys" (Komarovsky, 1962). What is distinct about the feminist version of this bond of support between mothers and daughters is both a recognition of women's relative lack of power and a demand that they *should* become more powerful.

Women-Are-Equal. From this perspective, women are viewed as much more similar to than different from men in terms of intellectual and creative abilities. The goal of feminism is equality in very basic ways. Women should have equal opportunity in all types of work. Women should *not* be limited by their biological functioning. In an article entitled "Motherhood: The Annihilation of Women," Allen (1984) wrote that "motherhood is dangerous to women" and that if women do not have children they can devote themselves to their creative development.

Actually, the beyond-motherhood feminist perspective has old roots. Historically, there have been many women who have chosen careers instead of marriage and motherhood. Before modern birth control, the choice for women was always careers *or* babies.

This perspective on power for women — power beyond motherhood — implicitly diminishes the importance of the mother-daughter bond by suggesting that daughters either should avoid the motherhood trap that constricted their mothers' lives or they should approach motherhood with a different value system. Under the "traditional" ideology of motherhood, mothering was seen as an all-consuming role, where the mother is an expert on the idiosyncratic needs of her child. One of the mothers in my sample, for example, described her daughter as a good mother because she could "anticipate" her child's needs. In other words, this young mother knew her child so well that she could read his mind! From a women-are-equal feminist perspective, however, such an all-consuming involvement in a child might well be seen as inappropriate.

A child should have multiple caregivers—a mother and father (equally involved and both reasonably familiar with the child) and other paid helpers. Under the ideology of equality, mothers and fathers should be equally invested in their careers and these careers should have comparable importance in family decisions.

One could imagine a chasm between mother and daughter when daughters insist on the ideology of equality. Some mothers may be profoundly disappointed when their daughters choose to forego motherhood in order to focus on their careers. Other mothers may find their grandmother role limited by the fact that the daughter and her husband jointly serve as gatekeepers vis-à-vis the grandchildren. Traditionally, maternal grandmothers have had an advantage because of their connection to the primary childcarer. With a truly egalitarian marriage, the mother's mother would not be any more privileged than the father's mother. And, in fact, both grandmothers might be seen as representing old-fashioned and unwelcome values in the new-style family life.

Of course, the fact that some daughters reject traditional mothering does *not* necessarily lead to misunderstanding with their own mothers. Clearly, many mothers want their daughters to have opportunities denied to themselves. There were hints of such feelings in my study—mothers who encouraged their daughters' professional pursuits and who vicariously enjoyed their daughters' successes (see also Hochschild, 1973).

A CONTINUING RESEARCH AGENDA

In the last few years, I have discussed my research on mothers and daughters in college classes, in lectures to community groups, and with readers of *Linked Lives*. In these discussions, women students and other non-professionals have pointed to ways that their mother-daughter relationships differed from the patterns described in my research. Such comments suggest a research agenda which includes comparative studies on variability in mother-daughter relationships by cohort, class, culture, and other variables.

Clearly, cohort is an important variable—as I have indicated in this essay. One proposed project is an historical study of mothers and daughters, using diaries and other written documents. It also would be interesting to compare research and even raw data from different decades. A replication of my mother-daughter project in the 1990s, using a comparable sample, might reveal if or how mother-daughter relationships may have changed since 1978, when I did my interviews.

Social class and cultural factors may have an impact on mother-daughter relationships. My sample was too small, and generally too homogeneous, to delineate such variables. The research evidence on variability in the mother-role by social class is mixed. While some studies have revealed class differences in certain childrearing techniques (see Kohn, 1977), other studies have pointed to the uniformity in the mother role across class boundaries (see Boulton, 1983). There is a paucity of data on cultural or ethnic differences in intergenerational relationships. A provocative article by Woehrer (1978) suggests that there may be very different family expectations and behaviors associated with ethnicity.

One reader wrote to me to complain that lesbian daughters and their mothers were not mentioned in my book. I responded that there were many types of family configurations that I left out of my research, such as divorced daughters, abusive mothers, and incestuous families. Some women who have read my book have commented that their mother-daughter bonds have always been distant. They could not relate to the special closeness that seemed to characterize most of the mother-daughter relationships in my study. Their insistence that their relationships do not fit the ideal expectations for the mother-daughter bond raises sociological and political issues. People never completely conform to the normative expectations of a social role; and it is important to recognize the distinction between person and role. It is also possible that serious deviation from the ideal-type mother-daughter relationship has "political" consequences. What happens when mothers are not very good at nurturing or daughters resent the expectation that they be parent-caregivers? I suspect that there are large numbers of such women and that they struggle against social expectations for mothering and daughtering behavior. An important agenda for future research will be to look beyond the stereotypes and gain a deeper understanding of both sources of variability and role strain in contemporary relationships between mothers and their adult daughters.

REFERENCES

Allen, J. (1984). Motherhood: The annihilation of women. In J. Trebilcot (Ed.), *Mothering: Essays in feminist theory*. Totowa, NJ: Rowman and Allanheld.

Adams, B. (1968). *Kinship in an urban setting*, Chicago: Markham Publishing Co.

Baruch, G. & Barnett, R.C. (1983). Adult daughters' relationships with their mothers. *Journal of Marriage and the Family*, *45*, 601-606.

Boulton, M.G. (1983). *On being a mother: A study of women with pre-school children*. London: Tavistock Publications.

Boyd, C.J. (1989). "Mothers and Daughters: A discussion of theory and research, *Journal of Marriage and the Family*, *51*, 291-302.

Cherlin, A.J. (1981). *Marriage, divorce and remarriage*. Cambridge, MA: Harvard University Press.

Chodorow, N. (1978). *The reproduction of mothering*. Berkeley: University of California Press.

Dinnerstein, D. (1976). *The mermaid and the minotaur*. New York: Harper and Row.

Fischer, L.R. (1986). *Linked lives: Adult daughters and their mothers*. New York: Harper and Row.

Fischer, L.R. (1983). Married men and their mothers. *Journal of Comparative Family Studies*, *14*, 393-402.

Freud, S. (1933). *New introductory lectures*. New York: Norton and Co.

Glick, P.C. (1984). Marriage, divorce, and living arrangements: Prospective changes. *Journal of Family Issues*, *5*, March, pp. 7-26.

Hagestad, G. & Snow, R. (1977). Young adult offspring as interpersonal resources in middle age. Paper presented at the annual meetings of the Gerontological Society of America.

Hagestad, G. (1981). Problems and promises in the social psychology of intergenerational relations. In R. Fogel, E. Hatfield, S. Kiesler & E. Shanas (Eds.), *Aging, stability and change in the family*. New York: Academic Press.

Hochschild, A.R. (1973). *The unexpected community: Portrait of an old age subculture*. Berkeley: University of California Press.

Kohn, M.L. (1977). *Class and conformity: A study in values*. Chicago: University of Chicago Press.

Komarovsky, M. (1962). *Blue collar marriage*. New York: Vintage.

Macke, A. & Morgan, W. 1978. Maternal employment, race and work orientation of high school girls. *Social Forces*, *57*, 187-204.

Oakley, A. (1981). *Subject women*. New York: Pantheon Books.

Pearson, J. (1983). Mothers and daughters: Measuring occupational inheritance. *Sociology and Social Research*, *67*, 204-217.

Rollins, J. & White, P. (1982). The relationship between mothers' attitudes and daughters' sex role attitudes and self-concept in three types of family environment. *Sex Roles*, *8*, 1141-1155.

Sussman, M.B. (1953). The help pattern in the middle class family. *American Sociological Review*, *18* (1), 22-28.

Townsend, P. (1957). *The family life of old people*. London: Routledge & Kegan Paul.

Walker, A. & Thompson, L. (1983). Intimacy and intergenerational aid and contact among mothers and daughters. *Journal of Marriage and the Family*, *45*, 841-849.

Weitzman, L.J. (1985). *The divorce revolution: The unexpected social and economic consequences for women*. New York: Free Press.

Werlock, A. (1989). A profusion of women's voices: Mothers and daughters redefining the myths. In M. Pearlman (Ed.), *Mother puzzles: Mothers and daughters in contemporary American fiction*. Westport: Greenwood Press.

Willmott, P. & Young, M. (1960). *Family and class in a London suburb*. London: Routledge & Kegan Paul.

Woehrer, C.E. (1978). Cultural pluralism in American families: The influence of ethnicity on social aspects of aging, *The Family Coordinator*, *27*, 329-338.

Fathers and Their Adult Sons
and Daughters

Corinne N. Nydegger
Linda S. Mitteness

We live most of our lives as adult children and as parents to adult children, yet we know least about this lengthy phase of the parent-child relationship. For over two decades, interactions between the old and their offspring have been studied intensively. We know a great deal about visiting patterns, satisfaction with contacts, caretaking, and consensual agreement across generations. We can say with confidence that "intergenerational linkages have proved to be the most salient component . . . of the kin network" (Sussman, 1985, p. 429), that "parent-child solidarity appears to consistently represent an important interpersonal bond" (Troll & Bengtson, 1979, p. 155) and "both aged parents and their adult children express high levels of regard for one another" (Bengtson, Cutler, Mangen & Marshall, 1985, p. 321).

What we cannot speak about with confidence are the content and shape of these relations outside the limited context of caretaking. Reports are impoverished substantively. We know there must be many different *kinds* of satisfactory relations between parents and children as adults; folklore, literature, and our own experience provide an enormous variety of prototypes, scarcely touched by the single dimension of satisfaction. The challenge is to explore the quality of parent-child relations among adults (as in Mitteness and Nydegger's 1982 and Walker and Thompson's 1983 factor-analyses of parent-child relationships, and Hagestad's 1984 multigenera-

Corinne N. Nydegger is Professor and Linda S. Mitteness is Associate Professor of Medical Anthropology, University of California, San Francisco, CA 94143.

tional thematic study) and to identify the sources of differentiation among these relations.

This paper will focus on how the sex of the child affects parent-adult child relations. The family literature documents its importance in early childhood and adolescence in determining parental patterns of belief and behavior consonant with socially sanctioned gender stereotypes. It also suggests that fathers play a major role in gender socialization for daughters as well as sons (e.g., Block, 1973, 1979; Lynn, 1974). Beyond the period of childhood, information about differential relations due to the sex of children has been largely literary or clinical, except for studies of caregiving daughters.

THE FATHERHOOD PROJECT

Early research on parents and children was almost exclusively on mothers and young children; interest in fathers focused on their absence. This imbalance is being rectified, although: "Only in the early 1970s did the father emerge as an object worthy of direct study" (Hanson & Bozett, 1985, p. 9). Despite the burgeoning literature on fathers in recent years, the age imbalance present in parent-child research remains: The primary focus is on families with young children, currently supplemented by an interest in the families of the old. In both cases, the emphasis is on caretaking and support, with the responsibility of parents on the one hand and that of adult children on the other. The Fatherhood Project[1] was undertaken to investigate the middle years of parent-*adult* child relations and especially the quality of these relations.

The project focused on the relationship as experienced and interpreted by the actors. This approach, commonly termed *emic*, does more than document subjective perceptions. It shows how individuals "give meaning to those perceptions by culturally appropriate ways of organizing, thinking, and feeling about them; literally, the phenomenology of culture" (Nydegger, 1983, p. 452). In this study, the goal was to describe the cultural phenomenology of the reciprocal roles of father and adult son, adult daughter. To this end, we posed "naive" questions: What does it mean to be an adult son or daughter? The father to such a child? What issues are salient? In what terms are common experiences interpreted? What criteria determine one's success?

To obtain the information required, we used an eclectic mix of methodological tools, but we relied most on lengthy, semi-structured taped interviews. Where possible, these raw materials were reduced to coded categories by an iterative process of cautious response-grouping, at increasing levels of abstraction. This method enabled us to retain those distinctions which were meaningful to our informants (and maintain coding reliabilities of .90 or better). This technique is well-described, though lacking a consistent terminology (e.g., Bernard, 1988; Clark & Anderson, 1967; Nydegger, Mitteness & O'Neil, 1983).

The Samples

The first phase of the Fatherhood Project involved 267 men, aged 45 to 80 years (stratified into three age cohorts). These respondents had a total of 582 children eighteen years or older, of whom almost 60% were married. Initially, the men were identified via random-digit dialing within the greater San Francisco Bay area. In order to minimize intergenerational differences in education and socioeconomic status, stringent criteria of inclusion were followed: All had some college, had been functioning fathers in their first families until the children were in their teens, and all participants were native-born and non-Asian.

These men were largely advantaged middle-class: Occupations ranged from minor civil service jobs to high level professional and managerial positions, the majority being businessmen. They had traditional marriages, with few wives working while their children were young. Thus, in terms of family, the informants represented the most stable portion of middle class fathers; they also are the last cohorts whose members could take "traditional" gender roles for granted (Lewis, 1986). For the children's study, we drew a random sample from the pool of respondents' children living within sixty miles of San Francisco. We interviewed one child per family, 62 sons and 62 daughters, ranging in age from the 20s to the 50s (median age 31 years). Sixty percent of this sample were married.

In the Fatherhood Project we rejected the one child per family tradition in order to capture the full experience of fathering. We asked fathers about relations with *all* their children. The data fully justify our decision: dyadic father-child relations are so varied within families that it is impossible to predict from one dyad to another except in the extreme cases. However this approach also means that many of the parent-child relations to be discussed are not truly independent. For the analyses presented here, this is not a serious fault: for example, we do not correlate relations to fathers' characteristics.

A NOTE ON THE LANGUAGE OF FATHERING

Our interviews with fathers began with an overview of their careers. This allowed the men to comfortably discuss the least private parts of their lives, after which we could ease into more intimate questions about family relations. This proved to be a very successful strategy. Occupationally representative samples of men, even of the well-educated, include very few men with psychological or social science backgrounds and only a handful with a penchant for the humanities. Primarily businessmen, adult elaboration of vocabulary is narrowly focused on their occupational concerns. Moreover, they feel discomfort when talking about emotions and generally avoid such topics. Not surprisingly, they possess a minimal terminology in which to speak about interpersonal relations, and probably misinterpret many phrases habitual in family research.

When we asked the men in our study to discuss family relations in their own terms, we posed a difficult problem for them. Most men found it awkward; some were literally inarticulate. This was especially true in regard to terms of affection: "They described good relations in terms of interest in the child and his/her activities, encouragement of plans, etc. Our common terms for loving relationships were very seldom used" (Mitteness & Nydegger, 1982, p. 1). Paternal devotion was often expressed in the form of a supervisor's evaluation.

However, there was no misinterpreting the glow of pleasure or expansiveness of pride which so often accompanied superficially prosaic, even meager, descriptions. But only clinical research customarily takes body language into account; it cannot appear in self-

ratings or checklists. Thus, accounts of fathers' emotional investment in children often have been distorted by persistent neglect of
their distinctive mode of talking about relations. This error is less
common in research in other cultures (e.g., Lamb, 1987).

SONS VERSUS DAUGHTERS

Being a father to a daughter and to a son are profoundly different
experiences. This is the conclusion of virtually every man who had
experienced both relationships. Fathers report the convergence of
their own distinctive fathering functions with those of mothers as
children reach adulthood (Nydegger & Mitteness, 1979), but distinctive relations with sons and daughters persist throughout life.

Given such emphatic statements, we would expect significant
differences in regard to sons and daughters to loom large in our
data. And such differences are prominent. Nevertheless, they are
easy to miss, for these differences are seldom matters of "How
much?" Typically, they appear as responses to "In what way?" or
"For what reason?" That is, they are predominantly *qualitative*.
And most often, difference underlies superficial similarity. Thus,
depending on the kind of questions asked, research can yield con-
flicting results. A few examples will make this point.

Nature of Differences

Is it more difficult to be a father to a son than to a daughter?
Seemingly not: Over half (54%) reported no difference; the remainder split almost evenly, 24% singling out daughters, 22% sons.
Similarly, accounts of problems caused by children's behavior in
adolescence and adulthood were rated on a 5-point scale of severity
as experienced by the father: Adult problems are strongly correlated
with ratings of fathers' satisfaction ($r = -.51$, $p < .0001$) and the
overall quality of their relationship ($r = -.35$, $p < .0001$) as indicated by five and seven point scales respectively.[2] But there are no
significant differences between sons and daughters in number or
severity of problems at either time period.

However, the *kinds* of problems and difficulties typically presented by sons and daughters show virtually no overlap. They faith-

fully mirror prevalent "sugar 'n spice" versus "puppy-dog tail" sex stereotypes. Briefly, sons are harder to control, more assertive and defiant in testing limits and pushing for independence; proving their masculinity can lead to serious trouble. Daughters are more sensitive and emotionally labile, but less defiant and easier to control, in part because they mature earlier than boys; but maturation entails worry about early pregnancy.

Although some fathers attribute these differences to innate characteristics of males and females, while others note the role of social expectations, most are not concerned about questions of source. For the most part, sex-role stereotypy has been a fact in these men's personal lives and social landscapes from the time they were children. However, they are by no means unaware of current efforts toward redefining sex roles. Many fathers, particularly in the youngest cohort, are experiencing the effects of this movement.

The sex stereotypes have one particularly important consequence: They lead to differing priorities of fathers' responsibilities.[3] In regard to a son, the generally held view is that a father's main responsibility is to foster his son's independence and ensure the basis for his future in social and economic terms. Daughters, on the other hand, are seen as open and trusting, rather than defensive, and are considered emotionally, as well as physically vulnerable. Thus, a father's foremost responsibility is perceived as protecting his daughter and ensuring her welfare. Therefore, those fathers who reported no difference in relative difficulty occasioned by sons and daughters did not do so because the sex of the child is irrelevant. Rather, they compared two distinct kinds of difficulty and concluded that they posed roughly equivalent—but not the same—problems.

Do children also perceive sex-related differences? We asked the adult children to describe each sibling's current relations with their father as to its similarity to their own and to rate the similarity on a four-point scale. Over half of the children report dissimilarity: Sons, 60%, daughters, 58%. The presence of opposite sex children in the family increases the sense of differentiation, as shown in Table 1 (the scale is collapsed for clarity). Of the reasons given for dissimilarities in mixed sex families, the most prominent is a sibling's sex and its correlates such as shared activities, especially in

Table 1. Siblings' Relations with Father

	Similar	Dissimilar	
Daughters			
With Brothers (N=78)	36%	64	100%
No Brothers (N=19)	47%	53	100%
Sons			
With Sisters (N=86)	38%	62	100%
No Sisters (N=30)	43%	57	100%

the views of daughters (50% to sons' 35%). Thus, children give even greater weight to sex as a differentiator than do their fathers.

Sharing a World

One point which emerged during discussions of raising sons and daughters represents a key element in shaping adult relations between fathers and their children. Fathers not only socialize sons into their male world, but also share it with them. Thus, they find it easy to understand sons, which facilitates the development of common interests and mutual empathy. In one father's words, "It was easy to find a common denominator with the boys. We had interests in common from early on and still do."

To the contrary, daughters have a different perspective and inhabit a different, female, world. Fathers find it difficult to understand them: Girls are described as being "complex," "baffling," and "harder to understand their feelings." As one father put it, "I felt it was easier with a boy because I was a boy. But I was never a girl and I didn't really know how fathers and girls *should* respond to one another." Children agree that, in adolescence and adulthood, fathers understand sons better than daughters.

For both fathers and sons, this sense of sharing a world and a distinctively male perspective grows stronger as sons enter their careers, establish their own families, and move through adulthood. Regardless of the quality of relations, it provides a commonality between sons and fathers that is not available to daughters.

Quality of Relations

Because the scope of "quality of relations" is broad, with few guideposts to its assessment, we used multiple approaches. In general, qualitative approaches were more meaningful than quantitative measures. For example, the simplest was to have fathers identify the "closest" child and to explain their choice. In contrast to many studies which found daughters more often considered close (e.g., Lowenthal, Thurnher & Chiriboga, 1975), sons and daughters were named in approximately, equal numbers. But explanations of why a particular child was chosen are more revealing. Some are sex-irrelevant, such as having a similar personality or special characteristic (e.g., the child who helped with a disabled sibling). But the most frequently mentioned reasons for being "closest" are virtually sex-specific: Shared activities or interests are mentioned almost exclusively for sons; being open and communicative is a category primarily used for daughters. In families having only daughters or sons, this sex-specificity tends to break down, but the sexes never approach equality in these categories.

Global ratings (on a seven-point scale) of the quality of the father-child relationship show sex differences varying with children's ages and marital status. Overall, 74% of the relations with adult daughters are judged very good in contrast to 64% for sons. As mentioned previously, the children noted stronger effects of sex: Their ratings of relative closeness to each parent in childhood and adulthood (Table 2) show that sons report a much stronger movement toward parental equality than do daughters. Although the bond between mothers and daughters persists, sons' ties with mothers weaken over time. This contrasts with some earlier studies (notably Adams, 1968 and Lowenthal et al., 1975) and may reflect either the older age of children in the Fatherhood Project or the relative salience to sons of the advantaged fathers in this project.

In a detailed factor-analysis of twenty-two dimensions of father-

Table 2. Closest Parent in Childhood and Adulthood

	Childhood		Adulthood	
	Son (N=61)	Daughter (N=59)	Son (N=55)	Daughter (N=55)
Mother	59%	76%	24%	60%)
Same	15	7	47	31
Father	26	17	29	9
	100%	100%	100%	100%

child relations (Mitteness & Nydegger, 1982), two of the three relationship factors differ significantly by sex of the child: While warmth/involvement shows no difference, fathers are more negative about sons than daughters (more dissatisfied, worried, angered, etc.). However, they also are more reflective about a son's perspective and better able to specify a son's characteristics. Modest though these differences appear, when coupled with the sex distinctions in fathers' responsibility and shared perspective, they point to the nature of fathers' more complex relations with their sons.

FATHER-SON RELATIONS

Relations between fathers and sons are the more complex of the father-child dyads. They involve more dimensions, greater change over time, and inherent, sustained tensions. Their potential for drama has been a mainstay of literature for centuries. But are such dramas inherent in the roles once children have traversed adolescence and grown into adulthood? Our data show that tension and potential conflict continue for some time, but that most fathers and sons in these families ultimately attain relations they regard as good.

We cannot deal with these relations fully here, and therefore will limit discussion to those aspects most salient in the interviews. In regard to good father-son relations, the most important characteristic is respect. Fathers hope for their sons' respect and sons want to earn the respect of their fathers. But each wants to gain it on his own terms, that is, to be respected on the basis of his own values, not the other's. Attaining this goal is a slow, lengthy process, with tension typically unresolved until the son is well into his 30s.

Independence

Although fathers have varying responsibilities for young sons, it is long range goals that occupy most of their attention. The responsibility is explicit: A father must guide his son safely toward independence, and he must ensure that his son has a sound social and economic base on which to build his future. Thus, fathers' responsibilities continue well into sons' adulthood.

Fathers' relinquishing of authority and the growing independence of sons have been well documented through the college years (e.g., Greene & Boxer, 1986). The usual problem is to brake sons' determined drive towards independence. Occasionally a son poses the opposite problem and his father must encourage independence. In line with sex stereotypes of limit-testing boys, the former is anticipated; the latter is not and conventional parenting wisdom does not address it. As Greenberg and Becker (1988) also report, dependency in adult sons (but not daughters) is particularly stressful for fathers.

In most families, battles in the war of independence are outgrown and forgotten as sons achieve maturity. In accord with the conclusions of intergenerational research, that the more benign view is generally held by the older generation (Bengtson et al., 1985), we find that sons report independence conflicts as more severe than do their fathers.

Career

Tensions that result from a father's attempts to ensure his son's future are more serious. Such decisions have lifelong consequences and the parent cannot assume these tensions will be outgrown. For families in our study, downward mobility is a major fear. A son is not expected to do better than his father, but at least should do as well. A college education is only the beginning: Fathers' oversight extends through subsequent entry on a "sensible" career path.

What constitutes a "sensible" career is a frequent source of contention. We will not deal with this issue here, except to note that, although fathers may encourage one career rather than another, very few try to impose a choice. The latter course is disastrous. However, paternal concerns are forcefully voiced if a son delays for too long his career decision.

The fathers in our sample are well qualified to evaluate sons' careers and they keep a sharp eye on their sons' progress, poised to offer opinion, advice, and assistance. Thus, because being kept fully informed is important, fathers' ratings of sons as less open than daughters take on significance. Sons, interpreting fathers' behavior as critical and intrusive, either learn techniques of information management (Nydegger & Mitteness, 1988) or curtail visiting. The tendency of sons to distance themselves from the family during the early years of career and marriage is widely reported (e.g., Fischer, 1983a; Greene & Boxer, 1986; Lowenthal et al., 1975). Avoidance of oversight is one motive.

A son's steady career achievement is the surest sign that his future has been ensured. Fathers' concern is demonstrated in the kinds of complaints they make about married sons, as shown in Table 3: Achievement concerns dominate. But defining achievement can be problematic. Sons in atypical career paths, for example, reject conventional criteria of success. Therefore, varying life-styles and

Table 3. Fathers' Complaints about Married Children

	Sons (N=123)		Daughters (N=129)	
Marriage	20%		31%	
Parenting	4	24%	9	40%
Lack of Achievement		28		20
Goals/Lifestyle		19		19
Personal Qualities		11		11
Lack of Maturity		7		3
Relations with Parents		6		5
Other		5		2
		100%		100%

goals, with their differing criteria of success, can cause persistent tensions.

Marriage is another welcome marker of full maturity but may also create strains (Table 3). Strong mother-daughter bonds and wives' kin-keeping function result in a de facto asymmetry that tends to weaken the ties between sons and their parents (Fischer, 1983a, 1983b; Greene & Boxer, 1986; Nydegger, 1986). In extreme cases the son's family ties may be severed.

Maturation

Tense relations are commonly reported between fathers and sons into their 30s, but most agree that as sons mature, tensions abate and relations greatly improve. Conflict reducing mechanisms help, such as conversational "demilitarized zones" (Hagestad, 1984). But sons' maturity is the main reason for improvement. At this point, fathers believe they have fulfilled their obligations, even if they are not completely satisfied with the outcome. Being no longer responsible for their sons, they are better able to accept and respect sons on their terms, and to express unqualified affection. One father provides a good illustration: "He's never going to make money teaching, but he's really good at it, loves working with those kids. So, as long as he's happy, I am too."

Among sons, it is the youngest who most resent paternal criticism and, in turn, are most critical of their parents. As they settle into careers, become fathers themselves, and mature toward middle age, sons commonly develop a better understanding of their fathers' backgrounds and perspectives. Disdained attitudes and opinions can be excused as relics of a father's past social world (Nydegger et al., 1983). Sons too are freed to accord their fathers respect and affection.[4]

Good adult relations between fathers and sons are facilitated by establishing some basis of commonality beyond the family tie. In this sample, socioeconomic status is fairly stable across generations. Therefore, fathers and sons are very likely to fully comprehend each other's occupational successes and setbacks. Many share other interests or participate in the same activities. These commonalities encourage empathy and a sense of closeness. But they are not essential. Some fathers and sons who are very close share nothing but a deep affection for each other.

FATHER-DAUGHTER RELATIONS

First, we will discuss daughters experiencing or anticipating traditional roles: a job (rather than a career), marriage and children. Career-oriented daughters will be discussed separately.

Fathers' relations with traditional daughters are less complex and more relaxed than relations with sons. In most of these families, fathers and daughters have developed good relations early in adulthood. Their most important characteristic is affection: each wants the other's love.

Vulnerability

During the interviews, we were struck by fathers' affection for their daughters. They find it more difficult to describe daughters than sons, but nonetheless, they glow with pride. Although intelligence and beauty are often mentioned, the most prized attributes seem to be the personal qualities of warmth, affection, and kindness. Moreover, a favorable bias toward daughters appears throughout the study. Fathers are less critical of daughters than sons and readier to make excuses for daughters' mistakes. The pattern of assigning blame for divorce is an example of this bias: Sons are blamed in 18% of the cases to 2% for daughters; at most, daughters share the blame with their husbands (Nydegger, 1986, p. 103).

Perceived sex differences are at the root of this bias. As we have noted, daughters are considered vulnerable. This may be seen as an inherent quality or the result of social gender roles. It matters little, for both points of view define daughters as vulnerable, especially in regard to significant men in their lives: boyfriends, husbands, employers. Many men also include fathers, noting that daughters' sensitivity compels fathers to exercise more care when angry than is necessary with sons.

Because of this vulnerability, fathers' primary responsibility is to protect daughters.[5] The men in our study accept traditional gender-based division of responsibility: While mothers handle daughters' socialization, fathers are responsible for their protection. Freed of the necessity for critical oversight of a daughter's progress, a father can relax and enjoy her.

The only predictable source of tension is marriage or serious involvement. Although daughters' marriages confer social adulthood, the protective concern of fathers is not reduced. To the contrary, it is aroused and now directed toward sons-in-law. As Table 3 shows, marriage (here including divorce and disapproval of the child's spouse) is almost twice as likely to occasion dissatisfaction with daughters than with sons. And in 50% of these cases, the son-in-law is faulted for being a poor provider for the daughter (Nydegger, 1986). For most men, "a son makes his own mistakes in marriage, but a daughter's marital problems raise the spectre of her father's inadequate protection—his failure in fathering" (Nydegger, 1986, p. 109).

Fathers' concerns can create tension. From the daughters' point of view, protection may be seen as control and criticism of sons-in-law as unwarranted interference. But, unlike strains in relations with sons, these tensions seldom disrupt family bonds. Daughters' ties to family are strong and tensions with sons-in-law can be handled by quasi-avoidance. Thus, asymmetrical (i.e., matrifocal) kin involvement accounts for modal tensions arising in regard to sons-in-law, as well as maintenance of family bonds despite tension (Nydegger, 1986; Troll, 1986).

Different Worlds

Fathers and traditional daughters inhabit different social worlds. Fathers are more prone to exaggerate this difference than to minimize it. They perceive daughters as delightful, but mysterious creatures. Daughters are likely to find fathers equally incomprehensible. Insofar as closeness involves some understanding, it is not surprising that daughters' most common complaint is that they are misunderstood and that they do not feel close to fathers (Table 2). Some circumstances make for a better understanding or a more substantive relationship. For example, a particular shared interest or a father's assistance with problems outside the family such as college, jobs, and finances. And daughters' maturity, marriage, and parenting may bring about a deeper understanding of fathers. But this is idiosyncratic. Only a few traditional daughters develop a strong commonality with their fathers.

Despite the lack of closeness, daughters are less critical of their fathers than are sons. Rather than using occupational achievement criteria, daughters assess fathers in terms of family performance: They value affection and consideration most highly. Good traditional father-daughter relations are based on uncritical, mutual affection to which incomprehension seems to be no hindrance.

Nontraditional Daughters

Current trends in women's lives are markedly altering father-daughter relations, and in predictable directions. As daughters move into the occupational world of men, their relations with their fathers are recast into a shape more like that between fathers and sons. Fathers still feel the need to protect, but expand their responsibility to include socializing daughters into the male world of work, easing their career entry, and overseeing their progress. Virtually all fathers find this very rewarding even if they are skeptical of daughters' longterm commitment. For, as with sons, the shared work-world promotes commonality: Daughters and fathers report a new, fuller understanding and respect for each other and their achievements.

However, these daughters lose their immunity from criticism. A career-oriented daughter and her father now meet on his ground and she is subject to his critical appraisal, evaluated by criteria developed in his world. The tensions typical of father-son relations now also appear in father-nontraditional daughter relations. Nevertheless, among families in this category in our sample, both fathers and daughters find the advantages outweigh the disadvantages.

SUMMARY

Sex of children is a major source of variation in father-child relations. Perceived sex differences shape adult relations in two respects. First, fathers share with sons a male world that provides a commonality not available to daughters. Second, fathers have different responsibilities towards sons and daughters: Sons are guided and advised; daughters are protected.

Relations between fathers and sons are complex. They involve many dimensions, changes over time, and sustained tensions, which typically remain unresolved until sons are in their 30s. The key to achieving good relations is mutual respect.

Fathers' relations with daughters are less complex, more relaxed, and more stable. Mutual affection is the basis of their good relations. However, current trends are altering this picture: Career-oriented daughters develop relations with their fathers more like those of sons than traditional daughters. In future, we can anticipate an increase in fathers' involvement in daughters' lives, thus provoking tension, but also promoting better understanding.

ENDNOTES

1. The Senior author acknowledges the support of NIMH (MH29657) and NIA (AG00097 and AG03871); the junior author acknowledges the support of NIA (AG00274).

2. These relationships are stronger than those reported for similar varilables by Greenberg and Becker (1988) in a small sample of older couples. In that study, children's problems were more broadly defined, including those for which the child could not be held responsible, such as illness.

3. Despite the passage of a quarter of a century of major social changes, our data on differential responsibilities toward sons and daughters is in close agreement with Benson's (1968) description of the father's role.

4. The key role that children's comprehension of parents plays in the development of filial maturity is discussed in Nydegger (in press).

5. Studies concluding that fathers feel more (rather than different) responsibility for sons than for daughters (such as Gilbert et al., 1982) do so without including protection or provision, which fathers regard as their most important responsibilities (Nydegger & Mitteness, 1979).

REFERENCES

Adams, B. (1968). *Kinship in an urban setting*. Chicago: Markham.

Bengtson, V., Cutler, N., Mangen, D. & Marshall, V. (1985). Generations, cohorts, and relations between age groups. In R. Binstock & E. Shanas (Eds.), *Handbook of aging and the social sciences* 2nd Ed. (pp. 304-338). New York: Van Nostrand Reinhold.

Benson, L. (1968). *Fatherhood: A sociological perspective*. New York: Random House.

Bernard, H. (1988). *Research methods in cultural anthropology*. Newbury Park: Sage.

Block, J. (1973). Conceptions of sex role. *American Psychologist, 28*, 512-526.

Block, J. (1979). Socialization influences on the personality development of males and females. Master Lecture, presented at annual meeting, American Psychological Association, New York.

Clark, M. & Anderson, B. (1967). *Culture and aging*. Springfield: Charles Thomas.

Fischer, L. (1983a). Married men and their mothers. *Journal of Comparative Family Studies, 14*, 393-402.

Fischer, L. (1983b). Mothers and mothers-in-law. *Journal of Marriage and the Family, 45*, 187-192.

Gilbert, L., Hanson, G. & Davis, B. (1982). Perceptions of parental role responsibilities. *Family Relations, 31*, 261-269.

Greenberg, J. & Becker, M. (1988). Aging parents as family resources. *The Gerontologist, 28*, 786-791.

Greene, A. & Boxer, A. (1986). Daughters and sons as young adults. In N. Datan, A. Greene & H. Reese (Eds.), *Life-span developmental psychology: Intergenerational relations* (pp. 125-149). Hillsdale: Erlbaum.

Hagestad, G. (1984). The continuous bond. In M. Perlmutter (Ed.), *Minnesota symposia on child psychology*, Vol. 17. (pp. 129-158). Hillsdale: Erlbaum.

Hanson, S. & Bozett, F. (1985). *Dimensions of fatherhood*. Beverly Hills: Sage.

Lamb, M. (1987). *The father's role: Cross-cultural perspectives*. Hillsdale: Erlbaum.

Lewis, R. (1986). Men's changing roles in marriage and the family. In R. Lewis & M. Sussman (Eds.), *Men's changing roles in the family* (pp. 1-10). New York: Haworth.

Lowenthal, M., Thurnher, M. & Chiriboga, D. (1975). *Four stages of life*. San Francisco: Jossey-Bass.

Lynn, D. (1974). *The father: His role in child development*. Belmont: Wadsworth.

Mitteness, L. & Nydegger, C. (1982). Dimensions of parent-child relations in adulthood. Paper presented at the annual meeting, Gerontological Society of America, Boston.

Nydegger, C. (1983). Introduction. In C. Nydegger (Ed.), Anthropological approaches to aging research [Special issue]. *Research on Aging, 5*, 451-453.

Nydegger, C. (1986). Asymmetrical kin and the problematic son-in-law. In N. Datan, Greene, A. & Reese, H. (Eds.), *Life-span developmental psychology: Intergenerational relations* (pp. 99-123). Hillsdale: Erlbaum.

Nydegger, C. (in press). The development of paternal and filial maturity. In K. Pillemer & K. McCartney (Eds.), *Parent-child relations across the lifespan*. Hillsdale: Erlbaum.

Nydegger, C. & Mitteness, L. (1979). Transitions in fatherhood. *Generations*, *4*, 14-15.

Nydegger, C. & Mitteness, L. (1988). Etiquette and ritual in family conversation. *American Behavioral Scientist*, *31*, 702-716.

Nydegger, C., Mitteness, L. & O'Neil, J. (1983). Experiencing social generations: Phenomenal dimensions. *Research on Aging*, *5*, 527-546.

Sussman, M. (1985). The family life of old people. In R. Binstock & E. Shanas (Eds.), *Handbook of aging and the social sciences* 2nd Ed. (pp. 415-449). New York: Van Nostrand Reinhold.

Troll, L. (1986). Introduction: parent-child relations. In L. Troll (Ed.), *Family issues in current gerontology* (pp. 75-83). New York: Springer.

Troll, L. & Bengtson, V. (1979). Generations in the family. In W. Burr, G. Nye, R. Hill & I. Reiss (Eds.), *Contemporary theories about the family*, Vol. 1 (pp. 127-161). New York: Free Press.

Walker, A. & Thompson, L. (1983). Intimacy and intergenerational aid and contact among mothers and daughters. *Journal of Marriage and the Family*, *45*, 841-850.

The Grandparent-Grandchild Connection

Vira R. Kivett

The grandparent-grandchild connection is second only in biological linkages to the parent-child dyad. The tie provides a clue to family integration, especially in the face of social change (Troll, 1980). Increases in the number of older adults and new rhythms in the family life cycle have contributed to a vertical expansion of the family (Barranti, 1985). Approximately 75% of adults over 65, for example, are grandparents (Shanas, 1979; Troll, 1983). Nearly 40% of older adults are greatgrandparents (Cherlin & Furstenberg, 1986; Kivett, 1985). Within the last 50 years a ten year old child's chances of two living grandparents have risen from 40 to 50%. The chances of three living grandparents have increased from 10 to 38% (Brody, 1979). It is anticipated that today's children will spend approximately 50% of their life in the grandparent role. Hagestad (1982) referred to this phenomenon as "life overlaps" or the increased possibility of the coexistence of three or four generations of parents and children. She labelled this important but potentially confusing array of parent-child units the "alpha-omega chain."

Differences may be seen in satisfaction with the grandparent role. Considerable satisfaction, however, is reported (Crawford, 1981; Neugarten & Weinstein, 1964; Robertson, 1977; Thomas, 1986). Variations also exist in frequency of association. While some have observed frequent grandparent-grandchild interaction (Harris & Associates, 1975; Kahana & Kahana, 1971; Tinsley & Parke, 1987) others have reported only intermittent contact (Cherlin & Furstenberg, 1986; Kohnhaber & Woodward, 1981). Differences may be seen in the prominence of the grandparent role. The role is more

Vira R. Kivett is Professor, School of Human Environmental Sciences, University of North Carolina at Greensboro, Greensboro, NC 27412-5001.

salient for the working class, for widows, for the less educated, for those who are older, for those who are unemployed or retired, and for those who are not involved in community affairs (McPherson, 1983). The diversity of grandparenting is consistent with the American family system. Relationships are optional, discretionary, and individually specified.

The grandparent-grandchild link is an increasingly important focus of study. There have been few attempts, however, to integrate this knowledge either conceptually or empirically. This article provides insight into the research and conceptual issues surrounding the grandparent-grandchild connection.

LITERATURE ON THE GRANDPARENT-GRANDCHILD CONNECTION

Most information on the grandparent-grandchild link has emerged since the 1950s and has followed thematic paths. Research has been both qualitative and quantitative. Disciplinary differences have occurred mainly in methodology rather than in concept. The majority of articles on grandparenthood during the last three decades has been empirical in nature (e.g., Apple, 1956; Cherlin & Furstenberg, 1985; Fischer, 1983; Johnson, 1983; Kahana & Kahana, 1970; Kivett, 1985; Kivnick, 1983; Kornhaber & Woodward, 1981; Matthews, 1984; Neugarten & Weinstein, 1964; Robertson, 1977; Wood & Robertson, 1976). Most of this research is from the perspective of both grandfather and grandmother. Major themes from grandparents' perspectives have centered on role meanings, perceptions, and behaviors. An emerging theme is the impact of divorce on the grandparent-grandchild connection (e.g., Blau, 1984; Gladstone, 1988; Johnson, 1983; Kalish & Visher, 1981; Matthews, 1984). Other less frequent perspectives include those of grandparent-grandchild, grandchild, grandparent-parent-child, and grandparent-parent. Several studies have included five and six generations (Albrecht, 1954; Burton, 1985; Kruse, 1984). Principal themes from intergenerational perspectives have centered upon role conceptions and meanings, outcomes of role timing, and intergenerational transfers. A significant proportion of articles on the grandparent-grandchild connection have been conceptual in nature (e.g., Baranowski, 1982; Barranti, 1985; Hagestad & Burton, 1986; Kahana & Kahana, 1971; Robertson, 1975; Sprey & Matthews, 1982; Tinsley & Parke, 1982; Troll, 1980; Wood & Robertson, 1976). Major themes include the value and function of grandparents, and theoretical perspectives of the connection.

Most of the initial research on the grandparent role was ethnographic in type (Apple, 1956; Nadel, 1951; Radcliff-Brown, 1952). Research mainly focused upon the relationship between friendly equality and informality in the grandparent-grandchild relationship. Research since the 1950s has shown several distinctive themes. These include: socialization processes; reciprocity and mutuality in intergenerational interactions; personhood, individual or personality dimensions of grandparenthood; and values and the process of transmission (Robertson, Tice, & Loeb, 1985; Troll, 1983).

Theoretical Approaches

Similar to other research on the family, investigations of the grandparent-grandchild connection have been largely atheoretical. Sociological and developmental theories have been used most frequently. Some of the earliest studies of grandparenthood were based upon psychoanalytic theories. Most of this research emphasized the negative aspects of the role upon the psychological development of the child (Abraham, 1955; Rappaport, 1958). Kahana and Kahana (1970) incorporated Piaget's developmental perspective and examined the changing meaning of grandparent for grandchildren according to age. Their results showed the importance of level of cognitive maturity to children's perceptions of grandparents. Similarly, Neugarten and Weinstein (1964), Robertson (1977), and Wood and Robertson (1976) used a psychodynamic framework and found developmental differences in the meaning of the grandparent role. These findings support Hagestad and Burton (1986) who emphasized the importance of psychodynamic theories in the grandparent-grandchild interpretive process. Psychosocial frameworks have also been used in studies of grandparenthood. Kivnick (1982), using a deprivation-compensation model, found that adults enhanced their mental health through the grandparent role. The role assisted them in maximizing psychological and circumstantial strengths, in reworking psychosocial deficits, and in compensating for circumstantial weaknesses.

Sociological theory has served most frequently as the theoretical base for research on the grandparent-grandchild connection. Included here is role theory (Fischer, 1983) and socialization theory (Neugarten & Weinstein, 1964; Robertson, 1975). The results of several studies suggest the utility of other sociological theories in grandparent research. These include exchange theory (Johnson, 1983) and attribution theory (Bengtson & Kuypers, 1971).

In summary, few studies of the grandparent-grandchild connection have been theoretically based. Theories most frequently used have been developmental, psychosocial, and sociological in type. There is considerable support for the increased use of developmental and socialization frameworks. Bengtson and Dowd (1980) noted the lack of articulation between mainstream sociological theory and the work of social gerontologists. They recommended the importance of sociological theories such as structural-functionism and exchange theories in explanations of life course phenomena and especially as they apply to intergenerational relationships.

The Grandparent Role

Norms of Familism

Grandparenthood is frequently referred to as a roleless role because of its absence of overtly prescribed functions (Troll, 1983). This assumption is perpetuated by a wide diversity of grandparenting styles. Role norms are present but they vary in specificity and strength relative to other family norms (Johnson, 1983). Johnson, in her cultural analysis of grandmothers of divorced children, found explicit norms of grandparenting. However, unlike norms associated with more primary family roles, they were proscriptive rather than prescriptive. Grandmothers usually juxtaposed prescriptions with proscriptions and weighed what they should do against what they should not do. Johnson attributed this observation to the auxiliary and subordinate functions grandparents have relative to parental responsibilities. She found norm specificity was further confused by a lack of directives as to who allocates the functions of the grandmother's role.

Several family researchers have suggested how families deal with the lack of norm specificity. Albrecht (1954) identified a "hands off" policy among grandparents. This she attributed to the perspective that grandparents have neither the right nor the obligation to take an active part in the socialization of grandchildren. Grandparents and parents also deal with sensitive areas, or normless domains, by declaring "demilitarized zones" that ward off grandparent intrusion (Hagestad, 1978). Cherlin and Furstenberg (1986) described this phenomenon as the "norm of noninterference." They suggested that the power of the norm reflects the ascendancy of the husband-wife bond over the parent-child bond. Kornhaber and Woodward (1981) referred to a new "social contract." Implicit here is the understanding that grandparents and children will not interfere in the lives of the other. Kornhaber (1985) blamed this covenant, as did Albrecht (1954), for creating an emotional disconnection between generations. Kornhaber attributed this disconnection to role abdication by grandparents through their emphasis on individualism and narcissism and their lack of commitment to grandchildren.

Socialization to the grandparent role, is particularly weak in American society (Johnson, 1983). Conditioning to the role has been found to be primarily based upon exposure to a grandparent. This modelling is thought to be more positive if the grandparent model is active and contemporary in type. Neugarten and Weinstein (1964) and Cunningham-Burley (1985) observed anticipatory socialization to the grandparent role, especially among women. Adult children, too, serve as important socializing agents to the grandparent role through their mediation of the grandparent-grandchild relationship (Robertson, 1975).

Norms are especially unclear for certain variant grandparent roles. Primary among these roles is that of stepgrandparents. Kalish and Visher (1981) discussed in detail numerous scenarios in which stepgrandparents may become confused as to their function and role. Role norms lack clarity, too, among greatgrandparents. Greatgrandparents must stand aside and make way for the new grandparents, their children, who in turn try to maintain the norm of noninterference. With each successive generation, expectations, responsibility, and credit for the youngest generation become more relaxed.

Role Interpretations

Concepts and Meaning

Concepts of the grandparent role have come from four sources: informal norms and myths, ex post facto research data, the clinical literature, and studies focusing directly on the role (Robertson, 1977). Early concepts of the role projected images of aged, loving, bespectacled adults (particularly grandmothers), and stern and authoritative grandfathers. Grandparents were also seen as overbearing individuals exerting negative influences on the development of grandchildren (Abraham, 1955; Kahana & Kahana, 1971; Rappaport, 1958).

Kivnick (1983) showed the multidimensional meaning of grandparenthood. Elaborating on Kahana and Kahana's (1971) earlier conceptual model of levels of analyses of grandparenthood, she found five dimensions of grandparent meaning. These included: centrality of meaning, valued elder, immortality through clan, reinvolvement with personal past, and indulgence (of grandchildren). Wentowski (1985) observed that meanings of immortality through clan were especially strong among greatgrandparents. Greatgrandchildren were viewed as a validation of family success and vitality.

Others, too, have demonstrated the important psychological dimensions of grandparenthood. Neugarten and Weinstein (1964) observed five psychological meanings of grandparenthood among middle-class adults. These were biological renewal, emotional self-fulfillment, vicarious accomplishments through grandchildren, resource person (satisfaction accruing from), and remoteness. The overall feeling or meaning of grandparenthood is thought to be a feeling generalized from the quality of the relationship with one or more grandchildren (Cherlin & Furstenberg, 1986).

There is little information on the role concepts of grandfather, stepgrandparent, and greatgrandparent. Several problems contribute to this observation. They include restricted subject types, difficulties in operational definitions, and diversity of constructs. Only a narrow range of dimensions of the grandparent role, mostly styles of interaction, have been examined (Blieszner, 1986). Few results or viewpoints are comparable. Some of the problems in conceptualizing grandparent roles are methodological. Johnson (1983) had considerable difficulty in formulating questions to capture perceptions of the role. Sprey and Matthews (1982) concluded that role clarification would be increased if interpreted in the context of family structure and life cycle transition.

In sum, concepts of both roles in the grandparent-grandchild connection are lacking in dimensions, context, and comparability. Vagueness in role concept may also lie in inappropriate methodology and conceptual designs.

Value

There are differences in opinion about the importance of the grandparent-grandchild connection. Fischer (1983) attributed part of this confusion to the multiple connotations of the grandparent term. She found at least four meanings attached to the role: older women, generation, prescriptions for behavior, and grandparenthood as a social status or a position in society. Conclusions regarding the value depend upon the definition used. Most studies devaluing the role appeared in the earlier literature and are described by Robertson (1977). Research through the 1970's indicated only limited significance of the role for most persons (Wood & Robertson, 1976). Troll warned of problems associated with "too much grandparenting" or "Goldilocks effect" (Hess & Waring, 1978). She reported that too much may be associated with "family troubles." Similarly, Tinsley and Parke (1982) indicated that a high degree of connection is not necessarily always positive for grandparents, especially when they are the recipients of frequent contact from their adult children. More recently, the literature has spoken to the value of the connection. Most sociologists and psychologists who stress the importance of the connection focus on either a symbolic, supportive, or interactive dimension (Fischer, 1983). Values are cited in gains to the grandparent, parents, and grandchild. Both grandchildren and grandparents generally assign importance to their connection.

Grandparenthood would appear to have both social and personal values. The grandparent role provides a primary group reference for many adults (Wood & Robertson, 1976). It also serves as a vehicle for expansion of self and social identity, especially for grandmothers (Timberlake, 1981). Timberlake found that the role filled a need for creativity, accomplishment, and competence among women and added structure and stability to life. Others, too, have made the point that grandchildren serve to anchor older adults in the social structure from which they are losing hold (Kahana & Coe, 1969). Some have observed that grandparenthood may have a compensatory function. It offers individuals, especially men who were busily involved in earlier years, a second chance at parenting (Nahemow, 1985). The grandchild role may also take on symbolic importance, especially among greatgrandparents (Fischer, 1983; Wentowski, 1985). Hagestad and Burton (1986) pointed out that an important value of the grandparent-grandchild connection may be the model the grandparents (especially the very old) establish for the resolution of late life tasks. Others have accredited grandparents as providing the final validation of life (Taylor, 1948). Grandparents, too, stand as "symbols of change" to the younger generations. They add continuity between the past and future through oral and written history (Mead, 1970). They are important in value transmission (Bengtson & Kuypers, 1971).

There is considerable evidence of the value of grandparents to the family. Grandparents are valued for their backup, watch dog, safety valve, and stabilizing functions in divorce and other family disruptions (Albrecht, 1954; Hagestad, 1985; Johnson, 1983; Troll, 1983). They are also valued as preservers of family ties (Troll, 1983) and as "wardens of culture" (Gutmann, 1985). Grandparents are one of the few constant objects in the lives of some children (Kornhaber & Woodward, 1981). Hagestad (1985) pointed out the "elusive being" function of grandparents. This function she saw as a type of comforting presence that grandparents provide families. Kornhaber and Woodward (1981) supported this view through their observation that no matter how grandparents act, they affect the emotional well-being of their grandchildren, for better or worst, simply because they exist (p. xii). Grandparents may play important "surrogate parent" roles during economic and historical distress. Grandparents, too, are valued for their gifts. They, in certain economic situations, have been found to maintain family living standards when grandchildren are young (Wilson, 1987). Grandmothers, however, are more important than grandfathers in continuity of support (Wilson, 1987). Some studies have shown the important confidant or arbitrator role that grandparents play in adolescent-parent relations (Baranowski, 1982; Stevens, 1984). Others have discussed the emotional support that grandmothers provide parents (Tinsley & Parke, 1982).

The interactive value of the grandparent role is also important to the cognitive development of young children (Tinsley & Parke, 1982). Some have addressed the significant mediating role of grandmothers in the successful functioning of the mother-child unit (Troll, 1983). Positive perceptions of the elderly have also been attributed to grandparent-grandchild interaction.

In summary, most literature on the grandparent-grandchild connection points out the value of the role to both grandparents, adult children, and grandchildren. Values derived from the connection vary greatly in type, depending upon the developmental needs of the individual, family dynamics, and family resources. The value from the connection may be either direct or indirect to the grandparent, adult child, or grandchild. There is some indication that there may be less value in the role of grandfather than grandmother. This observation, however, may be related to a lack of sensitivity to gender differences in the measurement of intergenerational interaction and exchanges.

Styles

Several factors interact with one another to determine grandparenting styles. These factors also affect life styles, an important predictor of the saliency of the grandparent role. They include: employment, age, education and marital status of the grandparent, number of grandchildren, and number and types of competing roles (Robertson, 1977; Wood & Robertson, 1976). A wide variety of styles exist on a continuum of heavy involvement to remoteness. Three typologies of note are found in the literature. Several parallels may be seen between them in extent and type of involvement with grandchildren and normative expectations. Neugarten and Weinstein (1964) observed five grandparenting styles among upper-middle and lower-middle class adults aged 50 to 60. These included: formal type, fun seeker, surrogate, reservoir of family wisdom, and distant figure. Formal types followed strict prescribed roles, fun seekers emphasized informality and mutual satisfaction in interactions. The surrogate type (mostly grandmothers) replaced mother roles which were usually started by the younger generation. The reservoir of wisdom type represented a distinctly authoritarian grandparent-grandchild relationship (usually grandfathers), and the distant figure type played only an intermittent role. Age was an important factor in grandparent styles.

Robertson observed a somewhat wider age range (40 years and over) of only grandmothers and found four distinct types of grandparenting according to role meaning (1977). She found an apportioned type who was equally divided between "doing what was right" for their grandchildren and placing emphasis on personal satisfaction. They were also more likely to be indulging grandparents. The second type, symbolic, placed little emphasis on the personal dimensions of the relationship but much on the sources of satisfaction of the role. The third type, individualized, had little regard for normative expectations and placed emphasis on grandparenthood as a source of satisfaction. The fourth type, which resembled Neugarten and Weinstein's (1964) distant figure type, was seldom involved with grandchildren. Similarly, they placed little emphasis on either the social or personal aspects of the relationship. Robertson's grandparenting styles, similar to those of Neugarten and Weinstein (1964), were associated with age of grandparent. They were, however, more associated with normative expectations than those of Neugarten and Weinstein. Cherlin and Furstenberg's (1985) data on 510 men and women 45 years and older showed three grandparent types: detached, passive, and active. Most grandparents fell into the active group which contained three styles of interaction: supportive, authoritative, and influential. Their research supported others' findings of the wide range and quality of the grandparent-grandchild connection.

In conclusion, several typologies of grandparenting styles have been identified. There is no single dominant style. Considerable variation is found between typologies. Each typology differs in number of styles identified. Styles are similar in the extent to which each varies on a continuum of high to low involvement with grandchildren.

FACTORS MEDIATING
THE GRANDPARENT-GRANDCHILD
CONNECTION

Several factors influence the grandparent-grandchild nexus. These effects account in large measure for the diversity of findings in the literature regarding the link and the loose structure of the connection.

Age and Role Timing

The median age of grandparenthood in the United States is 45 years (Sprey & Matthews, 1982) and it has remained fairly consistent throughout this century (Hagestad, 1985). Ranges, however, may be from approximately 25 years to 100 or more years. It is possible for grandchildren to range from newborn to 60 or more years of age. As these ranges might suggest, the ages of grandparent and grandchild are among the most frequently cited factors influencing the linkage. In general, the grandparent becomes less actively involved with age (Johnson, 1983; Sprey & Matthews, 1982; Thomas, 1986). Grandparenthood has been likened to occupational careers. It, for example, has distinctive stages related to the ages of the grandparent and to the grandchild (Cherlin & Furstenberg, 1986). The first stage of grandparenthood spans from birth to the teenage years when grandparents are most involved. The second stage, the teenage years is characterized by less involvement. The last stage, adulthood, may bring about more involvement if grandchildren live nearby (Sprey & Matthews, 1982). Other than diminishing energy levels, age differences in grandparenting behaviors have been attributed to cohort variations in grandparenting behaviors (Neugarten & Weinstein, 1964). Age related differences also have been associated with competing extrafamilial roles, such as those of friend (Johnson, 1983), work, and community (McPherson, 1983). Shifts in grandparenting styles according to children's age are thought to occur as a result of grandchildren's changing developmental needs. These needs, in turn, influence their perceptions of grandparents (Kahana & Kahana, 1970). The important mediating function of parents in the grandparent-grandchild connection also is seen to decrease with the age of the grandchild (Sprey & Matthews, 1982).

The timing of grandparenthood is associated with differences in grandparenting. When the role is "on schedule," individuals have time to prepare for the anticipated transition by reorienting their expectations (Hagestad & Burton, 1986). The "on schedule" role is also less likely to conflict with the age identity of the adult and with other of his or her developmental needs (Burton, 1985). In this regard, some have referred to the importance of interacting timetables in the family (Hagestad & Burton, 1986). When the grandparent role is on schedule, more social support is available through peer and cultural approval (Hagestad & Burton, 1986). The chronological occurrence of grandparenthood would seem to be of less importance than its expected sequence in the life course.

Ethnic and Racial Diversity

Wide cultural differences may be observed in the grandparent-grandchild relationship. Apple (1956), in an analysis of 75 societies, found that cultural factors were paramount to the grandparent-grandchild connection. Relationships were structured upon the degree of authority held by the grandparent, especially by grandfathers. Friendly equality increased with decreased authority.

The grandparent role is more salient in ethnic groups than in the dominant culture (Barresi, 1987). Examples can be seen in the traditional structure of ethnic families. The saliency of the grandparent role can also be observed in the surrogate parental role frequently assumed by older Native Americans, Blacks, and Hispanics (Cherlin & Furstenberg, 1986; Lee, 1980; Lubben & Becerra, 1987; Markides & Mindel, 1987). Similarly, older Amish grandparents remain active participants in the running of the family farm and in the management of the extended household (Brubaker & Michael, 1987). These ethnic elders as well as Mexicans and Chinese are also more likely than whites to live in the household with grandchildren

(Lubben & Becerra, 1987). All groups vary, however, in amount of contact with grandchildren and types and patterns of exchange. Ethnic grandparents frequently assume functional centrality in the family out of economic necessity of one or both generations. Role centrality, nonetheless, cannot be attributed in total to social class differences (Lee, 1980).

The important function of the black family as a social and psychological refuge for individual members is a common theme in the literature (Markides & Mindel, 1987). Black grandmothers are more likely to take on a parent role with grandchildren than white grandmothers. The more important functional role of black grandmothers over that of white grandmothers is suggested by differences in household structure. For example, 40% of families headed by black elderly compared to 10% of families headed by older white women take in dependent children under 18 years of age (Tate, 1983). Data show that as many as two-thirds of black children under 18 living with relatives (approximately 11%) are grandchildren (Tate, 1983). Many black grandparents have been found to serve as a point of anchorage. They are less likely than whites to adopt norms of noninterference, especially when children are single parents (Kornhaber & Woodward, 1981). Frequently they operate as individual departments of welfare by providing supports for grandchildren unavailable from their own families (Cherlin & Furstenberg, 1986). Considerable reciprocation of goods, services, and emotional support is thought to occur between young and old blacks. Reciprocation is especially frequent in absorbed households, for example, exchanges of services and goods for shelter. There have been tendencies to romanticize the role of the black grandmother (Black Granny). The stereotyped matriarchal image of the black grandmother who dominates all family roles also has been criticized (Jackson, 1986).

Social Class

The few specific studies looking at the importance of social class to grandparenting have shown little relationship. Cherlin and Furstenberg (1985) found little evidence of socioeconomic differences in grandparenting styles. No class differences were found in the extent of contact, service exchange, or value transmission. The absence of class differences pointed to several factors: the continuing strength of the grandparent-grandchild connection, the erosion of class differences in family life, and the levelling effects of dominant life events such as geographical moves, divorce, and war. Cherlin and Furstenberg's finding relative to the erosion of class differences supported an earlier observation by Clavan (1978). She reported a moving of middle-class attitudes and behaviors patterns towards those traditionally associated with families of lower socioeconomic status.

Geographical Distance

There is considerable support for the important relationship between amount of family contact, support, and geographical distance. Cherlin and Furstenberg (1986) found that distance accounted for 62% of the variance in number of visits per year between grandparents and grandchildren. Kivett (1985) observed that proximity was the most important predictor of association between grandfathers and grandchildren. Similarly, Wilson (1987) and Tinsley and Parke (1982) reported a relationship between support received and geographical distance. In general, contact and support decrease with increased distance. The distance-contact relationship illustrates both the strengths and vulnerability of the grandparent-grandchild connection (Cherlin & Furstenberg, 1986). Few studies have examined the effect of distance on the quality of grandparent-grandchild relationships.

Gender Differences

Information on gender differences in the grandparent-grandchild connection supports the long tradition of sociological research in the family. These findings show the relative importance of female roles over those of males. Included here are the significance of the mother-daughter bond and the importance of women as "kin keepers" and "lineage bridges." The implication for the grandparent-grandchild connection is that grandchildren become more involved with maternal than paternal grandparents. Matthews and Sprey (1985) found gender differences in kin position to be more important to the grandparent-grandchild connection than gender differences per se. Relationships were closer with maternal grandparents.

Similarly, Fischer (1983) observed that grandmothers favored a daughter's child over that of a son. Still others have found that young adult grandchildren rate their relationship with maternal grandmothers higher than that with other grandparent-grandchild links (Hartshorne & Manaster, 1982). Maternal grandmothers, regardless of social class, have been reported to give more assistance than other grandparents.

Sex role differences also have been cited in the grandparent-grandchild linkage. Most of these have to do with sex role orientation and type of help provided. Cherlin and Furstenberg (1986) found gender differences in grandparenting. They observed these to break down along sex-typed traditional lines with grandfathers providing more instrumental help and grandmothers giving more expressive assistance. These findings supported earlier reports of Hagestad (1985). Compatible with this observation is the finding that grandmothers have warmer, more expressive relationships with grandchildren than grandfathers (Cherlin & Furstenberg, 1986). There is some support for the psychodynamic view of age-related increases in nurturance among men and the increasing instrumentality of women with age. Thomas (1986) found high levels of responsibility for grandchildren among grandfathers. Gender role differences in grandparenting might be expected among current cohorts of middle aged and older adults given their earlier socialization. Despite recent changes in sex distribution of work, traditional differences would seem to be maintained in grandparents as they are in parents (Troll, 1983).

Some studies have shown the importance of the sex of the grandchild to the grandparent relationship. Cherlin and Furstenberg (1986) and Hagestad (1985) found that sex of grandchild meant more to grandfathers than to grandmothers, especially in exchanges. Grandfather-grandson exchanges were more frequent and instrumental in nature.

Parental Mediation

The grandparent-grandchild connection is closely related to the mediating role of the middle generation. Parents specify both grandparent and grandchild roles by setting conditions and providing the structure for their relationship. Feelings of affect between generations impact parents' mediation. Cherlin and Furstenberg (1986) observed that grandparents tend to "selectively invest" in one or more grandchildren. This process was based, among other factors, on their feelings of closeness to the parent of the grandchild. The quality of relations between a grandparent and a daughter or daughter-in-law (gatekeepers) can be a major factor in the grandparent-grandchild relationship. Lopata (1973), found that widows' tensions with the middle generation diminished their satisfaction with the grandmother role. Similarly, Bengtson, Olander, and Haddad (1976) spoke to the threatening nature of cohort or lineage gaps to the intergenerational family bond.

The mediating function of parents varies in some situations. Parental mediation has been found to decline with the increasing age of a grandchild (Sprey & Matthews, 1982), and to be less important in adult granddaughter to grandmother connections than in other connections (Thompson & Walker, 1987). The amount of grandchild-grandparent contact, too, affects the mediating role of parents. Thompson and Walker (1987) found that mothers served as mediators of young adult-grandmother relations only under low contact situations. That is, when contacts were high, young adult granddaughters mediated their own relationship with grandmothers. Robertson (1975), using socialization theory, identified eight dimensions of mediation which socialize both grandparents and grandchildren to their respective roles. The majority of the dimensions was perceptual on the part of the parents. They included their perceptions of: the significance of grandparenthood, appropriate grandparent behaviors, appropriate initiator of grandparent behavior, and extent of equity in mediation. Other dimensions included the means, frequency, and focus of mediation, and attitude toward mediation.

Disruptive Life Events

Divorce

Thirty-three percent of persons 65 years and older are stepgrandparents (Cherlin & Furstenberg, 1986). Increasing divorce rates have significantly heightened interest in grandparenthood. Divorce disrupts established intergenerational links by changing the balance of resources within the extended family. As a result, established bonds must be renegotiated (Matthews, 1984). Several factors figure into successful renegotiation. These include: who is the custodial parent, outcomes of the new grandparent role in remarriage, and perceptions of the grandchildren of the reconstituted family (Kalish & Visher, 1981). The grandparent-stepgrandchild connection is stronger if the children are young when they become members of the family (Sanders & Trygstad, 1989). It is stronger also if stepgrandchildren live full-time with the grandparents' adult child (Cherlin & Furstenberg, 1986). The grandparent-grandchild connection is threatened when the custodial parent is affinal kin.

There has been a strong movement during the past two decades toward legal rights for grandparents in cases of family disruption (Bean, 1986; Blau, 1984; Foster & Freed, 1981; George, 1987; Kalish & Visher, 1981; Shandling, 1986; Wilson, 1982). This action is due to growing divorce rates and the increasing numbers of older adults and their associated political power. Courts are also recognizing grandparents as providing an important sanctuary for children. Nearly every state has adopted statutory provisions for court-ordered grandparent or third party visitation (Bean, 1986). States vary considerably, however, in provisions. Grandparent visitation legislation only assures grandparents the legal right to be heard in court. Most court decisions are based upon the court's determination of whether visitation is in the child's best interest. What constitutes a child's best interest remains a controversial legal and clinical question. Current issues facing courts in visitation rights decisions include: animosities of adult parties; effects of adoption, especially by stepparents; the legal rights of biological grandparents; centrality of the grandchild in intrafamilial disputes; and judicial prudence in intrusion into intact families. An overall issue is the impact of court-awarded visitation rights on parental authority. Custody, too, is an issue facing the courts. In such cases, parents must be declared as unfit or unable to meet the child's basic needs. In these instances, it is usually the non-parent who has had *de facto* custody or *in loco parentis* who gains custody (Foster & Freed, 1981).

Contacts with grandchildren have been found to increase among grandmothers following a child's separation or divorce (Gladstone, 1988). In general, high levels of contact are maintained with consanguinal relatives while a decrease occurs with affinal kin. Maternal grandmothers are especially active (Sprey & Matthews, 1982). Johnson (1983) found that when children divorced, grandmothers' role potentially functions in several directions (or coalitions): between grandmothers and the divorced child, between grandchild and the parent, and even between her child and his or her spouse. Frequently, grandmothers' ambivalence in knowing "how much to do" presented a major personal dilemma.

Other Disruptive Events

Poor health of grandparents also can affect the grandparent-grandchild connection through a lessening of contacts and instrumental exchanges (Cherlin & Furstenberg, 1986). Institutionalization, especially, has been observed to reduce the importance of the grandparent role (Kahana & Coe, 1969; McPherson, 1983). In contrast, historic events often serve to heighten the role of grandparent. Examples may be seen during war and post-war crises which frequently precipitate divorce, spousal desertion, and shortage of resources (Von Hentig, 1946). Critical life events such as widowhood also may increase the saliency of the grandparent role (McPherson, 1983).

In summary, the grandparent-grandchild connection is largely indirect. The many factors mediating the relationship account for the difficulty in articulating norms of behavior, functions, and role value and meaning. In addition, several factors interact adding increased complexity to the interpretation of the relationship.

CONCLUSIONS

Grandparenthood is characterized by its diverse and its symbolic and functional qualities. The grandparent-grandchild connection plays a pivotal role in bridging generations. It is less defined and more poorly understood, however, than other more primary family connections. This occurrence is related to its largely voluntaristic and subordinate nature. Yet its discretionary and individualistic character is not unlike that of other contemporary American family linkages. The meaning, function, and value of grandparenthood must be interpreted in context of: whether the role is expected or anticipated, if it is appropriately timed (on schedule), and if it is synchronous with other life events or circumstances. A multiplicity of factors mediate the grandparent-grandchild connection which serve to add diversity and tenuousness to the link. Role expectations for the grandparent-grandchild connection are unclear except, perhaps, when the resources of either party are called upon. The grandparent-grandchild link, becomes more heightened during family crises. At these times the role provides important and unique insights into family organizational processes.

Despite increasing research on the grandparent-grandchild connection, the dynamics and functions of the link are poorly understood. This is due to its atheoretical, noncumulative, and fragmentary nature. Conceptual issues include the need to examine the connection within a broader system of relationships; to conceptualize the link as indirect, particularistic bonds rather than as roles; to focus on grandparents' relationships with specific children (or sets) rather than on the global significance and meaning of the role (Sprey & Matthews, 1982); and to base studies upon a life span perspective. Conceptual issues also center around the increased use of theoretical frameworks, and the development of mid-range theories. Other theoretical issues deal with instrumentation and the ability to pose questions or structure observations that adequately measure role perceptions.

Little is known of the relative contribution of grandparents to that of other members of the extended family. Further research is needed on the impact of the grandparent on children's social and cognitive status at different points in development (Tinsley & Parke, 1982). Of empirical interest also is the effect of the grandchild upon the grandparent's continuing development, especially as it relates to the completion of final life tasks. Research is needed, too, on the nature and quality of grandparent-grandchild connections arising from newer family forms.

There is increasing acknowledgement of the importance of the grandparent-grandchild connection and of the subsequent need to enhance natural grandparenting. Examples are seen in increased legislation to secure grandparents' rights, the proclamation of Grandparents' Day, and the establishment of foundations for grandparents (Robertson et al., 1985). Several intergenerational programs have incorporated the socializing function of grandparents in educational institutions and other agencies of socialization (Tice, 1982). The major premise underlying these efforts is the need to enhance and maintain the integrating function of grandparent-hood — a significant factor in the bridging of generations and the transmission of culture and values.

REFERENCES

Albrecht, R. (1954). The parental responsibilities of grandparents. *Marriage and Family Living, 16,* 201-204.

Apple D. (1956). The social structure of grandparenthood. *American Anthropologist, 58,* 656-663.

Baranowski, M. D. (1982). Grandparent-adolescent relations: Beyond the nuclear family. *Adolescence, 17,* 575-584.

Barranti, C. C. R. (1985). The grandparent/grandchild relationship: Family resource in an era of voluntary bonds. *Family Relations, 34,* 343-352.

Barresi, C. M. (1987). Ethnic aging and the life course. In D. E. Gelfand & C. M. Barresi (Eds.), *Ethnic dimensions of aging* (pp. 18-34). New York: Springer Publishing Company.

Bean, K. S. (1986). Grandparent visitation: Can the parent refuse? *Journal of Family Law, 24,* 393-449.

Bengtson, V. L., & Dowd, J. J. (1980). Sociological functionalism, exchange theory and life-cycle analysis: A call for more explicit theoretical bridges. *International Journal of Aging and Human Development, 12,* 55-73.

Bengtson, V. L., & Kuypers, J. A. (1971). Generational differences and the developmental stake. *Aging and Human Development, 2,* 249-259.

Bengtson, V. L., Olander, E. B., & Haddad, A. A. (1976). The generation gap and aging family members: Toward a conceptual model. In J. G. Gubrium (Ed.), *Times, roles, & self in old age* (pp. 237-263). New York: Human Sciences Press.

Blau, T. H. (1984). An evaluative study of the role of the grandparent in the best interests of the child. *The American Journal of Family Therapy, 12,* 46-50.

Blieszner, R. (1986). Trends in family gerontology research. *Family Relations, 35,* 555-562.

Brody, E. (1979). Aged parents and aging children. In P. K. Ragan (Ed.), *Aging Parents* (pp. 267-287). Los Angeles: University of Southern California Press.

Brubaker, T. H., & Michael, C. M. (1987). Amish families in later life. In D. E. Gelfand & C. M. Barresi (Eds.), *Ethnic dimensions of aging* (pp. 106-117). New York: Springer Publishing Company.

Burton, L. M. (1985). Early and on-time grandmotherhood in multigenerational black families. *Dissertation Abstracts International, 46,* 1409A-1410A.

Cherlin, A., & Furstenberg, F., Jr. (1985). Styles and strategies of grandparenting. In V. L. Bengtson & J. F. Robertson (Eds.), *Grandparenthood* (pp. 47-116). Beverly Hills, CA: Sage Publications, Inc.

Cherlin, A., & Furstenberg, F., Jr. (1986). *The new American grandparent*. New York: Basic Books, Inc.

Clavan, S. (1978). The impact of social class and social trends on the role of grandparents. *The Family Coordinator, 27*, 351-357.

Crawford, M. (1981). Not disengaged: Grandparents in literature and reality, an empirical study in role satisfaction. *Sociological Review, 29*, 499-519.

Cunningham-Burley, S. (1985). Constructing grandparenthood—anticipating appropriate action. *Sociology, 19*, 421-436.

Fischer, L. R. (1983). Transition to grandmotherhood. *International Journal of Aging and Human Development, 16*, 67-78.

Foster, H. H., Jr., & Freed, D. J. (1981). Grandparent visitation: Vagaries and vicissitudes. *Journal of Divorce, 5*, 79-100.

George, J. (1987). Children and grandparents: The right to visit. *Children's Legal Rights Journal, 8*, 2-8.

Gladstone, J. W. (1988). Perceived changes in grandmother-grandchild relations following a child's separation or divorce. *Gerontologist, 28*, 66-72.

Gutmann, D. L. (1985). Deculturation and the American grandparent. In V. L. Bengtson & J. F. Robertson (Eds.), *Grandparenthood*, (pp. 173-181). Beverly Hills, CA: Sage Publications.

Hagestad, G. (1978). *Patterns of communication and influence between grandparents and grandchildren in a changing society*. Paper presented at the World Congress of Sociology, Sweden.

Hagestad, G. (1982). Parent and child: Generations in the family. In T. M. Field, A. Huston, H. C. Quay, L. Troll, & G. E. Finley (Eds.), *Review of human development* (pp. 485-499). New York: Wiley.

Hagestad, G. (1985). Continuity and connectedness. In V. L. Bengtson & J. F. Robertson (Eds.), *Grandparenthood* (pp. 31-48). Beverly Hills, CA: Sage Publications.

Hagestad, G. O., & Burton, L. M. (1986). Grandparenthood, life context and family development. *The American Behavioral Scientist, 29*, 471-484.

Harris, L., & Associates (1975). *The myth and reality of aging in America*. New York: National Council on Aging.

Hartshorne, T. S., & Manaster, G. J. (1982). The relationship with grandparents: Contact, importance, role conception. *International Journal of Aging and Human Development, 15*, 233-245.

Hess, B., & Waring, J. M. (1978). Parent and child in later life: Rethinking the relationship. In R. M. Lerner & G. B. Spanier (Eds.), *Child influences on marital and family interaction: A life span perspective* (pp. 241-273). New York: Academic.

Jackson, J. (1986). Black grandparents: Who needs them? In R. Staples (Ed.), *The black family: Essays and studies* (pp. 186-194). Belmont, CA: Wadsworth Publishing Company, Inc.

Johnson, C. (1983). A cultural analysis of the grandmother. *Research on Aging*, *5*, 547-568.

Kahana, E., & Coe, R. M. (1969). Perceptions of grandparenthood by community and institutionalized age. *Procedures of the 77th Anniversary Convention of the American Psychological Association*, *4*, 735-736.

Kahana, B. & Kahana, E. (1970). Grandparenthood from the perspective of the developing grandchild. *Developmental Psychology*, *3*, 98-105.

Kahana, E. & Kahana, B. (1971). Theoretical and research perspectives on grandparenthood. *Aging and Human Development*, *2*, 261-268.

Kalish, R. A., & Visher, E. (1981). Grandparents of divorce and remarriage. *Journal of Divorce*, *5*, 127-140.

Kivett, V. R. (1985). Grandfathers and grandchildren: Patterns of association, helping, and psychological closeness. *Family Relations*, *34*, 565-571.

Kivnick, H. Q. (1982). Grandparenthood: An overview of meaning and mental health. *Gerontologist*, *22*, 59-66.

Kivnick, H. Q. (1983). Dimensions of grandparenthood meaning: Deductive conceptualization and empirical derivation. *Journal of Personality and Social Psychology*, *44*, 1056-1068.

Kornhaber, A. (1985). Grandparenthood and the "new social contract." In V. L. Bengtson & J. F. Robertson (Eds.), *Grandparenthood* (pp. 159-171). Beverly Hills, CA: Sage Publications.

Kornhaber, A., & Woodward, K. (1981). *Grandparents/grandchildren: The vital connection*. Garden City, New York: Anchor Press/Doubleday.

Kruse, A. (1984). The five-generation family: A pilot study. In V. Grams-Homolova, E. M. Hoerning, & D. Schaeffer (Eds.), *Intergenerational relationships* (pp. 115-125). Lewiston, NY: C. J. Hogrete.

Lee, G. R. (1980). Kinship in the seventies: A decade review of research and theory. *Journal of Marriage and the Family*, *42*, 923-934.

Lopata, H. Z. (1979). *Women as widows: Support systems*. New York, New York: Elsevier North Holland, Inc.

Lubben, J. E., & Becerra, R. M. (1987). Social support among Black, Mexican, and Chinese elderly. In D. E. Gelfand & C. M. Barresi (Eds.), *Ethnic dimensions of aging* (pp. 130-144). New York: Springer Publishing Company.

Markides, K. S., & Mindel, C. H. (1987). *Aging and ethnicity*. Beverly Hills, CA: Sage Publications.

Matthews, S. H. (1984). The impact of divorce on grandparenthood: An exploratory study. *Gerontologist*, *24*, 41-47.

Matthews, S. H., & Sprey, J. (1985). Adolescents' relationships with grandparents: An empirical contribution to conceptual clarification. *Journal of Gerontology*, *40*, 621-626.

McPherson, B. D. (1983). *Aging as a social process*. Toronto, Canada: Butterworths.

Mead, M. (1970). *Culture and commitment: A study of the generation gap*. New York: Basic Books.

Nadel, S. F. (1951). *The social foundations of social anthropology*. Glencoe, IL: The Free Press.

Nahemow, N. (1985). The changing nature of grandparenthood. *Medical Aspects of Human Sexuality, 19,* 175-190.

Neugarten, B. L., & Weinstein, K. K. (1964). The changing American grandparent. *Journal of Marriage and the Family, 26,* 199-204.

Radcliffe-Brown, A. R. (1952). *Structure and function in primitive society*. London: Cohen and West.

Rappaport, E. A. (1958). The grandparent syndrome. *Psychoanalytic Quarterly, 27,* 518-538.

Robertson, J. F. (1975). Interaction in three generation families, parents as mediators: Toward a theoretical perspective. *International Journal of Aging and Human Development, 6,* 103-110.

Robertson, J. (1977). Grandmotherhood: A study of role conceptions. *Journal of Marriage and the Family, 39,* 165-174.

Robertson, J. F., Tice, C. H., Loeb, L. L. (1985). Grandparenthood: From knowledge to programs and policy. In V. L. Bengtson & J. F. Robertson (Eds.), *Grandparenthood* (pp. 211-224). Beverly Hills, CA: Sage Publications.

Sanders, G. F., & Trygstad, D. W. (1989). Stepgrandparents and grandparents: The view from young adults. *Family Relations, 38,* 71-75.

Shanas, E. (1979). The family as a social support system in old age. *The Gerontologist, 19,* 169-174.

Shandling, J. L. (1986). The constitutional constraints on grandparents visitation rights. *Columbia Law Review, 86,* 118-138.

Sprey, J., & Matthews, S. H. (1982). Contemporary grandparenthood: A systemic transition. *Annals of the American Academy of Political & Social Science, 464,* 91-103.

Stevens, J. H., Jr. (1984). Black grandmothers' and black adolescent mothers' knowledge about parenting. *Developmental Psychology, 20,* 1017-1025.

Tate, N. (1983). The black aging experience. In R. L. McNeely & J. L. Colen (Eds.), *Aging in minority groups* (pp. 95-107). Beverly Hills, CA: Sage Publications.

Taylor, K. W. (1948). The opportunities of parenthood. In H. Becker and R. Hill (Eds.), *Family, marriage, and parenthood* (pp. 454-492). Boston: D. C. Heath.

Thomas, J. L. (1986). Age and sex differences in perceptions of grandparenting. *Journal of Gerontology, 41,* 417-423.

Thompson, L., & Walker, A. J. (1987). Mothers as mediators of intimacy between grandmothers and their young adult granddaughters. *Family Relations, 36,* 72-77.

Timberlake, E. M. (1981). The value of grandchildren to grandmothers. *Journal of Gerontological Social Work, 3,* 63-76.

Tice, C. (1982). Linking generations. *New Designs for Youth Development, III,* 1.

Tinsley, B. R., & Parke, R. D. (1982). Grandparents as support and socialization agents. In M. Lewis (Ed.), *Beyond the Dyad* (pp. 161-194). New York: Plenum.

Tinsley, B. R., & Parke, R. D. (1987). Grandparents as interactive and social support agents for families with young infants. *International Journal of Aging and Human Development, 25,* 259-277.

Troll, L. (1980). Grandparenting. In L. Poon (Ed.), *Aging in the 1980's: Psychological issues* (pp. 475-481). Washington, DC: American Psychological Association.

Troll, L. (1983). Grandparents: The family watchdogs. In T. Brubaker (Ed.), *Family relationships in later life* (pp. 63-74). Beverly Hills, CA: Sage.

Von Hentig, H. (1946). The sociological function of the grandmother. *Social Forces, 24,* 389-392.

Wentowski, G. W. (1985). Older women's perceptions of great-grandmotherhood: A research note. *Gerontologist, 25,* 593-596.

Wilson, G. (1987). Women's work: The role of grandparents in intergenerational transfers. *The Sociological Review, 35,* 703-720.

Wilson, K. B. (1982). Legal rights of grandparents: A preliminary discussion. *Gerontologist, 22,* 67-71.

Wood, V., & Robertson, J. F. (1976). The significance of grandparenthood. In J. Gubrium (Ed.), *Times, roles and self in old age* (pp. 278-304). New York: Behavioral Publications.

Sibling Relationships in Adulthood

Victor G. Cicirelli

WHAT IS MEANT BY A CONNECTION BETWEEN SIBLINGS?

The term "siblings" refers to individuals who share common biological parents; when stepsiblings, half-siblings, and adoptive siblings are discussed, they will be referred to specifically as such. (See also Cicirelli, 1985b.) The term "sibling connection" refers to the total of the interactions (actions, verbal and nonverbal communication) of two (or more) individuals who share common parents, as well as their knowledge, perceptions, attitudes, beliefs, and feelings regarding each other from the time when one sibling first became aware of the other. The term "sibling connection" will be used interchangeably with the term "sibling relationship"; it is regarded as having behavioral, cognitive, and affective components and as existing over an extended time period.

Although sibling connections share many characteristics of other human relationships, there are several important differences. Siblings share a common biological heritage from their parents, having from 33% to 66% of their genes in common (Scarr & Gracek, 1982); thus, most sibling pairs are more alike than are unrelated pairs of individuals. Because the sibling relationship is based on a fundamental biological relationship (and is ascribed rather than voluntary), most siblings have a commitment to maintain their relationship. The sibling connection has a longer duration than most other kinds of connections, continuing from birth of the younger member of the pair until the end of the life span. Finally, siblings

---

Victor G. Cicirelli is Professor of Developmental and Aging Psychology, Department of Psychological Sciences, Purdue University, West Lafayette, IN 47907.

291

share a long history of intimate family experiences; although this shared intimacy is true of other family connections as well, the connection between siblings is both more egalitarian and long-lasting.

DO SIBLINGS MAINTAIN A CONNECTION IN ADULTHOOD?

The fact that most older people have at least one living sibling and continue to remain in some kind of contact with that sibling until nearly the end of life is well known. Data have been amply summarized in a number of reviews and will not be repeated here (Cicirelli, 1980, 1985b; Scott, 1983; Troll, 1971).

Sibling relationships are likely to become more important in the years to come as the members of the "baby boom" generation proceed through adulthood and into old age. Not only does this group have a larger number of siblings than do cohorts preceding them, but it is likely that they may come to depend more on the connections with siblings than do the preceding groups as a result of having less stable marriages and fewer children of their own. Thus the sibling connection could conceivably assume a central position in their lives.

SIBLING STRUCTURE

Beyond merely knowing that an individual has a sibling, it is important to know how many children in the family make up the sibship and how the individual is placed within the entire sibling group. The sibling structure is typically described by such variables as the number of siblings, the age, sex, and birth order of each, and the age spacing between them. The more specific one can be about the sibling structure, the better one can understand the connection between an individual and a sibling. Simply identifying a brother-sister connection, for example, conveys far less information than knowing the relationship is between a first-born older brother (aged 45) from a family of five and his last-born and only sister who is 15 years younger.

THE SIBLING SUBSYSTEM

The connection between members of a sibling pair does not occur in isolation, but takes place within the larger context of a family system and the society where it takes place. The sibling subsystem is one of three major subsystems making up the family (the spousal subsystem, the parent-child subsystem, and the sibling subsystem); family systems theory maintains that what happens within any subsystem affects and is affected by events within the other subsystems. In addition, within the family system, more or less stable coalitions of two or more members may be formed based on mutual interests, similar temperament, or power considerations. A sibling coalition constitutes a mini-subsystem within the sibling system as a whole (see Bank & Kahn, 1982a, 1982b; Schvaneveldt & Ihinger, 1979). Finally, it must be remembered that the sibling subsystem is never static but evolves over time as members of the family system are born or die and as individual roles in the system change (Cicirelli, 1985a, 1988).

METHODS OF STUDYING SIBLING CONNECTIONS

Because sibling structure introduces many complexities into the study of sibling connections, a rigorous analysis which takes the effects of sibling structure variables into account should be restricted to subjects of a single family size (e.g., two-child families or three-child families). To represent all the possible sex combinations of siblings in a two-child family as well as the relative age of the siblings (older, younger) involves eight subgroups of siblings; the number goes up geometrically as more sibling structure characteristics (e.g., age spacing) and larger family size are considered in the analysis (Sutton-Smith & Rosenberg, 1970). Such analyses become highly impractical for all but small family sizes; however, ignoring the sibling structure variables means that some confounding will be introduced into the analysis.

Although carefully controlled studies investigating all sibling structure variables are common in the child development literature, studies of adults tend to consider the four sibling sex combinations while the remaining sibling structure variables are free to vary. One reason for this is that larger family sizes are common among older people. Another reason is that significant numbers of older people have at least one dead sibling. On the average about forty percent of the siblings of the elderly are dead, so that only a fragment of the original sibship can be studied.

A problem in deciding the proper unit of analysis arises when an investigator collects data from an individual subject regarding connections with all siblings in a family. If the sibling dyad is taken as the unit of analysis, each individual contributes data regarding more than one dyad; the dyads are not completely independent. Further, a large sibship is represented by more data points than is a small sibship. One way to avoid such a problem is to select only one sibling dyad per subject for use in the analysis. However, devising a consistent criterion for selection of the dyad to be included (e.g., the sibling closest in age) is difficult in actual practice, particularly when some siblings may have died. Another approach is to construct an average score for measures of a subject's connections with all siblings; this is proper only if it can be demonstrated that the average does not mask great disparities between measures for each of the dyads in a family.

It is clear that no analytic procedure is without methodological problems. At the very least, an investigator should make clear how the data are gathered and treated in the analysis so that resulting sources of bias can be recognized.

DIMENSIONS AND TYPES
OF SIBLING CONNECTIONS

Two approaches to the study of sibling connections are found. The first is to describe particular dimensions or qualities of the relationship, while the second is to identify types of sibling relationships. Since connections between siblings are quite variable, depending on the particular individuals involved, the question is not whether variations in sibling connections exist, but what is the most fruitful way to describe them.

Dimensions of Sibling Connections

Closeness and rivalry are the two most intensively studied dimensions of sibling connections. Previous reviews of this literature (e.g., Cicirelli, 1980, 1982, 1985b; Ross & Milgram, 1982) have concluded that the majority of adults feel close or very close to their siblings, with the greatest closeness between sisters and the least closeness between brothers. Closeness to siblings increases through adulthood and into old age. The situation is less clear-cut in regard to sibling rivalry. Rivalry appears to be greatest between pairs of brothers and least between pairs of cross-sex siblings. Further, sibling rivalry declines among the older age groups. Overall, sibling rivalry appears to be relatively low in adulthood, at least when direct measurement is used.

However, studies using more clinical methods of investigation have reported rivalry to be more prevalent in later life than direct reports indicated. Using a volunteer sample of 75 middle-class adults aged 22-93, Ross and Milgram (1982) conducted clinical group interviews to uncover rivalry, arguing that many people find it difficult or shameful to admit to feelings of sibling rivalry in adulthood. They found that 71% of their interviewees admitted feeling rivalry with siblings at some point in their lives, with 45% still feeling rivalry in their adult years. By old age, the renewal and repair of sibling relationships had assumed considerable salience. In extended interviews with 60 men and women over age 65 identified through senior centers, Gold (1989) found some evidence of resentment and envy in approximately half of her sample. Bedford (1989a), using an adaptation of the Thematic Apperception Test to measure rivalry in 60 men and women aged 30-69, found that older adults revealed as many themes of sibling rivalry in their responses as did younger adults, and that women expressed more conflict in their relationships with siblings than did men. She concluded that the projective methodology was tapping feelings not typically reported. Although some feelings of rivalry may indeed persist into old age, the evidence indicates that siblings value their connection highly in the later years and seem to have developed ways of interaction that avoid conflict and overt rivalry.

Sibling connections vary in the degree of the siblings' emotional involvement or indifference. Johnson (1982) found that emotional involvement in the sibling connection was greater among Italian-American adults than those of European Protestant backgrounds. Cicirelli (1985a) found greater indifference to the sibling connection among middle-aged adults than among the elderly, while Gold (1989) found considerable variation in involvement among the sibling dyads she studied. Clinical data (Bank & Kahn, 1982a, 1982b) observed very high levels of emotional involvement among some sibling pairs, with attendant adjustment problems. Certainly this dimension of a sibling connection deserves more serious attention in view of its value in interpreting an individual's position on other dimensions.

The sibling connection has also been characterized by value consensus (Cicirelli, 1979; Ross & Milgram, 1982; Suggs & Kivett, 1987) and by compatibility (Cicirelli, 1985b), with findings regarding both dimensions similar to those found for sibling closeness. A multidimensional approach (Mosatche, Brady, & Noberini, 1983; Noberini, Mosatche, & Brady, 1984) also has been used to describe the dimensions of the sibling connection. These authors found that a profile of several dimensions (e.g., sibling-related activity, admiration, positive affect, and emotional support) changed over the life span, with activity and admiration highest in young adulthood and positive feelings more important in later years.

Types of Sibling Connections

Another approach to the study of sibling connections is the identification of types of connections based on the combination of different variables. Early examples of typologies were those of Sutton-Smith and Rosenberg (1970) and Toman (1976) in which a set of characteristics were associated with a given combination of sibling structure variables, e.g., older sister of brothers.

More recently, Gold (1989) identified five types of sibling connections using constant comparative analysis of qualitative interview data. Based on patterns of psychological involvement, closeness, acceptance/approval, emotional support, instrumental support, contact, envy, and resentment, the five types were: the intimate, the congenial, the loyal, the apathetic, and the hostile. The intimate type is characterized by ardent devotion and psychological closeness, while the congenial type is characterized by friendship and caring, the loyal type by allegiance based on shared family background, the apathetic type by indifference, and the hostile type by resentment, anger, and enmity. Some 78% of all sibling connections studied by Gold fell into the loyal (34%), congenial (30%) and intimate types (14%), enjoying moderate to strong psychological involvement and emotional support. The remaining 22% were divided into the apathetic and hostile types. In a re-analysis of the same data (Gold, Woodbury, & George, 1988) using quantitative grade-of-membership methodology, the first three types were essentially upheld, while the apathetic and hostile types formed a single group. In a second study of sibling connections among blacks (Gold, 1988), 95% of all sibling connections fell into the loyal, congenial, and intimate types, with the loyal (55%) the most predominant.

Although typologies present appealing qualitative pictures of different sorts of sibling connections, they risk misclassifying particular relationships when characteristics making up the type are borderline. Further, overgeneralization may result when the characteristics of the type are uncritically applied to particular individuals. Investigations are needed that seek to determine the stability of type membership over time and the generality of the typology for larger samples and a greater variety of groups.

INFLUENCE OF SIBLINGS ON EACH OTHER

Since sibling connections continue to exist through adulthood, there is an opportunity for continued sibling influence on each other. Such influence can be an indirect expression of sibling structure variables or it can be the direct effect of interaction between the siblings.

Informal observations suggest that siblings can exert influence on one another by serving as models to emulate in dealing with such major life events as illness, retirement, and preparation for death, or by serving as teachers of particular skills and knowledge in certain situations. However, such effects have yet to be demonstrated systematically.

Siblings and Well-Being

Whether the sibling connection leads to greater well-being in old age is open to question. Both positive and negative evidence is present in the literature. In an early study, Cumming and Henry (1961) found that elderly people with living siblings had higher morale than those who did not. Cicirelli (1977, 1980) found that those elderly with more frequent interaction with siblings had a greater sense of control in life. Additionally, men with sisters had a greater sense of emotional security whereas women with sisters were stimulated and challenged in their social roles. However, a large-sample study (Lee & Ihinger-Tallman, 1980) failed to find a significant relationship between frequency of interaction with the sibling whom older people saw most frequently and a measure of morale, even when a large number of control variables were taken into account. A more recent study (McGhee, 1985) confirmed the negative findings of Lee and Ihinger-Tallman with regard to the effect of frequency of sibling interaction but found that the mere availability of a sister was related to greater life satisfaction. McGhee's results suggest that any positive effects of a relationship with siblings on morale and adjustment derives from the simple existence of the relationship and not from the frequency with which the siblings interact. O'Bryant (1988) examined sibling support and older widows' well-being and found that interaction with married sisters predicted higher positive effect among older widows. The relationship was more complex than it appeared on the surface, however, for those widows who received support from sisters when nearby adult children did not provide support perceived the sibling support negatively. In another study along these lines, Cicirelli (1989) found that the perception of a close bond to sisters by either men or women was related to well-being, as indicated by fewer symptoms of depression, while a close bond to brothers seemed to have little relevance for well-being. This finding may be explained by differing sex role expectations of relationships with sisters as compared to brothers.

Communication Between Siblings

Because siblings share a long and unique history, the communication between them is one avenue along which sibling influence can proceed. Yet there has been little study of the communication between siblings. Cicirelli (1985a) found that most communication centered around the discussion of family events and concerns and around old times. Such shared recollections appear to be a source of comfort and pride for many older people (Ross & Milgram, 1982). Further research is needed to learn how sibling communication changes in content and meaning over the many decades of the sibling connection and how these relate to the functions of the sibling connection.

SIBLING HELPING RELATIONSHIPS

Instrumental Help

Another major aspect of the sibling connection in old age is the help that siblings can provide for each other. In middle adulthood, siblings are seen as a source of aid in time of crisis (Troll, 1975), caring for children and sharing household responsibilities. For most, however, mutual aid is relatively infrequent (Adams, 1968). Among the elderly, instrumental help from siblings is also infrequent, since most older people depend on children for help. If the need for help becomes too great for the spouse or children to handle or if the normal scheme of family obligations is disturbed, siblings then tend to give help. Cicirelli (1979) found that the majority of older people regarded siblings as a source of support to be called on in a crisis, but only 7% regarded a sibling as a primary source of help. However, sibling help became more important among the oldest age groups (Hoyt & Babchuk, 1983), and when the brother or sister fell ill, needed transportation, needed household repairs, or lost a spouse (Cicirelli, 1979, 1985a; Goetting, 1986; Kivett, 1985; Lopata, 1973; Scott, 1983). In addition, those who have never married tend to receive more assistance from siblings (Johnson & Catalano, 1981; Troll, 1982).

Psychological Support

Although instrumental support from siblings is relatively small, psychological support is much more important. Providing companionship, serving as a confidant, giving advice, aiding in decision making, and boosting morale all serve as examples of sibling psychological support. Scott (1983) reported that visiting, various recreational activities, and miscellaneous other activities with siblings were on a level that compared quite favorably with companionate activities with children when proximity was controlled. Cicirelli (1982) reported high degrees of sibling compatibility both in middle adulthood and old age. While relatively fewer siblings talk over important decisions with a sibling or disclose feelings and personal problems, this is not surprising in view of the fact that most friendships are also conducted at a superficial level and without great intimacy (Duck & Miell, 1986). Sibling effects on the morale of older people have already been discussed, with the conclusion that simply being available and not any particular level of interaction was most important. In a recent study of hospitalized elderly (Cicirelli, 1990) the most frequently desired kind of support from siblings was psychological support, ranging from keeping in touch to simply thinking about, caring for, and praying for the hospital patient. Because siblings share common family values and perceptions, they may be uniquely suited for the provision of such support (Avioli, 1989; Dunn, 1985; Cicirelli, 1988).

Siblings and Psychotherapy

There are a number of situations when the sibling connection becomes important in dealing with the mental health problems of older people (Cicirelli, 1988). One such situation occurs when patients have had long-standing family problems stemming from their families of origin. There may be conflicts and estrangements from siblings persisting from childhood or from the time of certain critical incidents later on (Dunn, 1984; Ross & Milgram, 1982). Long-term dependencies between siblings who have had intensely loyal relationships or who have had sexual relationships can lead to maladjustment, guilt, fear, poor self-concept, and anxiety, (Bank &

Kahn, 1982a, 1982b; Finkelhor, 1980). Still another situation comes about when early rivalries and aggressions between siblings are reactivated in later adulthood and old age at times of crises or stress leading to conflicts and aggressive actions involving siblings or others outside the family (Berezin, 1977; Gully, Dengerink, Pepping, & Bergstrom, 1981; Laverty, 1962).

There are few existing guidelines for treatment of the elderly client with problems involving siblings. Therapeutic approaches range from probing sibling relationships in the course of psychoanalysis (Rosner, 1985), to individual therapy (Bank & Kahn, 1982b; Kahn, 1983), to inclusion of siblings in family therapy (Kahn & Bank, 1981; Palazzoli, 1985), and family counseling (Herr & Weakland, 1979). Therapy can include all living siblings, or only a subgroup of siblings. If the siblings are closeknit, they can be seen as a group; otherwise it may be more effective to see a sibling individually (Church, 1986; Kahn, 1988; Kahn & Bank, 1981; Toman, 1988).

The use of reminiscence as an approach to therapy with older people has gained favor in recent years with its use in the life review process. While reminiscence in itself is simply talking or thinking about the past, in the life review past experiences are analyzed, evaluated, and reintegrated in relation to present events, values, and attitudes in order to resolve old conflicts, come to grips with past mistakes, and achieve integrity in the latter portion of life (Butler, 1963; Molinari & Reichlin, 1985; Osgood, 1985). The therapist can use guided reminiscence to gain an understanding of the older client's life history and painful memories and to deal with it. There is little in the literature dealing with reminiscence of experiences with siblings. Gold (1986) used an extensive open ended interview technique to investigate reminiscences of sibling relationships over the life span and found that many interviewees felt that this process was in itself quite valuable to them. It helped them to put their current sibling connections in a meaningful context, to understand present events, and to appreciate the significance of siblings in their lives. Cicirelli (1985a) has noted similar themes expressed by elderly siblings. Certainly the persistence of the sibling connection and its value for the individual should not be underestimated.

Siblings in Family Businesses

For most siblings in adulthood, interaction consists of companionate activities and family occasions and concerns. However, for some siblings interaction also involves participation in a family-owned business. According to Carroll (1988), there are some 12 million family-owned businesses in the United States; the number of these in which adult siblings are partners and/or coworkers is not known. As yet, information about siblings in family businesses is anecdotal or clinical in nature. According to Carroll, family issues and business issues are inextricably interwoven. Siblings interact on day-to-day business matters which draw added meaning from existing family relationships, and against which themes of intimacy, dependency, rivalry, and fairness are enacted. Problems of power, responsibility, and succession in the business all depend on harmonious sibling connections for their satisfactory resolution.

Sibling Care of Elderly Parents

A major developmental task of adult siblings in midlife is to provide care for aging parents (Goetting, 1986); yet, most of what is known about care of elderly parents centers around the role of the primary caregiver, usually an adult daughter. How one child comes to assume a primary caregiver role, if such is the case, is less well understood. Even less is known about the support provided by siblings of the primary caregiver.

As parents grow older, adult children tend to increase their surveillance of their parents, being alert to any signs that help is needed (Bowers, 1987). The siblings may become closer to each other at this stage, discussing their parents' situation and various scenarios for their eventual care (Tonti, 1988). The adult children may conspire to shield the parents from consequences of physical decline and preserve a sense of psychological independence for as long as possible; a principle of least involvement in parents' lives seems to be followed which preserves the independence of both generations for as long as possible (Bowers, 1987; Matthews & Rosner, 1988). Only when care needs become too great for such an approach is more direct caregiving involved. It is in this stage that a principal caregiver emerges or some other means of dividing caregiving responsibilities is devised.

In many families, support to the elderly is a serial process with the primary caregiver giving support for as long as possible, followed by the next available person in the support hierarchy (Johnson, 1982). In others, adult children function as a cooperative group to divide tasks and agree on a plan for caregiving. Such sharing of caregiving responsibilities is more likely when adult daughters are employed, divorced, or both (Matthews, 1987; Cicirelli, 1984). Other families function in a looser way, with one or two adult children providing the bulk of care and remaining siblings offering occasional help, backup or respite help, or sporadic help (Matthews & Rosner, 1988). In such cases, there may be little discussion between the siblings, with each doing as he or she sees fit.

Matthews and Rosner (1988) identified five sibling participation styles in caregiving. In routine participation, regular help to the parent was incorporated into the child's ongoing activities. In backup participation, a sibling not routinely involved in care can be counted on when siblings routinely giving care ask for help. In circumscribed participation, an adult child gives predictable support to the parent, but help which is carefully bounded in scope and amount (e.g., a weekly phone call, or medical advice). In sporadic participation, an adult child provides services to the parent at his/her own convenience and without any coordination with siblings. Finally, in dissociation, the adult child cannot be counted on for any assistance in parent care; in many cases this adult child is dissociated from any contact with siblings as well.

Matthews (1987) found that pairs of adult sisters tended to share responsibility for tangible help as well as moral support to parents, with the division becoming more equal when both sisters were employed. In larger families, especially those including one or more brothers, support was less likely to be shared by all. Indeed, the majority of larger families contained an adult child who did not help in providing tangible services. In my own work (Cicirelli, 1981), adult daughters provided greater amounts of help in such areas as housekeeping and personal care while sons gave more help with household repairs and business matters, indicating that different kinds of support are provided by different family members depending on their situation. Preliminary results from an ongoing study indicate that most adult children understand and accept the unequal contributions of their siblings when a legitimate reason such as distance, employment, health, or competing responsibilities is apparent; only when there is an abdication of responsibility without a legitimate reason is there resentment of the sibling. Although participation in caregiving may be unequal, in most cases siblings participate in any needed decisions regarding the parent's care. An additional element of complexity in sibling participation in caregiving is introduced by Aldous' (1987) finding that older parents tended to be selective in their relationships with various children in terms of those they socialized with, assisted, or turned to for support. Such ongoing parental selectivity may fuel adult siblings' rivalry and conflict in a situation where parental caregiving is required. To deal with sibling discord, Tonti (1988) suggests improving communication between siblings and defining the parameters of care and commitment. Clearly, more study is needed to understand how an entire sibling subsystem functions to provide support, and how such support may depend on such factors as proximity, employment, other family commitments, and whether spouses are actively supportive, indifferent, or antagonistic to care for their mate's parents.

EXPLAINING SIBLING CONNECTIONS WITH THE ADULT ATTACHMENT THEORY

Most research on sibling connections in adulthood thus far has been atheoretical in nature, or one or another existing psychological theory is cited in an ad hoc explanation. Yet there is a need to explain the origins of bonds between siblings and the persistence of such bonds over time and distance into old age. Although there has been some use of generational solidarity theory from a sociological perspective (e.g., Gold, 1987) to explain sibling connections, using the notion of normative solidarity to account for the origin of the bond, it tends to be more descriptive than explanatory.

Life-span attachment theory (Bowlby, 1979, 1980) provides an explanation of the origin and persistence of sibling relationships. The interested reader is referred to Cicirelli (1983, 1985, 1989) for a fuller explanation. Briefly, attachment is an ethological-adaptational theory rooted in evolutionary biology and such concepts as biologically determined development of social attachments and the adaptational value for survival of family members sharing a common gene pool (Lamb, 1988; Nash, 1988; Scarr & Gracek, 1982). Attachment refers to an emotional or affectional bond between two people. It is essentially being identified with, having love for, and desiring to be with the other person, and represents an internal state within the individual. Somewhat later in time, a protective aspect of attachment develops in which the attached person takes measures to prevent the loss of the attached figure, e.g., preserving, and restoring. Such attachment extends to siblings in childhood and continues to adulthood and old age. Attachment behaviors in adulthood are manifested through periodic communication, visiting, and responses to reunions, whereas protective behavior is manifested in helping and caregiving behavior that attempts to maintain the survival of the attached figure. To explain the maintenance of the sibling bond over extended separations in space and time, it is argued that the need for closeness and contact with the sibling is satisfied on a symbolic level through the process of identification. A recent study (Cicirelli, 1989) found that sibling psychological support is related to the strength of the attachment bond, with a stronger relationship when attachment to a sister is involved.

FUTURE RESEARCH DIRECTIONS IN STUDYING SIBLING CONNECTIONS

Much further work needs to be done before sibling connections in adulthood are well understood. Further expansion of attachment theory and empirical tests of its implications are needed. In addition, changes in sibling connections over time need to be better delineated and explained, not only short-term changes such as those found in situation-specific ambivalence (Bedford, 1989b; Cicirelli, 1985b) but long-term changes such as those associated with sibling developmental tasks (Goetting, 1986). Ethnic and cultural differences in sibling connections need to be determined, with existing studies extended to apply to a wider representation of ethnic groups if such differences are to be explained.

Connections between adoptive siblings, half-siblings, and stepsiblings in adulthood and old age should be studied. In view of the increasing number of these changing family types, it is important to know the extent to which present findings about siblings apply to these connections.

If the family is truly a system, then further research needs to focus on the relationship between siblings and parent-child connections in adulthood and between different subgroups of the sibling subsystem. Dunn (1988) has shown how relationships with siblings in childhood are affected by parent-child relationships, while Aldous (1987) has suggested that the same might occur in adult caregiving relationships. Conidis (1988) found that relationships throughout the entire sibling network were shaped by the relationships with a sibling who was single, childless, or previously married. Many issues remain to be resolved: How do sibling coalitions affect other members of a sibling network? How do sibling relationships change when a parent dies? Do siblings draw closer together or drift apart over time? How do relationships with spouses affect relationships with siblings? The way a young sibling monitors the relationships between other family members, discusses them, and interprets them plays an important role in influencing the individual's own family relationships (Dunn, 1988). This may be a fruitful path to pursue in studying adult sibling connections.

REFERENCES

Adams, B. N. (1968). *Kinship in an urban setting*. Chicago: Markham.

Aldous, J. (1987). Family life of the elderly and near-elderly. *Journal of Marriage and the Family*, 49, 227-234.

Avioli, P. S. (1987). *The support relationship of elderly siblings: A research agenda*. Paper presented at the meeting of the American Psychological Association, New York.

Bank S., & Kahn, M. D. (1982a). Intense sibling loyalties. In M. E. Lamb & B. Sutton-Smith (Eds.), *Sibling relationships: Their nature and significance across the life span* (pp. 251-266). Hillsdale, NJ: Lawrence Erlbaum.

Bank, S. P., & Kahn, M. D. (1982b). *The sibling bond*. New York: Basic Books.

Bowers, B. J. (1987). Intergenerational caregiving: Adult caregivers and their aging parents. *Advances in Nursing Science*, 9(2), 20-31.

Bowlby, J. (1979). *The making and breaking of affectional bonds*. London: Tavistock.

Bowlby, J. (1980). *Attachment and loss: Vol. III. Loss, stress, and depression*. New York: Basic Books.

Bedford, V. H. (1989a). A comparison of thematic apperceptions of sibling affiliation, conflict, and separation at two periods of adulthood. *International Journal of Aging and Human Development, 28*, 53-66.

Bedford, V. H. (1989b). Ambivalence in adult sibling relationships. *Family Issues, 10*(2), 211-224.

Berezin, M. A. (1977). Partial grief for the aged and their families. In E. Pattison (Ed.), *The experience of dying* (pp. 279-286). Englewood Cliffs, NJ: Prentice-Hall.

Butler, R. N. (1963). The life review: An interpretation of reminiscence in the aged. *Psychiatry, 26*, 65-76.

Carroll, R. (1988). Siblings and the family business. In M. Kahn & K. Lewis (Eds.), *Siblings in therapy* (pp. 379-398). New York: W. W. Norton.

Church, M. (1986). Issues in psychological therapy with elderly people. In I. Hanley & M. Gilhooly (Eds.), *Psychological therapies for the elderly* (pp. 1-21). London: Croom Helm.

Cicirelli, V. G. (1977). Relationship of siblings to the elderly person's feelings and concerns. *Journal of Gerontology, 32*, 317-322.

Cicirelli, V. G. (1979, May). *Social services for elderly in relation to the kin network* (Report). Washington, DC: NRTA-AARP Andrus Foundation.

Cicirelli, V. G. (1980). Sibling influence in adulthood: A life span perspective. In L. W. Poon (Ed.), *Aging in the 1980s* (pp. 455-462). Washington, DC: American Psychological Association.

Cicirelli, V. G. (1981). *Helping elderly parents: Role of adult children*. Boston: Auburn.

Cicirelli, V. G. (1982). Sibling influence throughout lifespan. In M. E. Lamb & B. Sutton-Smith (Eds.), *Sibling relationships: Their nature and significance across the lifespan* (pp. 267-284). Hillsdale, NJ: Lawrence Erlbaum.

Cicirelli, V. G. (1983). Adult children's attachment and helping behavior to elderly parents: A path model. *Journal of Marriage and the Family, 45*, 815-825.

Cicirelli, V. G. (1984). Marital disruption and adult children's perception of their sibling's help to elderly parents. *Journal of Family Relations, 33*, 613-621.

Cicirelli, V. G. (1985a). The role of siblings as family caregivers. In W. J. Sauer & R. T. Coward (Eds.), *Social support networks and the care of the elderly: Theory, research, practice and policy* (pp. 93-107). New York: Springer.

Cicirelli, V. G. (1985b). Siblings relationships throughout the life cycle. In L. L'Abate (Ed.), *Handbook of Family Psychology* (pp. 177-214). Homewood, IL: Dorsey Press.

Cicirelli, V. G. (1988). Interpersonal relationships among elderly siblings: Implications for clinical practice. In M. D. Kahn & K. G. Lewis (Eds.), *Siblings in therapy* (pp. 435-456). New York: W. W. Norton.

Cicirelli, V. G. (1989). Feelings of attachment to siblings and well-being in later life. *Psychology and Aging, 4*, 211-216.

Cicirelli, V. G. (1990). Family support in relation to health problems of the elderly. In T. H. Brubaker (Ed.), *Family relationships in later life* (2nd. ed., pp. 212-228). New York: Sage.

Conidis, I. (1988, November). *Sibling ties and aging.* Paper presented at the meeting of the Gerontological Society, San Francisco.

Cumming, E., & Henry, W. (1961). *Growing old.* New York: Basic Books.

Duck, S., & Miell, D. (1986). Charting the development of personal relationships. In R. Gilmour & S. Duck (Eds.), *The emerging field of personal relationships* (pp. 133-143). Hillsdale, NJ: Lawrence Erlbaum.

Dunn, J. (1984). Sibling studies and the developmental impact of critical incidents. In P. B. Baltes & O. G. Brim (Eds.), *Life span development and behavior* (Vol. 6, pp. 335-353). Orlando, FL: Academic Press.

Dunn, J. (1985). *Sisters and brothers.* Cambridge, MA: Harvard University Press.

Dunn, J. (1988). Relations among relationships. In S. W. Duck (Ed.), *Handbook of personal relationships* (pp. 193-209). New York: Wiley.

Finkelhor, D. (1980). Sex among siblings: A survey on prevalence, variety, and effects. *Archives of Sexual Behavior, 9,* 171-194.

Goetting, A. (1986). The developmental tasks of siblingship over the life cycle. *Journal of Marriage and the Family, 48,* 703-714.

Gold, D. T. (1986). *Sibling relationships in retrospect: A study of reminiscence in old age.* Doctoral dissertation. Northwestern University, Evanston, IL.

Gold, D. T. (1987, August). *Generational solidarity: Sibling ties in late life.* Paper presented at the meeting of the American Psychological Association, New York.

Gold, D. T. (1988, November). *Late-life sibling relationships: Does race affect typological distribution?* Paper presented at the meeting of the Gerontological Society, San Francisco.

Gold, D. T. (1989). Sibling relationships in old age: A typology. *International Journal of Aging and Human Development, 28,* 37-50.

Gold, D. T., Woodbury, M. A., & George, L. K. (1988). *Relationship classification using grade of membership analysis: A typology of sibling relationships in later life.* Manuscript submitted for publication.

Gully, K. J., Dengerink, H. A., Pepping, M., & Bergstrom, D. (1981). Research note: Sibling contribution to violent behavior. *Journal of Marriage and the Family, 43,* 333-337.

Herr, J. J., & Weakland, J. H. (1979). *Counseling elders and their families: Practical techniques for applied gerontology.* New York: Springer.

Hoyt, D. R., & Babchuk, N. (1983). Adult kinship networks: The selective formation of intimate ties with kin. *Social Forces, 62,* 84-101.

Johnson, C. L. (1982). Sibling solidarity: Its origin and functioning in Italian-American families. *Journal of Marriage and the Family, 44,* 155-167.

Johnson, C. L., & Catalano, D. J. (1981). Childless elderly and their family supports. *Gerontologist, 6,* 610-618.

Kahn, M. D. (1983, December). Sibling relationships in later life. *Medical Aspects of Human Sexuality*, *17*(12), 94-103.

Kahn, M. D. (1988). Intense sibling relationships: A self-psychological view. In M. D. Kahn & K. G. Lewis (Eds.), *Siblings in therapy* (pp. 3-24). New York: W. W. Norton.

Kahn, M. D., & Bank, S. (1981). In pursuit of sisterhood. *Family Process*, *20*, 85-95.

Kivett, V. R. (1985). Consanguinity and kin level: Their relative importance to the helping network of older adults. *Journal of Gerontology*, *40*, 228-234.

Lamb, M. E. (1988). Social and emotional development in infancy. In M. H. Bornstein & M. E. Lamb (Eds.), *Developmental psychology: An advanced textbook* (2nd. ed., pp. 359-410). Hillsdale, NJ: Lawrence Erlbaum.

Laverty, R. (1962, January). Reactivation of sibling rivalry in older people. *Social Work*, *7*, 23-30.

Lee, G. R., & Ihinger-Tallman, M. (1980). Sibling interactions and morale. *Research on Aging*, *2*, 367-391.

Lopata, H. (1973). *Widowhood in an American city*. Cambridge, MA: Schenkman.

Matthews, S. H. (1987). Provision of care to old parents: Division of responsibility among adult children. *Research on Aging*, *9*, 45-60.

Matthews, S. H., & Rosner, T. T. (1988). Shared filial responsibility: The family as the primary caregiver. *Journal of Marriage and the Family*, *50*, 185-195.

McGhee, J. L. (1985). The effects of siblings on the life satisfaction of the rural elderly. *Journal of Marriage and the Family*, *47*, 85-91.

Molinari, V., & Reichlin, R. E. (1985). Life review reminiscence in the elderly: A review of the literature. *International Journal of Aging and Human Development*, *20*, 81-92.

Mosatche, H. S., Brady, E. M., & Noberini, M. R. (1983). A retrospective lifespan study of the closest sibling relationship. *Journal of Psychology*, *113*, 237-243.

Nash, A. (1988). Ontogeny, phylogeny, and relationships. In S. W. Duck (Ed.), *Handbook of personal relationships* (pp. 121-141). New York: Wiley.

Noberini, M. R., Mosatche, H. R., & Brady, E. M. (1984). *Qualitative alterations in adult sibling relationships*. Paper presented at the meeting of the Gerontological Society, San Antonio, TX.

O'Bryant, S. L. (1988). Sibling support and older widows' well-being. *Journal of Marriage and the Family*, *50*, 173-183.

Osgood, N. J. (1985). *Suicide in the elderly: A practitioner's guide to diagnosis and mental health intervention*. Rockville, MD: Aspen.

Palazzoli, M. S. (1985). The problem of the sibling as the referring person. *Journal of Marital and Family Therapy*, *11*, 21-34.

Rosner, S. (1985). On the place of siblings in psychoanalysis. *Psychoanalytic Review*, *72*, 457-477.

Ross, H. G., & Milgram, J. I. (1982). Important variables in adult sibling relationships: A qualitative study. In M. E. Lamb & B. Sutton-Smith (Eds), *Sib-

ling relationships: Their nature and significance across the lifespan (pp. 225-249). Hillsdale, NJ: Lawrence Erlbaum.

Scarr, S., & Gracek, S. (1982). Similarities and differences among siblings. In M. E. Lamb & B. Sutton-Smith (Eds.), *Sibling relationships: Their nature and significance across the lifespan* (pp. 357-381). Hillsdale, NJ: Lawrence Erlbaum.

Schvaneveldt, J. D., & Ihinger, M. (1979). Sibling relationships in the family. In W. R. Burr, R. Hill, R. I. Nye, & I. L. Reiss (Eds.), *Contemporary theories about the family. Vol. I. Research-based theories* (pp. 453-467). New York: Free Press.

Scott, J. P. (1983). Siblings and other kin. In T. H. Brubaker (Ed.), *Family relationships in later life* (pp. 47-62). Beverly Hills, CA: Sage.

Sutton-Smith, B., & Rosenberg, B. C. (1970). *The sibling.* New York: Holt, Rinehart, and Winston.

Suggs, P. K., & Kivett, V. R. (1987). Rural/urban elderly and siblings: their value consensus. *International Journal of Aging and Human Development, 24,* 149-159.

Tonti, M. (1988). Relationships among adult siblings who care for their aged parents. In M. D. Kahn & K. D. Lewis (Eds.), *Siblings in therapy* (pp. 417-434). New York: W. W. Norton.

Toman, W. (1976). *Family constellation: Its effects on personality and social behavior* (3rd ed.). New York: Springer.

Toman, W. (1988). Basics of family structure and sibling position. In M. D. Kahn & K. G. Lewis (Eds.), *Siblings in therapy* (pp. 46-65). New York: W. W. Norton.

Troll, L. E. (1971). The family of later life. A decade review. *Journal of Marriage and the Family, 33,* 263-290.

Troll, L. E. (1975). *Early and middle adulthood.* Monterey, CA: Brooks/Cole.

Troll, L. E. (1982). *Continuations: Adult development and aging.* Monterey, CA: Brooks/Cole.

The Intergenerational Family Roles
of Aged Black Americans

Linda M. Burton
Peggye Dilworth-Anderson

Older black men and women have historically been portrayed as the mainstay of kin networks, a monolithic institution in extended families over time. A number of changes, however, have occurred in recent years that suggest that the traditional perceptions of the family roles of the black elderly need reassessment. One concerns historical shifts in social definitions of elders' family roles. Another is demographic transition — specifically changes in patterns of mortality, fertility, and single parenthood. These factors have produced a variety of intergenerational family structures, norms, and role behaviors among aged black Americans.

This article examines the literature on the intergenerational family roles of elderly black men and women. Roles are defined as the set of behaviors or activities enacted within a particular status position in the family (Rosow, 1976). The discussion focuses on roles created by vertical ties in families — between aged parents and their adult children; grandparents and grandchildren; and older family members and extended kin. First, a discussion of the impact of historical shifts in social definitions of elder roles and demographic transition on family structure and the role of aged blacks is presented. Second, contemporary research on the black elderly as aged

Linda M. Burton is Associate Professor of Human Development, Department of Human Development and Family Studies, The Pennsylvania State University, University Park, PA 16802. Peggye Dilworth-Anderson is Professor of Child Development and Family Relations, University of North Carolina, Greensboro, NC 27412.

parents, grandparents, and kin-keepers in extended kin networks is reviewed.

TRADITIONAL FAMILY ROLES OF AGED BLACKS

The black elderly, from slavery to the present, have been described as the central stabilizing figures in extended black families (Bernard, 1966; Hill & Schackleford, 1977; Martin & Martin, 1978; Mindel, 1983). The role of family stabilizer is rooted in the age-graded family systems of West African culture and enacted by older blacks as a means of survival amid the social, political, and economic adversities experienced by black families throughout American history (Foster, 1983; Lesnoff-Caravaglia, 1982; Sudarkasa, 1981; Wylie, 1971).

Historically, the black elderly as family stabilizers have provided material and spiritual support for kin (Aschenbrenner, 1975; Martin & Martin, 1978; Mutran, 1985; Mutran & Reitze, 1984; Shimkin, Shimkin, & Frate, 1978); "prepared folk-remedies for the myriad illnesses which beset families" (Huling, 1978, p. 28); been the repositories and transmitters of family history and folklore (Huling, 1978; Troll, 1983); served as family advisors (Taylor, 1988); mediated disputes among family members (Gutman, 1976); and in many cases reared grandchildren, great-grandchildren, and the children of extended and fictive kin (Frazier, 1939; Jones, 1973; Tate, 1983; Wilson, 1986). Although these tasks are often considered synonymous with the family roles of black elderly, it is important to note that they are not exclusive to aged blacks (Jackson & Walls, 1978; Lesnoff-Caravaglia, 1982; Troll, 1983), but are performed by the elderly in other racial/ethnic groups as well.

Much of what we know about the roles of the black elderly is documented in historical and ethnographic studies of extended black family life (Aschenbrenner, 1975; Blassingame, 1972; Frazier, 1939; Genovese, 1974; Gutman, 1976; Stack, 1974; Wilson, 1983). Although these studies have made significant contributions to our understanding, when evaluated as a collective, they tend to present a static, homogenized view of older black Americans (Myers, 1982; Jackson, 1971). For example, black grandmothers of the 1980s are often depicted in the literature as having role attributes comparable to those of grandmothers of the 1800s (Burton, 1989). Two explanations may account for the similarities. Either there is, in fact, a high degree of cultural continuity in black families, reflecting consistency in the transmission of norms regarding family roles (McAdoo, 1978; Shimkin, Shimkin, & Frate, 1978; Martin & Martin, 1978), or current views, which are limited by research that has not systematically studied older blacks in varied socio-economic and cultural subpopulations, do not reflect existing differences (Jackson, 1988; Krauss, 1981).

Continuity in the roles of aged blacks through historical time has been challenged by a number of scholars (Blackwell, 1985). The basis of the challenge lies in the substantial changes that have occurred in American society and consequently in American families since the turn of the century. The evolution of American families in general, and black families specifically, is notable for changes in the norms that direct family life and the roles assigned family members (Wells, 1982). Jones (1973, p. 21), for example, argues that the role of black grandmothers has changed as black families "consciously or unconsciously adopted the values and life-styles of the white middle class." Huling (1978) notes that changes in the structure of extended black families, urbanization, and familial shifts to an individualistic value system have dramatically altered the traditional family roles of the black elderly. Staples (1985) indicates that socio-structural conditions, such as high rates of black male unemployment, have changed the structure of black families which consequently redefines family roles. These challenges underscore the effects of changing ideological and value orientations on family roles. Even more important, they reflect the impact that recent demographic changes in intergenerational family structure have had on the familial roles of aged black Americans (Treas & Bengtson, 1987).

DEMOGRAPHIC TRANSITION, FAMILY STRUCTURE, AND FAMILY ROLES

The Changing Demography of Intergenerational Family Life. Today's black elderly grow older in intergenerational families that are distinct from those of their predecessors (Wells, 1982; Billingsley, 1968). Aged blacks in the 1980s are more likely than their grandparents to be part of a four-, even five-generation extended family comprising smaller parent/child units (Hagestad, 1988). They are also more likely to be the oldest members of a kin network in which recent generations are composed of single parents (Fogel and Engerman, 1974; Furstenberg, Hershberg, & Modell, 1985; Gutman, 1976; Lammermeier, 1973; Smith, Dahlin, & Friedberger, 1979; Stampp, 1956).

Changes in the intergenerational family life of aged blacks can be attributed to the effects of three demographic trends: (1) declines in mortality—the life expectancy for black males and females at birth has increased approximately 20 and 30 years, respectively, in the last century (Farley & Allen, 1987); (2) declines in fertility—the number of children born per black female has decreased from 4.5 in 1940 to 2.2 in 1984; the rate of teenage childbearing among blacks has also declined but continues to remain high relative to other racial groups; the number of black women who delay childbearing or remain childless has increased slightly (Farley & Allen, 1987); and (3) the dramatic increase in single-parent female headed households—at present, half of black families with children are maintained by single women (Farley, 1988; McLanahan, 1988; U.S. Bureau of the Census, 1988).

The interaction of these trends has a complex influence on intergenerational family relationships and roles. Although changes in mortality, fertility, and single parenthood do not determine the interpersonal framework of family relations, they do create the parameters or context of family life—the family structure (Gee, 1987). These changes have produced a variety of black intergenerational family structures, varying in width, length, and composition of members, with distinct implications for the family roles of older black Americans.

Diversity in Family Structure. Family roles are a function of family structure. As structures change, roles change. To date, no empirical studies have examined the family roles of aged black men and women in the context of changing intergenerational family forms. The discussion presented here, then, reflects hypotheses concerning the types of families that contemporary elderly blacks are part of and the spectrum of family role behaviors they engage in.

At least three general types of intergenerational family structures can be found among contemporary older blacks (see Billingsley, 1968, and Kellam, Adams, Brown, & Ensminger, 1982, for a description of specific types of black family structures). Each one offers distinct alternatives for family roles. The first is the *verticalized intergenerational family*. This structure is a product of declining mortality and fertility. It is characterized by intergenerational extension, meaning that the number of living generations within a lineage increases, and intragenerational contraction, meaning that there is steady decrease in the number of members within each generation (Bengtson & Dannefer, 1987; Knipsheer, 1988).

The verticalized structure has several implications for the roles of older blacks. First, this family structure, which comprises multiple generations, offers a variety of vertical role statuses for older blacks to occupy simultaneously — aged parent, grandparent, and even great-grandparent. Second, although individuals within these family structures assume a greater variety of vertical roles, because of declines in fertility, they will have fewer children, grandchildren, great-grandchildren, and siblings (Pullam, 1982). With fewer family members per generation, older blacks have a greater opportunity to invest themselves more heavily within a kin group that is manageable in size. On the other hand, smaller numbers of kin reduce the size of the potential caregiver pool that older blacks may need to call upon for assistance in the future.

The *age-condensed structure* is a second intergenerational family form. This form, which is also a function of mortality and fertility trends, is found among families with consistent patterns of teenage childbearing (Ladner & Gourdine, 1984). It is a vertically compact structure, in which the age distance between generations in the family is roughly 12-17 years, compared to 20-26 years in young adult childbearing families and 30-40 years in delayed childbearing families.

In an exploratory study of the effects of teenage pregnancy on intergenerational family structure and the roles of black women, Burton (1985) demonstrated how adolescent childbearing can affect the family lives of older blacks. The study involved 41 four-, five-, and six-generation black female lineages from a large urban community. The sample included mothers age 11-18, grandmothers age 25-38, and great-grandmothers age 46-57.

Findings from this study indicated some striking effects of early childbearing on family structure and the roles of aging women. First, consistent teenage childbearing coupled with low mortality among older family members created even more levels of grandparenthood than the verticalized family form. Although such a situation is rare, Burton interviewed a 91-year-old woman who was the great-great-great-great-grandmother in her lineage (Burton & Bengtson, 1985; Burton & Martin, 1987). This woman had simultaneously occupied at least three vertical family roles for more than 60 years of her life.

Second, teenage childbearing created a context that increased the work load of older women in the family. In the majority of families that Burton studied, teenage pregnancy sparked early transitions to grandmotherhood that were not welcomed by the respondents (Burton & Bengtson, 1985; Elder, Caspi, & Burton, 1987). Most of the young grandmothers in the study refused to take on the role of surrogate parent to their grandchildren. The burden of care was pushed up the generational ladder to the great-grandmother in the lineage. In most instances, the young great-grandmother was responsible not only for the care of her great-grandchild, but for her adolescent granddaughter (the child's mother) and her own aged mother, as well.

Older women who assume responsibility for the care of grandchildren and great-grandchildren are also found in multi-generation single-parent families. The rise in out-of-wedlock childbearing, separation, and divorce among blacks has created intergenerational family structures where older blacks are called upon by their daughters and sons to serve as the "other parent" for grandchildren and great-grandchildren (Lindblad-Goldberg & Dukes, 1985; Wilson, 1986). The degree of grandparental involvement, however, depends on the grandparents' domicile. In a study of single parents in three-generation black families, Wilson (1984) found that grandmothers who lived with their daughters who were single parents were more involved in the parenting of their grandchildren than those who did not.

A third type of intergenerational family form is the *substitutional* (Johnson & Catalano, 1981; Shanas, 1979). This form evolves when the kin network of the older adult is notably small as a consequence of family patterns of delayed childbearing or childlessness. In substitutional family structures, older blacks become part of the support network of fictive or remote kin. The roles that older blacks play in these family structures vary depending on the degree to which they are absorbed in a network.

The number of family role statuses that older people occupy is contingent upon family structure, but it is important to note that a person's actual role behavior depends on a number of factors. These factors include: the economic (Harris, 1980), marital (Lopata, 1978), and health status of the aged individuals (Taylor, 1988) as well as the personal preferences, familial expectations, and cultural norms that guide their behaviors. The influence of these factors is duly noted in the black elderly's role behavior as aged parents, grandparents, and kin-keepers.

AGED PARENTS AND THEIR ADULT CHILDREN: THE SUPPORTIVE ROLE

The literature on aged parents and their adult children primarily focuses on role behaviors related to the family as a support system. In general, black elderly exercise two types of role behaviors within this system—they give support to their adult children and receive support from them (Yelder, 1979).

Several studies (Aschenbrenner, 1975; Martin & Martin, 1978; Seelbach, 1978; Stack, 1974) have provided a foundation for understanding what aged blacks do for their adult children. For example, Cantor (1979) and Mutran (1985) report that elderly blacks give advice and economic support to their adult children more often than do whites. Older blacks also help their offspring via the services they provide to their grandchildren (Gillespie, 1976; Ladner, 1971; Tinsley & Parke, 1984). Black grandparents provide temporary and sometimes permanent homes for their grandchildren, serve as co-parents in their socialization and rearing, and frequently support them financially. In a recent study by Slaughter and Dilworth-Anderson (1990) on family coping in the care of children with sickle-cell disease, the sick grandchildren received a range of instrumental and emotional support from their grandparents. In fact, the mothers of these sick children noted that after the fathers, maternal grandparents were their secondary caregivers.

In regard to older blacks as recipients of support, studies conducted over a decade ago (Cantor, 1979; Hays & Mindel, 1973; Jackson, 1971, 1972; Seelbach, 1978) as well as those in recent years (Chatters, Taylor & Jackson, 1986; Mitchell & Register, 1984; Mutran, 1985; Taylor, 1986) found that elderly blacks receive a great deal of support and caregiving from their children. For example, Mindel, Wright, and Starrett (1986) found that the family support system of elderly blacks provides the following in order of frequency: transportation, checking services, homemaker services, and administrative/legal services. In a study conducted by Dilworth-Anderson (1986), involving 123 black elderly parent-adult children dyads, the majority of elderly parents indicated that their adult children assisted them when they were sick, helped during financial crises and emergencies, and advised them on matters that impact their lives. In a recent review of the literature of intergenerational family support, Taylor (1988) notes, however, that there is a gender difference in the receipt of support from adult children. Older women have a greater probability of receiving support from their children than do older men (Chatters, Taylor, & Jackson, 1986; Wolf, Breslau, Ford, Ziegler, & Ward, 1983).

In addition to receiving direct assistance from their offspring, the elderly have a second advantage if they have adult children. Current research indicates that elderly blacks with adult children are more likely to have larger extended kin networks to provide support than those older blacks without children (Chatters, Taylor & Jackson, 1986).

Despite consistent positive findings concerning the tendency of black families to provide significant support and care to the elderly, some researchers have questioned the generalizability of these patterns to the black population as a whole. Jackson (1980) strongly encourages researchers to examine heterogeneous structures of caregiving in black families. She asserts that not all black aged are in an extended family and not all adult children can and want to provide support to their parents. She further suggests that a stereotypical view of the extended/intergenerational support system of caregiving has emerged from research that focuses primarily on intensive emotional attachment in black families. This focus prohibits researchers from exploring other factors related to the family roles and needs of the black elderly. Clearly, these remarks, made a decade ago, suggest a need for exploring variability in support patterns among elderly blacks of different socioeconomic and subcultural groups. Unfortunately, to date, these suggestions have not been adequately followed up.

GRANDPARENTHOOD

Although research on the grandparent role has grown considerably in the last decade (for a current overview see Barranti, 1985; Bengtson & Robertson, 1985), relatively little attention has been devoted to grandparenthood among blacks, particularly among black men. In general, the literature offers a tenuous perception of the role in contemporary society (Hagestad & Burton, 1986). Troll (1980) describes grandparenthood as a contingent role—a role in which what grandparents do with and for their grandchildren is modified by myriad factors including age at role entry (Burton & Bengtson, 1985), the developmental stage of the grandchild (Tinsley & Parke, 1984), residential proximity of grandparents to grandchildren (Hale, 1982; Shanas, 1979; Staples & Smith, 1954), the extent to which parents make grandchildren available to the grandparents (Robertson, 1975), gender (Kivett, 1985; Jackson, 1971), race (Cherlin & Furstenberg, 1986; Markides & Krause, 1983), and social class (Clavan, 1978). A number of scholars have developed typologies of grandparental role behaviors (Kivnick, 1983). Neugarten and Weinstein (1964) identified five styles of grandparenting: formal, fun-seeker, surrogate parent, reservoir of family wisdom, and distant figure. Wood and Robertson (1976) describe four: remote, symbolic, individualized, and apportioned. These typologies emerged from studies of grandparenthood in white populations. Their applicability to black grandparents has not been systematically studied.

What is known about the role that black grandparents play in the lives of their grandchildren is primarily limited to discussions of their role as surrogate parents and co-parents to their grandchildren. As mentioned earlier, historically, many black grandparents have served as surrogate parents to their grandchildren. This role was often enacted by older blacks in response to family needs. For example, during the "great migration" of young adult blacks from the South to urban centers in the North and West, grandparents kept their grandchildren until the parents were financially able to take care of them. There is evidence that a number of today's black grandparents, particularly maternal grandmothers, continue to assume the role of surrogate or co-parent to their grandchildren. What have changed, however, are the reasons why many assume the role. Teenage pregnancy and drug addiction among young black parents are often cited as factors that influence grandparental assumption of the surrogate and co-parent roles.

Although the precise number of grandmothers who are surrogate or co-parents for the children of adolescent mothers is not known, descriptive studies suggest that a significant proportion of grandmothers in early childbearing families assume this critically important role (Field, Widmayer, Stringer, & Ignatoff, 1980; Furstenberg & Crawford, 1978). Colleta and Lee (1983) reported that 66% of the black teen mothers they interviewed indicated that their mothers were the primary caretakers of their children. Chase-Lansdale, Brooks-Gunn, and Reiss (1989) note that three-quarters of the children of teen mothers live in households with their grandmothers during their first three years of life.

A number of studies have documented what grandmothers do as caregivers of the children of teen parents (Smith, 1975; Stevens, 1984; Wilson, 1986), but little has been written about the costs to the grandmother of assuming parental responsibilities. The life circumstances that surround the grandmother can determine whether or not the role is a positive experience. For example, grandmothers in teen childbearing families are often quite young and have parenting obligations of their own. Many may find themselves overburdened by juggling the care of their own children and grandchildren with work, school, and maintaining interpersonal relationships outside the family.

Grandmothers who assume the surrogate parent role because of their own children's drug addiction are faced with equally complex dilemmas. Burton's (1989) case study of a black grandmothers' support group illustrates the impact of drug dependency in families on the grandparental role. Burton reports that unlike the young grandmothers of teen pregnancies, the women in this study were great-grandmothers in their late 60s and early 70s who were in poor health. They assumed primary care for not one, but several of their grandchildren and great-grandchildren because the parents were chronic drug abusers. The respondents indicated that they attended the support group because they were overwhelmed with family responsibilities and needed help from formal social service agencies to continue in their role as surrogate parents. Six areas of needed social service support were identified by the women: (1) respite child care for their grandchildren and great-grandchildren; (2) physical and mental health care for themselves; (3) legal counseling concerning foster care and guardianship; (4) financial assistance; and (5) training programs for coping with family members who were drug dependents.

Although surrogate parenting by black grandparents has received the most attention from researchers, it should not be viewed as the normative grandparental role among older black Americans. Future studies of grandparenting among blacks must expand the current knowledge base by acknowledging heterogeneity in the role. Research must examine grandparenthood not only in highly dependent, at-risk intergenerational family networks, but also in families whose structure and composition offer alternative options for grandparental behavior.

THE ROLES OF AGED BLACKS IN THE EXTENDED KIN NETWORK

The existing literature indicates that aged blacks engage in one inclusively defined role in the extended kin network—kinkeeper. Researchers have described the kinkeeper role as including such activities as visiting, telephoning, letter writing, sharing a mutual aid system, and maintaining a sense of family through psychological support (Adams, 1968; Hagestad, 1986; Martin & Martin, 1978; Rosenthal, 1985). Rosenthal (1985) notes that kinkeeping is an infrequently studied family role. This is particularly true in the case of older blacks. The discussion of aged blacks as kinkeepers thus draws from a meager information base. As is true for most families in this society, women in black families are the kinkeepers. The majority have outlived their husbands, who had either shared in the kinkeeping role or served as the dominant figure in the family. General perceptions and stereotypes, however, do not promote the view that older black males are dominant family figures who serve as primary kinkeepers with the help of their wives.

Martin and Martin (1978) identified a number of characteristics of kinkeepers in black families. The kinkeeper typically is the most dependable and most respected family member. She sees her role as crucial to the maintenance and perpetuation of continuity and integrity in the extended kin network. Kinkeepers foster continuity and integrity in families by (1) passing on the history of the family; (2) living by and encouraging a family philosophy or theme, moral prescriptions, and general family ethos; (3) promoting family unity and confronting members who may disrupt it; and (4) helping with family responsibilities and encouraging others to do the same.

An important aspect of kinkeeping among black women also involves taking care of the children of extended and fictive kin. Stack (1974, p. 63), in her description of extended family life in a midwestern community, writes: "From the point of view of the children, there may be a number of women who act as mothers towards them. . . . A woman who intermittently raises a sister's, niece's or cousin's child regards their offspring as much her grandchildren as children born to her own son and daughter." Many of the women Stack refers to, especially the elderly women in the family, take care of the children of others at great expense to themselves. Nonetheless, their response to the needs of the children reinforces the kinkeeping philosophy that perpetuates continuity, integrity, and stability in families through investing in children.

CONCLUSION

The purpose of this article was twofold: (1) to discuss the impact of historical shifts in the definition of elder family roles and of demographic transition on the intergenerational family life of older blacks; and (2) to present an overview of literature on elderly blacks as aged parents, grandparents, and kinkeepers.

The adoption of mainstream values, urbanization, and changing social conditions have affected the family roles of older black Americans. In addition, intergenerational family structures — namely, the verticalized, age-condensed, and substitutional — which have evolved through demographic transition, provide a variety of contexts for the enactment of elder family roles. Although it is not clear how broad the spectrum of roles is in black families, two trends can be inferred. First, older blacks are more likely to be part of four- or even five-generation families and thus simultaneously to experience multiple vertical role statuses in the family. Second, grandparenthood, which has historically been an important role in extended families, may become increasingly significant as the number of single-parent households increases.

Despite some laudable research efforts, there remains a paucity of information on the family roles of black elderly, particularly older black men. As a consequence, several serious gaps in the literature can be identified. First, research that examines diversity in the roles of aged blacks is warranted. As indicated earlier, the limited body of existing research, which is primarily composed of ethnographic and historical studies, has tended to project homogenized views of elderly blacks. Studies that explore gender, socioeconomic, regional, and sub-cultural variation in roles within the black population would test the generalizability of existing perspectives.

Second, research that explores the costs as well as the benefits of elder family roles is needed (Wilson, 1986). For example, studies of grandparents as surrogate parents have tended to be uni-directional, focusing on benefits to the parents and grandchildren. Little attention has been given to the liabilities of the role for the aged grandparents.

The third area of needed research concerns the exchange of resources within extended families. Of particular importance is the study of the exchange of support between aged parents and their middle-aged adult children and its affect on role behaviors. Gibson (1986) points out that because of the growing crises of unemployment and underemployment of middle-aged blacks, their need for familial support increases at the same time younger and older generations in the family look to them for help. What are the implications of the life situation of middle-aged children for the types and frequency of support given and received by older blacks? What factors mediate the exchange of resources between the black elderly and their adult children?

Demographic profiles of older blacks point to a fourth area of needed research. Although one may speculate about the demography of intergenerational family life among aged blacks, as has been done in this article, reliable estimates would provide valuable information for policy makers, program developers, and social science researchers. Future demographic research efforts concerning the black elderly should include the following: (1) simulation studies of the duration of family roles that are comparable to the studies conducted about white females (Watkins, Menken, & Bongaarts, 1987); (2) estimations of the size and composition of intergenerational family structures, including the number of generations in families and within households; (3) prevalence studies of grandparenthood and surrogate parenting in extended kin networks; and (4) profiles of the kin networks of the childless elderly.

REFERENCES

Adams, B. (1968). *Kinship in the urban setting*. Chicago: Markham.

Aschenbrenner, J. (1975). *Lifelines: Black families in Chicago*. New York: Holt, Rinehart & Winston.

Barranti, C. C. R. (1985). The grandparent/grandchild relationship: Family resources in an era of voluntary bond. *Family Relations, 34,* 343-352.

Bengtson, V. L., & Dannefer, D. (1987). Families, work, and aging: Implications of disordered cohort flow for the 21st century. In R. A. Ward & S. S. Tobin (Eds.), *Health in aging: Sociological issues and policy directions* (pp. 256-289). New York: Springer.

Bengtson, V. L., & Robertson, J. (Eds.). (1985). *Grandparenthood: Research and policy perspectives*. Beverly Hills, CA: Sage.

Bernard, J. (1966). *Marriage and family among negroes*. Englewood Cliffs, NJ: Prentice-Hall.

Billingsley, A. (1968). *Black families in white America*. Englewood Cliffs, NJ: Prentice-Hall.

Blackwell, J. (1985). *The black community*. New York: Harper & Row.

Blassingame, J. W. (1972). *The slave community*. New York: Oxford University Press.

Burton, L. M. (1985). Early and on-time grandmotherhood in multigeneration black families. Unpublished doctoral dissertation. University of Southern California.

Burton, L. M. (1989). Black grandmothers as a family resource: Perspectives on social service needs. Paper presented at the National Conference on Mental Health and Aging, University of California, Los Angeles.

Burton, L. M., & Bengtson, V. L. (1985). Black grandmothers: Issues of timing and meaning in roles. In V. L. Bengtson & J. F. Robertson (Eds.), *Grandparenthood: Research and policy perspectives* (pp. 61-78). Beverly Hills, CA: Sage.

Burton, L. M., & Martin, P. (1987). Thematikin der mehrgenerationenfamilie: Ein beispiel. *German Journal of Gerontology, 20*, 275-282.

Cantor, M. H. (1979). The informal support system of New York's inner city elderly: Is ethnicity a factor? In D. Gelfand and A. Kutzik (Eds.), *Ethnicity and aging: Theory, research, and policy* (pp. 67-73). New York: Springer.

Chase-Lansdale, L., Brooks-Gunn, J., & Reiss, D. (1989). Developmental perspectives on grandmothers, young mothers, and children. Unpublished manuscript.

Chatters, L. M., Taylor, R. J., & Jackson, J. S. (1986). Aged blacks' choices for an informal helper network. *Journal of Gerontology*, 41, 94-100.

Cherlin, A., & Furstenberg, F. F. (1986). *The new American grandparent*. New York: Basic Books.

Clavan, S. (1978). The impact of social class and social trends on the role of grandparent. *The Family Coordinator, 27*, 351-358.

Colleta, N. D., & Lee, D. (1983). The impact of support for black adolescent mothers. *Journal of Family Issues, 4*, 127-143.

Dilworth-Anderson, P. (1987). Elderly blacks and relations with adult children. Paper presented at Purdue University, Department of Child Development and Family Studies, West Lafayette, Indiana.

Elder, G. H., Caspi, A., & Burton, L. M. (1987). Adolescent transition in development perspective: Sociological and historical insights. In M. Gunnar (Ed.), *Minnesota Symposium on Child Development, Vol. 21* (pp. 121-143). Hillsdale, NJ: Erlbaum.

Farley, R. (1988). After the starting line: Blacks and women in an uphill race. *Demography, 25*(4), 477-495.

Farley, R., & Allen, W. (1987). *The color line and the quality of life in America*. New York: Russell Sage Foundation.

Field, T. M., Widmayer, S. M., Stringer, S., & Ignatoff, E. (1980). Teenage, lower class, black mothers and their preterm infants: An intervention and developmental follow-up. *Child Development, 51*, 426-436.

Fogel, R. W., & Engerman, S. L. (1974). *Time on the cross: The economics of American negro slavery*. Boston: Little, Brown.

Foster, H. J. (1983). African patterns in the Afro-American family. *Journal of Black Studies, 14*, 201-232.

Frazier, E. F. (1939). *The Negro family in the United States*. Chicago: Chicago University Press.

Furstenberg F. F., Jr., Hershberg, T., & Modell, J. (1985). The origins of the female-headed black family: The impact of the urban experience. *Journal of Interdisciplinary History, 6*, 211-233.

Furstenberg F., & Crawford, D. B. (1978). Family support: Helping teenagers to cope. *Family Planning Perspectives, 10*, 322-333.

Gee, E. M. (1987). Historical change in the family life course. In V. Marshall (Ed.), *Aging in Canada* (2nd ed., pp. 120-132). Ontario: Fitzhenry and Whiteside.

Genovese, E. (1974). *Roll, Jordan, roll*. New York: Pantheon Press.

Gibson, R. C. (1986). Blacks in an aging society. *Daedalus, 115*, 349-372.

Gillespie, B. J. (1976). Black grandparents: Childhood socialization. *Journal of Afro-American Issues, 4*, 432-441.

Gutman, H. (1976). *The black family in slavery and freedom: 1750-1925*. New York: Pantheon Books.

Hagestad, G. O. (1986). The aging society as a context for family life. *Daedalus, 115*, 119-139.

Hagestad, G. O., & Burton, L. M. (1986). Grandparenthood, life context, and family development. *American Behavioral Scientist, 29*, 471-484.

Hale, J. (1982). *Black children: Their roots, culture and learning styles*. Provo, UT: Brigham Young University Press.

Harris, R. (1980). An examination of the effects of ethnicity, socioeconomic status, and generation of familism and sex role orientation. *Journal of Comparative Family Studies, 2*, 173-193.

Hays, W., & Mindel, C. H. (1973). Extended kinship relations in black and white families. *Journal of Marriage and the Family, 35*, 51-56.

Hill, R., & Schackleford, L. (1977). The black extended family revisited. *The Urban League Review, 1*, 18-24.

Huling, W. E. (1978). Evolving family roles for the black elderly. *Aging, 287*, 21-27.

Jackson J. J., & Walls, B. (1978). Myth and realities about aged blacks. In M. Brown (Ed.), *Readings in gerontology* (pp. 67-83). Saint Louis: C. V. Mosby Company.

Jackson, J. J. (1971). Sex and social class variation in black aged parent-adult child relationships. *Aging and Human Development, 2*, 96-107.

Jackson, J. J. (1972). Comparative life styles of family and friends relationships among older black women. *The Family Coordinator, 3*, 477-485.

Jackson, J. J. (1980). *Minority aging*. Belmont, CA: Wadsworth.

Jackson, J. J. (1988). Growing old in black America: Research on aging black populations. In J. Jackson (Ed.), *The black American elderly* (pp. 3-16). New York: Springer.

Johnson, C. L., & Catalano, D. J. (1981). Childless elderly and their family support. *The Gerontologist, 21*, 610-618.

Jones, F. C. (1973). The lofty role of the black grandmother. *Crises, 80*, 19-21.

Kellam, S. G., Adams, R. G., Brown, C. H., & Ensminger, M. E. (1982). The long-term evolution of the family structure of teenage and older mothers. *Journal of Marriage and the Family, 44*, 539-554.

Kivett, V. R. (1985). Grandfathers and grandchildren: Patterns of association, helping, and psychological closeness. *Family Relations, 34*, 565-571.

Kivnick, H. O. (1983). Dimensions of grandparenthood meaning: Deductive conceptualization and empirical derivation. *Journal of Personality and Social Psychology, 44*(5), 1056-1068.

Knipsheer, C. P. M. (1988). Temporal embeddedness and aging within the multigenerational family: The case of grandparenting. In J. E. Birren & V. L. Bengtson (Eds.), *Emergent theories of aging* (pp. 426-446). New York: Springer.

Krauss, I. K. (1981). Between- and within-group comparisons in aging research: In L. Poon (Ed.), *Aging in the 1980's* (pp. 542-551). Washington, DC: American Psychological Association.

Ladner, J. (1971). *Tomorrow's tomorrow: The black woman.* Garden City, NY: Doubleday.

Ladner, J. A., & Gourdine, R. (1984). Intergenerational teenage motherhood: Some preliminary findings. *SAGE: A Scholarly Journal on Black Women, 1*(2), 22-24.

Lammermeier, P. J. (1973). The urban black family of the nineteenth century: A study of black family structure in the Ohio Valley, 1850-1880. *Journal of Marriage and the Family, 35*, 440-456.

Lesnoff-Caravaglia, G. (1982). The black granny and the soviet babushka: Commonalities and contrast. In R. C. Manuel (Ed.), *Minority aging: Social and psychological issues* (pp. 109-114). Westport, CT: Greenwood Press.

Lindblad-Goldberg, M., & Dukes, J. L. (1985). Social support in black, low-income, single-parent families: Normative and dysfunctional patterns. *American Journal of Orthopsychiatry, 55*, 42-48.

Lopata, H. Z. (1978). Contributions of extended families to the support systems of metropolitan area widows: Limitations of the modified kin network. *Journal of Marriage and the Family, 40*, 355-364.

Markides, K. S., & Krause, N. (1983). Intergenerational solidarity and psychological well-being among older Mexican Americans: A three-generation study. *Journal of Gerontology, 40*, 506-511.

Martin, E. P., & Martin, J. M. (1978). *The black extended family.* Chicago: University of Chicago Press.

McAdoo, H. P. (1978). Factors related to stability in upwardly mobile black families. *Journal of Marriage and the Family, 40*, 762-778.

McLanahan, S. (1988). Family structure and dependency: Early transitions to female household headship. *Demography, 25*, 1-16.

Mindel, C. H. (1983). The elderly in minority families. In T. Brubaker (Ed.), *Family relationships in later life* (pp. 72-93). Beverly Hills, CA: Sage.

Mindel, C. H., Wright, R., & Starrett, R. (1986). Informal and formal social and health service use by black and white elderly: A comparative cost approach. *The Gerontologist, 26,* 279-285.

Mitchell, J., & Register, J. (1984). An exploration of family interaction with the elderly by race, socioeconomic status and residence. *The Gerontologist, 34,* 48-54.

Mutran, E. (1985). Intergenerational family support among blacks and whites. Response to culture or to socio-economic differences. *Journal of Gerontology, 40,* 382-389.

Mutran, E., & Reitze, D. (1984). Intergenerational support activities and well-being among the elderly: A convergence of exchange and symbolic interaction perspectives. *American Sociological Review, 49,* 237-263.

Myers, H. J. (1982). Research on the Afro-American family: A critical review. In B. A. Bass, G. E. Wyatt, & G. J. Powell (Eds.), *The Afro-American family* (pp. 35-68). New York: Grune & Stratton.

Neugartern, B. L., & Weinstein, K. K. (1964). The changing American grandparent. *Journal of Marriage and the Family, 26,* 199-204.

Pullam, T. W. (1982). The eventual frequencies of kin in a stable population. *Demography, 19,* 549-565.

Robertson, J. F. (1985). Interaction in three generation families, parents as mediators: Toward a theoretical perspective. *International Journal of Aging and Human Development, 6,* 103-110.

Rosenthal, C. J. (1985). Kin-keeping in the familial division of labor. *Journal of Marriage and the Family, 45,* 509-521.

Rosow, I. (1976). Status and role change through the life span. In R.H. Binstock & E. Shanas (Eds.), *Handbook of aging in the social sciences* (pp. 457-482). New York: Van Nostrand Reinhold.

Seelbach, W. (1978). Correlates of aged parents filial responsibility expectations and realizations. *Family Coordinator, 27*(4), 341-350.

Shanas, E. (1979). The family as a social support system in old age. *The Gerontologist, 19,* 169-174.

Shimkin, D., Shimkin, E., & Frate, D. (1978). *The extended family in black societies.* Chicago: Aldine.

Slaughter, D., & Dilworth-Anderson, P. (1990). Sickle cell anemia, child competence, and extended family life. In H. Cheatham & J. Stewart (Eds.), *Interdisciplinary perspectives on black families* (pp. 107-123). New Jersey: Transactions Publication.

Smith, D. S., Dahlin, M., & Friedberger, M. (1979). The family structure of the older black population in the American South in 1880 and 1900. *Sociology and Social Research, 63*(3), 544-565.

Smith, E. W. (1975). The role of the grandmother in adolescent pregnancy and parenting. *Journal of School Health, 45,* 278-283.

Stack, C. B. (1974). *All our kin: Strategies for survival in a black community.* New York: Harper and Row.

Stampp, K. M. (1956). *The peculiar institution.* New York: Vintage Books.

Staples, R. (1985). Changes in black family structure: The conflict between family ideology and structural conditions. *Journal of Marriage and the Family*, 1005-1013.

Staples, R. & Smith, J. W. (1954). Attitudes of grandmothers and mothers toward child rearing practices. *Child Development*, *25*, 91-97.

Stevens, J. H. (1984). Black grandmothers' and black adolescent mothers' knowledge about parenting. *Developmental Psychology*, *20*, 1017-1025.

Sudarkasa, N. (1981). Interpreting the African heritage in Afro-American family organization. In H. McAdoo (Ed.), *Black families* (pp. 27-53). Beverly Hills, CA: Sage.

Tate, N. (1983). The black aging experience. In R. L. McNeely & J. L. Colen (Eds.), *Aging in minority groups* (pp. 95-105). Beverly Hills, CA: Sage.

Taylor, R. J. (1986). Receipt of support from family among black Americans: Demographic and familial differences. *Journal of Marriage and the Family*, *48*, 67-77.

Taylor, R. J. (1988). Aging and supportive relationships. In J. Jackson (Ed.), *The black American elderly* (pp. 259-281). New York: Springer Publishing Company.

Tinsley, B. R., & Parke, R. (1984). Grandparents as support and socialization agents. In M. Lewis (Ed.), *Beyond the dyad* (pp. 161-195). New York: Plenum.

Treas, J., & Bengtson, V. L. (1987). Family in later years. In M. Sussman & S. Steinmetz (Eds.), *Handbook on marriage and the family* (pp. 625-648). New York: Plenum Publishing.

Troll, L. (1980). Grandparenting. In L. W. Poon (Ed.), *Aging in the 1980's: Psychological issues* (pp. 150-187). New York: American Psychological Association.

Troll, L. (1983). Grandparents: The family watchdogs. In T. Brubaker (Ed.), *Family relationships in later life* (pp. 63-74). Beverly Hills, CA: Sage.

U.S. Bureau of the Census (1988). Marital status and living arrangements: March 1987, *Current Population Reports* (Series P-20, No. 418). Washington, DC: U.S. Government Printing Office.

Watkins, S. C., Menken, J. A., & Bongaarts, J. (1987). Demographic foundations of family change. *American Sociological Review 52*, 346-358.

Wells, R. V. (1982). *Revolutions in Americans' lives*. Westport, CT: Greenwood Press.

Wilson, E. M. (1983). *Hope and dignity*. Philadelphia: Temple University Press.

Wilson, M. N. (1984). Mothers' and grandmothers' perceptions of parental behavior in three-generation black families. *Child Development*, *55*, 1333-1339.

Wilson, M. N. (1986). The black extended family: An analytical consideration. *Developmental Psychology*, *22*, 246-256.

Wolf, J. H., Breslau, N., Ford, A. B., Ziegler, H. D., & Ward, A. D. (1983). Distance and contacts: Interactions of black urban elderly adults and family and friends. *Journal of Gerontology*, *38*, 465-471.

Wood, V., & Robertson, J. (1976). The significance of grandparenthood. In J.

Gubrium (Ed.), *Time, roles, and self in old age* (pp. 46-59). New York: Behavioral Publications.

Wylie, F. M. (1971). Attitudes toward aging and the aged among black Americans: Some historical perspectives. *Aging and Human Development, 2,* 66-69.

Yelder, J. (1979). The influence of culture on family relations: The black American experience. Aging parents. Los Angeles: University of Southern California.

Puerto Rican Families
in New York City:
Intergenerational Processes

Lloyd H. Rogler
Rosemary Santana Cooney

Immigration has played an important role in the history of the United States, beginning with the early large-scale movement from Northwestern Europe and extending to today's influx from Latin America and Indochina. The integration of immigrant groups into American society has been widely researched, but little is known about the relationship between a migration-induced change in the sociocultural environment of parents and their children and intergenerational processes within the family.

This study examines the lives of 100 intergenerationally linked Puerto Rican families. Each family consists of two generations: the mothers and fathers in the parent generation and their married child and spouse in the child generation. Thus, the 100 intergenerationally linked families represent 200 married couples, making a total of 400 persons. In 56 of the families a daughter of the parent generation is the link between the parent and married-child generations; in 44 families a son represents the link. At the time we met and interviewed them members of the parent generation were in their mid-fifties; the majority had come to the continental United

The research reported here was supported by a grant from the William T. Grant Foundation and by Grants #R01 MH28314 and #R01 MH30569 from the National Institute of Mental Health, Minority Research Resources Branch.

With the exception of the introductory paragraphs, this paper represents the last chapter of the book by Lloyd H. Rogler and Rosemary Santana Cooney, *Puerto Rican Families in New York City: Intergenerational Processes*, Maplewood, NJ: Waterfront Press, 1984.

States as young adults in their mid-twenties and had lived on the mainland for nearly 30 years. Almost all of their children either were born on the mainland or had arrived during their preschool years. When interviewed, the members of the Puerto Rican child generation were young adults in their late twenties. Practically all of them live in New York City, mostly in the borough of the Bronx; a few live in the outskirts of the city. This study examines the experiences of the immigrant parent generation in their island-home, their migration and settlement in metropolitan New York City, and the experiences of their children, the child generation, raised in the United States. In addition, we investigate the impact of the two generations' different life experiences upon the transmission of sociocultural characteristics from parents to their children and upon the structure of the relationship between the parent and married child. Our research is premised upon the importance of examining the adaptation of immigrant groups from the perspective of generationally linked family units.

Before summarizing and interpreting our findings, we want to repeat the focus and limitations we set for this study. The 400 persons we studied were part of 200 nuclear families, which in turn were combined into 100 intergenerational families. The persons were all Puerto Rican by birth or parentage, and they all lived in New York City or adjoining areas, but mostly in the borough of the Bronx. The families were not selected by methods of probability sampling. Instead, we used census tracts of the Bronx which were at the top and at the bottom of a rank order developed according to the percentage of Puerto Ricans with a high school education, as reported by the 1970 Census. We visited schools, Catholic and Pentecostal churches, spiritualist centers, and Puerto Rican ethnic and civic organizations, and we approached households in door-to-door visits in selected neighborhoods. A 13-step screening sequence was required to fulfill the study's intergenerational family model. In terms of their greater residential and marital stability, these families differ from other Puerto Rican families wherever they may reside.

The parent generation was, in many important ways, typical of the large number of Puerto Ricans who were migrating to New York City. In the vanguard of the social transformation taking place in Puerto Rico from the Depression of the '30s to the industrialization of the '50s, they had a relatively high educational level and exposure to the conditions of urban life. Improving conditions on the island generated aspirations for a better life for themselves and their children, and to realize these aspirations they migrated to a sociocultural setting different from their own. Arrival in New York City formed the initial phase of yet another set of changes, this time experienced in the host society. The changes were economically troublesome but, in the long run, gratifying. The married-child generation became highly successful both educationally and occupationally. Their success represented a remarkable fulfillment of the aspirations which prompted their parents to migrate.

We knew very little about the lives of these families when we first met them. Although all of us in the field spoke Spanish and shared with them the many features of our Hispanic culture, we found that many of the parent generation in our study resisted the interviews, displaying more distrust than their adult children and their children's spouses. Still more marginal to the culture and with more modest educational attainments and jobs than their children, the parent generation was understandably less trusting of us as strangers during initial contacts. Thus, our field methods very early in the study had to take intergenerational differences into account. Because of the fundamental differences between generations, even within the same family lineage, our field workers had to make use of different techniques in interviewing the two generations. In shaping our efforts to collect data, therefore, we recognized at the very beginning of the study the importance of the main object of the research—intergenerational processes in immigrant Puerto Rican families.

The intergenerational differences between the parents and their married children were remarkably pervasive and strong. Originally, this pattern was revealed during the analysis of ethnic identity, a topic of compelling importance because of the study group's bicultural experience. The scope of our analysis was broadly conceived to include diverse elements of ethnic identity: mastery and use of Spanish and English; the extent of adherence to traditional Puerto Rican values and modernity scores; and subjective views of the self and the person's individualized preferences for aspects of both cultures. When educational and occupational characteristics were incorporated into the analysis, the same pattern of striking differences was evident: the married-child generation had substantially outdistanced their parents in terms of socioeconomic attributes.

The socioeconomic generational differences, taken in conjunction with the diverse items comprising ethnic identity, indicated, however, that intergenerational change was variable. The greatest intergenerational change occurred in socioeconomic status, then in the language used, then in values, and, finally, the least change occurred in the subjective elements describing self-concept and bicultural preferences. Immediately, the inference is that external elements, pragmatic in character, which were relevant to the immigrants' objective integration into the host society, were more susceptible to intergenerational change than the internal elements, subjective in character but of substantial symbolic importance. (Presently we shall reconsider these elements according to their "instrumental" and "expressive" meanings.) Both generations experienced the erosion of much that was associated with their lives as Puerto Ricans but internally, in the symbolisms linking them to the island, they experienced less change. Despite their remarkable upward mobility in the host society, the married-child generation still retained symbolic bonds with Puerto Rico, a place hardly known to them from direct experience.

We then turned to the important task of explaining variations in ethnic identity in each generation. Why were some persons more than others allied to their Puerto Rican heritage and cultural experiences? Rather than drawing up an *ad hoc* list of independent variables to explain ethnic identity, the choice of such variables, we believed, should reflect the person's receptivity to influences shaping ethnic identity and/or the degree of exposure to such influences. Although those we interviewed were all Puerto Rican by birth or parentage, they differed from each other in their receptivity and exposure to the bicultural environment in which they lived. The complexity of this problem required that we depart from the usual procedure of simple bivariate analysis and turn to multivariate techniques which would allow us to identify the independent sources of influences affecting ethnic identity. Two variables of single importance emerged in the analysis: the age at arrival in New York City and the level of education. Once these variables were taken into account as determinants of ethnic identity, the other independent variables added little or nothing to our understanding of ethnic identity.

Age at arrival in New York City and level of education, however, played sometimes similar and sometimes different roles in shaping ethnic identity, depending upon which elements of ethnic identity were being considered. Thus, each variable had an independent effect upon the language component of ethnic identity. As education increased, the knowledge of English and Spanish increased, but the daily use of Spanish decreased. Moreover, regardless of level of education, age at arrival was related to language ability and usage, with those who arrived at an older age reporting less ability and use of English than those who had arrived at a younger age. In turn, those with more years of education were less familistic, less fatalistic, and more modern than those with fewer years of education; age at arrival had no effect upon such variables. On the other hand, age at arrival was an important influence on ethnic self-identification, whereas education was not. The discovery of the importance of the sociocultural context of early socialization and of education programmatically shaped the way in which subsequent topics were examined. As used to examine ethnic identity, the variables provided the first clues as to how the experiences of migration and adaptation affected intergenerational family processes.

Before we discuss our analysis of the ways in which migration-induced changes were related to intergenerational continuity, we want to point out once again the meaning we have assigned to this concept. Simply put, intergenerational continuity refers to the presence of a statistically significant correlation between the parents and their children with respect to some characteristic chosen for analysis. The correlation is the operational counterpart to the concept of intergenerational continuity. It should be mentioned that the use of measures of association with less stringent assumptions than those of Pearson's product-moment correlation—which was used in this study—did not alter the pattern of findings relevant to intergenerational continuity. Nonetheless, in a cross-sectional study such as this one it is usually impossible to identify reliably and in detail the specific processes, including the intergenerational direction of influences, which create continuity. Our formulations regarding such processes represent informed speculations.

Early in the study we adopted the selective continuity approach because it left open to empirical demonstration the possible unevenness of intergenerational continuity. This approach, we believed, would have heuristic value but, as we proceeded to analyze the data with the objective of uncovering ways in which migration-induced change was related to intergenerational processes, the findings began to puzzle us. When the 100 intergenerationally linked families were analyzed, little if any evidence of intergenerational continuity was apparent. The ethnic characteristics of the children were unrelated to the corresponding ethnic characteristics of either parent. We began to wonder if the two generations, even though connected through family lineage, were utterly disconnected in terms of continuity. Perhaps the wrenching change produced by migration from one sociocultural system to another attenuated or dissolved the type of linkage which continuity entails. The puzzle prompted more refined questions: Are there conditions which underlie continuity that strengthen it under some circumstances and weaken it under others? Are some of the characteristics used to evaluate intergenerational continuity more likely to produce continuity than others? Findings relevant to intergenerational change in ethnic identity and to the determinants of ethnic identity provided a point of departure for reexamining the puzzle.

We began with the assumption that age at arrival in New York City signified the cultural context of the person's early socialization. If born in New York City or arrived before the age of 15, the context was New York City; if arrived at 15 or older, the context was Puerto Rico. With such distinctions, the intergenerationally linked families could be classified according to whether or not the parents and their children had a common cultural context in their early socialization. Thus, what was first taken as an attribute of persons, age at arrival in New York City, in the explanation of ethnic identity, was recast in broader terms as a joint attribute of the parents and their children. The logic of this procedure was applied to the other major determinant of ethnic identity, education. Parents and their children were classified according to similarity of educational level, with graduation from high school as the dividing point. Thus, in answer to our first question, the sharing of an early context of socialization and similarities in educational level represent the two underlying conditions thought to be relevant to intergenerational continuity.

Previously we made the point that even though intergenerational differences were strong and pervasive, the differences themselves were variable: they were greater with respect to elements which are external and pragmatic and less among elements which are internal and subjective. This distinction between elements, suggested to us by Hill's intergenerational research,[1] needs to be further developed as we turn to the second question of whether some characteristics are more conducive to intergenerational continuity than others. In this regard, Bales' distinction between "instrumental" and "expressive" acts[2] is pointedly relevant. He takes this distinction from our common everyday habits of speech but argues, at the same time, that the two types of acts are not sharply separable, their differences being a matter of the "proper weight of emphasis." Customarily, some activities are viewed as *goal-directed, the person performing the acts "in order" to realize an end*. These are *instrumental* acts, for they are directed toward some objective in the future. *Expressive* acts, on the other hand, are not explicitly directed toward an objective; rather, they are reactive to, or signs of, a person's "immediate pressure, tension, or emotion." Not being explicitly harnessed toward the attainment of an end, expressive acts are produced "because" of some internal emotion or feeling. Bales summarizes the differences between the two types of acts as resting upon "the degree to which anticipated consequences enter as a steering factor." Some of the elements used to evaluate intergenerational differences and continuities do not lend themselves clearly to the instrumental-expressive distinction because they represent an admixture of meanings or do not fit. Other elements clearly do, and it is upon them that we shall focus in order to complete our formulations regarding intergenerational continuity.

In the lives of the Puerto Rican immigrants and their children, the acquisition of the English language had instrumental significance to their adaptation to the host society. The acquisition of English presents an instrumental element *par excellence* because in a multitude of ways it determines the attainment of a multitude of objectives. Without it, the migrants' life space would have been constricted largely to the ethnic in-group, thereby preventing them from realizing the aspirations which led them to migrate.

As we move through the many elements we have used to demonstrate intergenerational differences, and away from those which are instrumental, such as the mastery and use of English, we come to elements designating subjective feelings. The rise of such feelings was not immediately or explicitly linked to the anticipation of future goals. Rather, they were the psychological residuals or by-products of the migrant's bicultural experience which came to be suffused with expressive meaning. They reflected preferences as to place of residence, maintaining Puerto Rican traditions, or the language of use. Subjective elements of even more evident expressive content were the person's views of himself/herself as Puerto Rican or North American in terms of the corresponding cultural values and the perceived degree of closeness to Puerto Ricans or North Americans. To recall Bales' definition of the expressive, such feelings arise "because" of emotions or sentiments rather than of explicit organization "in order" to attain external goals. The distinction between expressive and instrumental elements, nonetheless, is still a matter of degree.

When the answers to the two basic questions previously posed are brought together, many of the complicated findings on intergenerational continuity can be brought into order. In response to the first question, we found there are underlying conditions which promote intergenerational continuity: when parents and their children were socialized in the same culture or when they were similar in educational level, intergenerational continuity increased. The distinction between expressive and instrumental elements, although a matter of degree, is relevant to the second question because it serves to identify the elements likely to form part of intergenerational continuity. We found that when the parents and their children were socialized in the same culture, intergenerational continuity appeared among both instrumental and expressive elements: there was intergenerational continuity in the mastery and use of English and in the subjective bicultural preferences just discussed. When the parents and their children were similar in educational level, intergenerational continuity did not appear among the expressive elements but did appear among those which were instrumental such as the mastery and use of English. Selective continuity was operative but must be qualified according to both the underlying conditions linking the generations and the character of the element used to evaluate continuity.

The general effect upon continuity of parents and children sharing their early socialization in the same culture is understandable. Such sharing involved a total cultural environment, whether Puerto Rico or New York City, not preselected exposure to a narrow band of cultural stimuli. It occurred early in childhood, allowing the learning to take hold in diverse ways from the development of personality to the shaping of world views, attitudes, and skills. The shared learning, in brief, was so pervasive and wide-ranging as to provide a backdrop for intergenerational continuity without favoring instrumental over expressive elements or the other way around. When parents and children experienced such sharing, their level of acquisition of the English language was directly correlated. Also directly correlated was the strength of their respective preferences for things either Puerto Rican or North American. The sharing of a common cultural environment early in life enabled intergenerational transmissions to produce continuity in both instrumental and expressive elements. One of the most notable consequences of migration-induced changes is that in about three-fourths of the families migration itself kept the parents and their children from having a common culture during their early socialization. Among these families, there was no intergenerational continuity in either instrumental or expressive elements. Put metaphorically, the children were orphans to family legacies which, for better or for worse, were truncated by migration.

We have seen that the sharing of educational levels between the two generations had a more specific impact: it promoted intergenerational continuity in instrumental but not expressive elements. Again, this finding can be rendered understandable if we keep in mind that educational similarities were instrumental in character, and thus narrowed the focus of intergenerational transmissions to other similar elements, purposively oriented, such as the acquisition of the English language. Against the backdrop of similar education for the two generations, the transmissions decisively favored instrumental elements. But in most of the families, in fact, in about two-thirds of them, no such similarities were found, since the child generation's upward mobility created sharp dissimilarities between the generations in education. In these families there was no continuity in either instrumental or expressive elements. To use the same metaphor, the child generation was rendered an orphan to family legacies, this time because of its own extraordinary socioeconomic success in adapting to the host society.

The pieces of the puzzle previously discussed now fall into place. The pervasive absence of intergenerational continuity at the level of the entire study group, with no subdivisions, is the result of the preponderant number of families in which the parents and their children did not share the culture of their early socialization and were strongly dissimilar in their educational levels. Migration and social mobility, therefore, play a significant role in shaping the important intergenerational processes of continuity.

Extending the pattern of intergenerational findings already presented, notable intergenerational differences were demonstrated once again in the examination of spouse relations. This analysis focused upon the sharing of household tasks, decision-making, and leisure activities. We found that in each generation there was more sharing in decision-making and leisure activities than in the performance of household tasks. The overall thrust of change from parent to child was, however, in the direction of stronger egalitarian relations. Our data, for the first time, resoundingly confirm what other observers of stateside Puerto Ricans have speculated, but the specific meaning of this change must be taken into consideration. Thus, of the three functions mentioned above, the greatest intergenerational change toward egalitarianism occurred in the sharing of household tasks, resulting from the wife taking on traditional male tasks and not from the husband performing traditional female tasks.

Our findings, based upon a more comprehensive set of cultural elements than had been used in prior research on spouse relations in immigrant families, are consistent with the findings of others: culture does not directly affect the sharing of household functions. However, we did not conclude from such findings that culture is irrelevant. Rather, we undertook the challenging task of uncovering the role culture plays in shaping factors relevant to the sharing of functions. Rodman's cross-national theory[3] of spouse decision-making was singularly useful even though we focused upon cultural differences in the generations and not upon the culture of nations at different levels of economic development, as Rodman had done. In the parent generation, which was still demonstrably enmeshed in the cultural norm of a modified patriarchal society, the higher the husband's occupational status, the greater the sharing of decision-making. In the child generation, which adhered to the cultural norms of a transitional egalitarian society, the higher the husband's occupational status, the less the sharing of decision-making. The different cultural norms the generations represented conferred different meanings upon the husband's occupational status, thus showing the important indirect role culture plays in shaping husband and wife decision-making. Another set of findings strikingly revealed the general importance of the wife's education: in each of the two generations, the higher the wife's education, the less the role segregation in each of the three functions.

The distinction between expressive and instrumental elements, so useful to the understanding of intergenerational continuity with respect to selected elements forming part of ethnic identity, was not applied to the analysis of intergenerational continuity in the three spouse functions. We believed it would be difficult, indeed, to decide how the functions reflect the meaning of the expressive-instrumental distinction and concluded it would be logically inappropriate to attempt the distinction. Thus, the analysis of intergenerational continuity of the three functions used only the two underlying conditions stipulated before: sharing of a common culture by parent and child during their early socialization, and the similarity of their educational attainments. One modification was introduced, namely the use of the wife's education instead of the husband's, because the strength of the findings indicated the general importance of the wife's education in influencing the spouses' sharing in the performance of the three functions. The findings followed the predicted path. A common context of early socialization was conducive to intergenerational continuity with respect to the sharing of household tasks, decision-making, and leisure activities. The other underlying condition, namely, similarity of educational attainments, was also conducive to intergenerational continuity with respect to the three marital functions. Once again, such continuity was wiped out at the level of the entire study group, with no subdivisions, because most of the parents and children in the families were not socialized in the same culture and because of dissimilarities in their education. We should bear in mind that the factors used to evaluate intergenerational continuity represent the degree of sharing between husbands and wives in a complex set of marital functions. This highlights the powerful influence of migration-induced changes in early socialization and social mobility in shaping intergenerational continuity, even when such continuity involved the husbands and wives negotiating their own special marital arrangements.

Historically, the parent generation, in comparison to the total Puerto Rican population, enjoyed at an early age a set of advantages which favored them in the context of modernization occurring on the island, but they were more or less comparable to the many other migrants in the 1950s who came to New York City. However, their children's socioeconomic success in the host society far exceeded the success of an appropriately designated comparison group. Socioeconomic success was examined also from the perspective of family lineage, tracing back to the parents of our parent generation, the grandparents. The movement across the three generations, from the grandparents to the parents, and from the parents to their married children, described a clear sequence of upward mobility. Intergenerational upward mobility, however, has been uneven: although the parent generation was upwardly mobile, their married children's upward mobility was substantially greater. Tracing mobility through lineage also revealed another important facet of the generations' experiences: there had been intergenerational continuity in socioeconomic status between the grandparents and the parents, but no such continuity between the parents and their married children. The pattern of findings for the parent generation fit the status attainment model which affirms intergenerational continuity in socioeconomic status. Indeed, one of the most consistent findings of research on social mobility in the United States indicates that the educational attainments of children are directly related to the socioeconomic characteristics of their parents. The parents transfer their socioeconomic advantages or disadvantages on to their children. Moreover, an earlier study of Puerto Ricans demonstrated intergenerational continuity in socioeconomic status between the parents of first-generation migrants and the first-generation migrants themselves,[4] but the findings pertaining to the child generation strongly departed from the model. Once again we found ourselves in an intergenerational puzzle: the substantial educational attainments of the child generation were unrelated to the socioeconomic achievements of their parents.

Intergenerational continuity in socioeconomic status is shaped by the setting in which it occurs. Years before, in pre-industrial Puerto Rico, even small variations in socioeconomic resources at an even more modest level had been sufficient to create intergenerational continuity between the grandparents and the parent generation. The migration experience ruptured intergenerational continuity in socioeconomic status because of the increasingly higher educational requirements of New York City's labor force, with accompanying rapid erosion of employment opportunities at the bottom of the occupational hierarchy. The parent generation did not transmit their socioeconomic advantages or disadvantages to their children because the variations in their humble socioeconomic resources did not meaningfully coincide with the more elevated labor market opportunities of the host society.

To develop this point further, we turned once again to one of the underlying conditions which the preceding data analysis had shown to be relevant to intergenerational continuity, the sharing by parent and child of the same culture in their early socialization. The pattern of correlations substantiated our expectations. Although the educational attainments of the parents were at their lowest in families where both the parent and child generations were born and raised in Puerto Rico, intergenerational continuity was higher among them than among families in which the generations did not share an early context of socialization or shared it in New York City. The higher educational attainments of the latter two types of families must be seen in the context of decreasing opportunities for low-skilled jobs in New York City. Thus, the impact of migration upon intergenerational continuity is complex. It creates a sharp change in the context of early socialization between the immigrant parents and their children. Additional differences are introduced by the children's upward social mobility. Among immigrants with marginal labor market skills, intergenerational processes are further complicated because the parents are unable to draw upon their labor market skills to advance their children's achievements. Research on the impact of migration upon intergenerational continuity must be sensitive to the degree of congruity between the migrants' socioeconomic resources and the labor market structure of the host society.

In sum, the extensive application of the status attainment model to the study's data revealed new and unsuspected findings. Continuity can occur in one generational sequence but not in the next generational sequence. Migration had a critical effect upon such transmissions, operating through the disjunctions it induced. The parents' socioeconomic attributes were not helpful in understanding the exceptional upward mobility of the younger generation we studied. One variable forming part of the status-attainment model, namely, the number of siblings, was inversely related to the child generation's educational attainments, thus suggesting its influential role. If the migration experience serves as a necessary qualifier to the status-attainment model, other findings compel an expansion of the model. The parent generation's degree of adherence to the traditional values of familism and fatalism also was inversely related to the child generation's educational attainments. When released from the force of such values, the parents were able to induce in their children greater educational achievements. The role traditionally derived cultural factors played in the child generation's educational attainments foreshadowed the need to incorporate the relevance of culture into status-attainment models of social mobility.

One point which we have not discussed previously should be mentioned here. In our analysis, we were sensitive to the possible importance of gender in the parent and child generations. In general, we found that there were more differences between husbands and wives in the parent generation than in the child generation. We also divided the 100 intergenerational families into two groups: in 56 families the daughter was the connecting link and in 44, the son was the connecting link. There were no differences between these two groups with respect to the three major components of intergenerational processes: intergenerational differences and similarities, continuities and discontinuities, and the degree of integration. In sum, none of the intergenerational processes we analyzed was influenced by whether the married child was a son or a daughter.

We then turned to the examination of another major component of intergenerational processes: intergenerational integration. This analysis was based upon the statistical patterns of visitations and reciprocal help exchanges between the parents and their married children. The use of such patterns has the advantage of rooting the concept of integration in objective measures which had been used in another major study of intergenerational processes.[5] By replicating the measures, a basis for interstudy comparisons was established. The comparisons amply justified the use of the concept of a modified extended family in characterizing our Puerto Rican families, that is, if the strength of intergenerational integration is taken as the deciding criterion. The human picture underlying such integration was one of almost incessant interaction between the parents and their married children.

Once we combined the findings demonstrating strong integration with the other findings pertaining to intergenerational differences and discontinuities, we were then able to focus upon a major conclusion of the intergenerational research literature, that of Troll and Bengtson: ". . . high levels of intergenerational cohesion do not necessarily reflect high levels of similarity. . . ."[6] Our findings require that such a concluding statement be followed by the emphasis of an exclamation point, since it states weakly the decisive and preponderant pattern we found. Step by step, our study has demonstrated a strong and pervasive pattern of intergenerational differences and discontinuities among the 100 families taken as a whole. It found also that the two underlying conditions inducing discontinuity, intergenerational differences in the settings of early socialization and in educational attainment, had no effect upon the strength of intergenerational integration. Metaphorically, it seems as if the parents and their married children, having come through the vicissitudes of a rapidly modernizing pre-industrial Puerto Rico, the migration experience, and almost three decades of a changed life style in New York City, were still bound together in an almost-sacred agreement: "No matter what potentially divisive elements and influences may impinge upon us, we shall retain our unity." In this context, the portrait of intergenerational solidarity was of compelling importance.

Such findings, taken together, led to an important implication. Intergenerational transmissions which created continuity were no more inducing of family solidarity than were those interactions between generations which failed to produce continuity. The implication can be more clearly focused if early socialization context is taken as an example. When the parents and their children shared the early context of their socialization, intergenerational continuity in education was greater than when there was no sharing. The parents' educational advantages or disadvantages were transmitted to their children, which could lead one to suppose a greater intergenerational solidarity, but that supposition is patently erroneous. Erroneous, too, would be any inference that the magnitude of educational differences between the generations affected intergenerational integration. Whether or not such transmissions occurred, and no matter the degree of educational differences, intergenerational solidarity was uniformly retained, almost as if there had been a primitive bonding between the generations.

At first, the findings surprised us. Upon reconsidering them, however, our surprise diminished. To examine the issue we focused upon intergenerational differences, although a similar argument could have been developed with respect to intergenerational continuity. From the very moment of the child's birth and on through his/her socialization into adulthood, differences between parents and children were intrinsic to the relationship. Though bound together into complex reciprocal patterns, the parents and children were enmeshed into a partnership of persons who necessarily and habitually differed in a multitude of ways but, no matter the differences between them, the Puerto Rican value of familism strongly sanctified and reinforced the mutual commitment of the parents and children to their enduring familial bond. Suffused with an almost sacred character, the commitment underlies the statistical patterns demonstrating strong intergenerational integration. Thus, the intergenerational integration observed in the present, which has retained solidarity in the face of so many pervasive differences, is an up-to-date instance of a life-long acceptance of differences in the interest of parent-child unity.

A further observation should be made. Many of the differences between the parents and their children derived directly or indirectly from the child generation's superior educational attainments. Their higher education, in turn, led to better occupations and larger incomes. Upward social mobility was viewed as desirable by both generations. Instead of being divisive to intergenerational integration, the children's exceptional social mobility was the object of parental pride. It also buttressed parental feelings that the sacrifices and hardships they endured in leaving the island were now being recompensed.

Intergenerational differences, or the "gulf" between generations, are often taken to signify the loss of family heritage. The view is that something of considerable value has been lost, but an alternative view should be advanced if the issue is one of determining that the direction of intergenerational change fits many of the requirements of the sociocultural environment where the change occurred. In this study, the married children's socioeconomic attributes exceed those of their parents. The general pattern of intergenerational change, which created such a wide gulf between the generations, at the same time enabled the children to function more effectively and successfully in the host society without the loss of intergenerational family solidarity.

The prevailing pattern of intergenerational integration varied from one extreme in which the child generation was fully submerged into the parent generation's household, totally dependent upon it, to the other extreme of distinctly separate, economically autonomous nuclear units. Although the children commanded more human and economic resources, the prevailing flow of help still moved from the parents to the children as a continuation of previous life-cycle experience. The matriarchy and the team structure represented variant forms of intergenerational integration. In the matriarchal structure, the husband-father was relegated to a marginal role while the wife-mother dominated help-giving transactions at the sociometric core of family life. Team structures entailed the mobilization of the entire family in the interest of a common goal; sometimes, this involved the construction of a new set of corporately organized roles; other times it involved the extension and reshaping of usual family roles. Each variant form of intergenerational integration can be viewed as oriented toward social survival or social mobility.

It is important to note that the role changes associated with the development of a matriarchy paralleled intergenerational changes in the roles of husband and wife in the performance of household tasks. In those exceptional cases where a matriarchy did arise, the direction of intergenerational family change was congenially related to the rise. Consistent with this interpretation is the finding that not one intergenerational family, out of the 100 studied, had a husband-father performing both socioemotional and instrumental functions while relegating the wife-mother to a peripheral family role. The woman's family role was bound and locked into socioemotional functions which were not easily relinquished to the man and, culturally, the husband's performance of traditional women's tasks was tinged with stigma. The inverse of this pattern carried with it no culturally induced stigma. In combination with such cultural factors, the intergenerational social change the Puerto Rican families experienced through urbanization, migration, and increasing levels of education consistently and decisively favored the acquisition, by women, of competency in areas of performance customarily associated with the male role or representing an extension of it.

The prevailing patterns of intergenerational integration and their two variant forms revealed how the Puerto Rican families are organized and how they functioned while making their way in the society to which they migrated in the face of pervasive intergenerational differences and discontinuities. We believe their strong intergenerational integration and the stability of their intact marital unions enabled them to confront the problems of social change from yesterday's Puerto Rico to today's New York City and buttressed the younger generation's drive toward success.

REFERENCES

1. Hill, R. (1970). *Family development in three generations*. Cambridge, MA: Schenkman Publishing Co., p. 386.

2. Bales, R.F. (1950). *Interaction process analysis: A method for the study of small groups*. Cambridge, MA: Addison-Wesley Press, Inc., pp. 50-51.

3. Rodman, H. (1967). "Marital power in France, Greece, Yugoslavia and

the United States: A cross-national discussion.'' *Journal of Marriage and the Family*, *30* (May): 321-324.

4. Rogler, L.H. (1972). *Migrant in the City: The life of a Puerto Rican action group*. New York: Basic Books, Inc., pp. 212-225.

5. Hill, R., see note 1.

6. Troll, L. and V. Bengtson (1979). ''Generations in the Family,'' in Wesley R. Burr et al. (eds.), *Contemporary theories about the family*, Vol. 1. New York: The Free Press.

Continuity and Change:
Intergenerational Relations in Southeast Asian Refugee Families

Gail Weinstein-Shr
Nancy Z. Henkin

INTRODUCTION

Chou Chang and Sai Vang met at Ban Vinai refugee camp in Thailand. They were among thousands of other Hmong refugees who survived the trek from Laos. Moving first through the mountains and then through the jungle by night for nearly a month, they finally swam across the Mekong river to safety. The two young people married and had their first child at the camp. Sai became very sick after childbirth. Her first son died before they were granted asylum.

By their fourth year in Philadelphia, Sai had borne the couple's fourth child. The first was a son, and the next three were daughters. Sai wanted to stop having children, but Chou was still anguished over the loss of parents, brothers, sisters and a majority of his own generation that, like him, became soldiers at the age of 12. He says he wants to be surrounded again by Hmong people and to have sons who will bring new strength to his clan.

Sai's mother Joua is the only elder from their collective family

Gail Weinstein-Shr teaches English as a Second Language at Temple University College of Education, Ritter Hall 003-00, Philadelphia, PA 19122. Nancy Z. Henkin is Director of the Center for Intergenerational Learning at Temple University Institute on Aging, 1601 N. Broad St., Philadelphia, PA 19122.

This paper benefited greatly from the knowledge and experiences of Elzbieta Gozdziak of Refugee Policy group, and Nora Lewis who works in Philadelphia's Southeast Asian refugee community.

that survived the journey from Laos. Joua stays home most of the day to provide childcare. Because the household is located in a poor black area of the city where drug activity is constant, Joua is frightened and keeps the blinds drawn, staying inside all day. She complains of loneliness. Her frustrations grow, she says, when the older children come home from school and want to speak only English to one another and to their younger siblings. She fears that her grandchildren will forget how to speak Hmong and she will lose even her "small place in the big city."

Jimmy is the eldest son. When his mother cannot get permission to leave the factory where she works, Jimmy sometimes misses school to translate for his grandmother at the doctor's office. When he falls behind at school, he cannot turn to his parents for help since their own language and literacy skills are so limited. His older cousin, Moua helps when he can. Like other older Hmong children that Jimmy knows, Moua Pao is anxious to be as "American" as possible. With his punk hairstyle and leather clothing, he spends much of his time with other young teens listening to heavy metal music.

Chou and Sai are anxious for their children to succeed. They are also worried about Joua, and how they will care for her as she gets older. With two factory jobs and occasional double shifts, they can barely make ends meet. They hope for the day when their lives will be easier.

THE REFUGEE EXPERIENCE

The United States government defines a refugee as any person who "flees his [her] country to escape persecution based on race, religion, nationality, membership in a particular social group or political opinion." Since the end of World War II, the United States has provided haven for about two million refugees who have been involuntarily displaced from their homelands. In the last decade alone, some 800,000 Southeast Asians, 100,000 Soviet Jews and 125,000 Cubans have been accepted for resettlement in this country (Office of Refugee Resettlement 1986). While these three groups represent the largest recent refugee populations, others have been admitted from Afghanistan, Ethiopia, Iran, Iraq, Poland, Rumania and elsewhere. It is not known how many undocumented or "illegal" refugees are living within United States borders.

In all families, members derive some support from one another. They also share the stresses of growing older and of coping with an ever-changing world. For families that come from other countries, cultural differences intensify the environmental changes that they will experience and the resulting impact on values that influence the behavior of each generation. Unlike both native born and immigrant families who have resettled voluntarily in the United States, refugees who have been involuntarily displaced from their homelands have unique experiences which shape their responses to life in a new country and to relationships within their families.

To explore issues that affect intergenerational relationships in refugee families, it is helpful to take note of common features that are unique to the refugee experience. Like others who have come to the United States from around the world, refugees are faced with enormous change in adapting to a new cultural setting. However, unlike immigrants who have resettled voluntarily, refugees have certain experiences that create unique challenges for their adjustment. First, because refugees often leave in circumstances of forced departure, little preparation is possible. Liu (1979) found, for example, that 85% of Vietnamese refugees made the decision to flee two days to two hours before their departure. Belongings are left behind and planning or preparation for life in the new country is often non-existent. The journey, itself, is one that often entails tremendous loss not only of possessions, but of human life. Tales of Vietnamese "boat people" tell of people risking rape, piracy and death as they set off in tiny fishing boats with hopes of reaching sanctuary. Hmong survivors tell of their treks through minefields and jungle, losing family members to sickness along the way (Weinstein-Shr, 1986). Few Cambodians who survived the journey to America have been spared witnessing the starvation of family members before and during their grueling marches to reach the border for safety.

Depending on the time of escape, informal support systems (i.e., kin from earlier migrations) may or may not be available to welcome the newcomer and ease adjustment. The second wave of Southeast Asian refugees who were mostly peasant farmers before resettlement, face enormous educational and cultural gaps between their original home and current host environments.

While voluntary immigrants may save and prepare for their journey with optimism for a better life in America, refugees come with little choice, little preparation, and frequently experience terrible material and human loss. Kunz (1973) suggests that the immigrant is "pulled" to the host country by various promises of a better life, while refugees are "pushed" from their own countries by powerful forces that are beyond their control. Immigrants may visit their native country as they please, while refugees may only dream of returning to a country they did not choose to leave. While both immigrants and refugees must adjust to radical life and culture changes, clearly, refugees begin their new lives with a different set of experiences. Consequently, there is a large difference in the material and psychological resources that both groups bring to the task of adapting to life in their new home.

In this paper, we examine intergenerational relationships of Southeast Asian refugees who have come to the United States over the last decade. We begin by examining some of the difficulties faced by refugees of each generation, as well as the tremendous resources these survivors bring to adapting to life in the United States. Next, we look at changing roles in refugee families in light of experiences and expectations each family member is likely to bring to familial interaction. While literature on intergenerational relationships in refugee families is scarce, we draw upon research that has focused on particular age groups in refugee communities, on changing role relations in other immigrant groups, as well as on our experiences in Philadelphia's refugee community.[1] Lastly, we suggest directions for future research and for policies that strengthen refugee families as units for adaptation to their challenging new environment.

ADAPTING TO AMERICAN LIFE: PROBLEMS AND RESOURCES

In order to gain insight into the nature of intergenerational relationships in refugee families, it is helpful to understand the context within which these families operate. This section examines problems that need to be solved by typical refugee families as well as the resources that have been developed and/or tapped for solving them.

General Difficulties

The first and most basic challenge facing refugees is the pursuit of financial security. By coming into exile, refugee families lose land, possessions or financial comfort accumulated over generations in their native countries. It is unlikely that skilled professionals will be able to find equivalent jobs in their new settings. Farmers and other unskilled migrants are even less prepared to find and keep work that provides adequate resources for maintaining their families. Among those who come from agricultural societies like the Hmong family described earlier, large households with many children is the norm. With many household heads earning minimum wage in factories and other low-paying positions, inner-city life characterized by poverty, inadequate housing and associated problems is a common experience for refugees (Gozdziak, 1988).

A second set of challenges facing recent refugees is the maintenance of physical and mental health. Life in impoverished areas is often characterized by inadequate access to health care for native and non-native residents alike (Hullet, 1989). For refugees, health conditions of flight including war wounds, undernourishment and rampant disease, coupled with poor sanitation and medical care received in refugee camps exacerbate other health problems (Gozdziak, 1988). Lack of familiar medicines and medical practices may result in refugees avoiding even those health resources that are available.

Each generation has its share of mental stresses to cope with. Anxiety and depression have been well documented among refugee elders (Hayes, 1984; Gozdziak, 1988; Sue and Morishima, 1982). They have often experienced loss of loved ones, trauma of war, and tremendous shifts in role relationships. Young adults who are raising their own families are faced with supporting their children and their parents despite limited resources for ensuring financial stability. This generation is also the most torn between the culture of the homeland where they were born, and the new culture that their children will need to adopt for future success.

Lastly, research shows that forced resettlement creates enormous mental stress for youth, from adolescents who experience physical changes within two sets of cultural rule systems (Goldstein, 1985), to 1-year-olds, who have their early language development disrupted at a critical stage. For these children, because the trauma of war occurred in a pre-verbal stage of development, associated anxieties cannot be verbalized and may become manifest in nightmares and other developmental problems (Ascher, 1985). In cultures where mental health is seen as an issue of spiritual balance and of family or community harmony, Western models of help are often not appropriate.

A third set of issues facing refugees in their adaptation to life in the United States is the critical role of language and literacy. Refugee adults report that their difficulties in adapting to American life are critically linked to their lack of English language skills (Hayes; 1984, Reder, 1982, 1985; Downing and Dwyer, 1981; Downing and Olney, 1982). Language plays an obvious role in eligibility for jobs, gaining access to community resources and negotiation of relationships both within and outside of families.

For those who come from agricultural societies such as the Hmong, the Cambodians and the second wave of rural Vietnamese, native language literacy is often not the norm. The Hmong language did not exist in a written form until approximately 20 years ago when missionaries in Laos created an alphabet and dictionaries for purposes of evangelization. For adults who are not literate in their native language, learning English in the traditional literacy-oriented classroom may be frustrating and unproductive (Weinstein, 1984), while helping children with homework can be a source of embarrassment and frustration for both the well-meaning parents and their disappointed children.

Financial security, physical and mental health, and language and literacy, create challenges for refugees that have a strong impact on the nature and quality of intergenerational relationships within families. Fortunately, the fact that these refugees are here at all indicates that they are resilient, resourceful survivors. Some of these survival resources are examined below.

Resources for Adaptation

Families

While refugees often arrive in America with few possessions, they are far from empty-handed. Escaping their native country, arriving in a second country of temporary refuge, and progressing through the immigration process into a third country of permanent resettlement, requires strategic planning and sharp wits. Refugees in America have been enormously resourceful in drawing on family, clan, and community, even when these have had to be reconstructed in the face of death and decimation.

For all the stresses a refugee family experiences, that unit is one of strength and support for its members. Maintenance of set roles in families has been demonstrated to provide stability, order, predictability and security in chaotic times (Devos, 1978). Studies of Chinese immigrants, for example, show that the family acts as an anchor in a strange environment, providing a sense of belonging and continuity (Hsu, 1971). Further studies document the "cushioning" effect provided by family for the first jarring years in a new culture (Torgoff, 1983). In addition, patterns of assistance and aid among family members in the form of services such as babysitting, shopping or house cleaning, or in material goods like money and gifts have been well documented (e.g., Troll, Miller and Atchley, 1979). Gelfand (1982) points out that mutual assistance among generations is a common family pattern among most minority populations in the United States.

Kinship

As long as there has been interest in other cultures, there has been interest in the ways that members of such cultures see themselves in relation to one another. While the notion of what constitutes kinship is not the same from culture to culture, the ascription of kinship relations by some set of principles is universal.

While American sociologists have long been interested in the family, until about forty years ago little attention was paid to the prevalence of extended kin groups in modern urbanized society.

Beginning in the 1950s, the attention of sociologists began to turn to kinship groups and social networks (e.g., Sussman 1953, 1959). Since that time, a plethora of studies have documented the existence of such networks and the vitality of their functions in both longtime resident groups as well as among more recently arrived immigrants (i.e., Moore, 1971 on Mexican Americans; Stack, 1974 and Liebow, 1967 on Blacks; Gans, 1962 on Italian-Americans).

Although Southeast Asian refugees have been arriving steadily in the United States over the last decade, the interest in their family and social structure is only recent. United States resettlement policy has been to separate extended kin groups, reflecting, in part, the view that separation facilitates assimilation. Studies emerging over the decade of resettlement have shown ways in which initial dispersion strategies have caused hardship. While resettlement workers and policy-makers have concentrated primarily on the nuclear family, studies show why this focus can be problematic. Among Vietnamese refugees, for example, husband-wife ties are not nearly as important as parent-adult children ties (Haines, Rutherford and Thomas, 1981). Haines et al. note that parents are the people who will become the ancestors, an important concept for a culture which is partially shaped by Confucian tradition.

Haines et al. also found that extended family members contribute in important ways to the economic well-being of the larger family unit (1981, p. 515). The importance of recognizing the vital functions of the larger kin group is echoed by Dunnigan (1982), who recommends working with extended kin groups among the Hmong in all matters of resettlement, including, for example, the administration of health care.

Among the Hmong refugees, patrilineal descent principles continue to play a major role in adapting to life in the United States. There are 20 clans, each of which traces its origin to a common mythological ancestor. Even strangers who share a clan name are considered to be siblings, and signal this relationship with the form of address *kuv ti/kuv tyo* literally meaning elder/younger sibling. A man in Laos could depend on his clan members for hospitality when travelling from village to village in the mountains. A woman was able to depend on clan ties to defend her rights in a marital dispute if she did not have close relatives nearby (Barney, 1981).

Many of these rights and obligations continue to operate today as Hmong adapt to life in America. Hang Chai, president of Philadelphia's Hmong Association, reports that when he went to a conference in San Francisco, he simply opened the phone book to the H's when he arrived at the airport. He reached the first "Hang" listed. They picked him up, housed and fed him for the duration of his stay (personal communication to G. Weinstein-Shr). Although he had never met these people before, they were acting on the reciprocal rights and obligations of clan brothers.

Units of kinship have become flexible and resilient in light of the terrible decimation of war. In Laos, the *pawg neeg* or sub-lineage that traces its roots to a common real ancestor, was the primary helping unit whose members traditionally lived in one village or cluster of proximate villages (Reder, 1985). Ties to this group were the most durable and dependable relationships that a Hmong individual had over his/her life.

In face of many changes wrought by war and relocation, traditional kin groups are being constituted in new ways to solve problems collectively. In Philadelphia, one *pawg neeg* now consists of a group of young orphans who take turns pooling their money to raise the bride price for one another as they marry in turn, since none have blood kin to help them (personal communication with G. Weinstein-Shr).

Community Organizations

In addition to corporate kinship structures, many refugee groups have created local community organizations that function to serve members of the community while interfacing effectively with the American bureaucracy. Mutual Assistance Associations (MAAs) have sprung up across the country, channeling resettlement monies, assisting mainstream organizations in doing case work, and setting up their own indigenous programs for their constituents. Among the services that MAAs around the country have provided for their members include English classes for adults, senior support or recreation groups (often beginning as burial societies), and native language classes for children. In addition, some MAAs have facilitated the development of other community organizations. In Philadelphia, for example, the Cambodian Association was instrumental in setting up a Buddhist temple, a project which involved buying a building, negotiating zoning issues with the city, and bringing monks in from Virginia. The temple has become a vital gathering place and spiritual center for thousands of members of the community.

In order to understand families, then, it is necessary to understand the contexts in which they operate. While statistics compiled by social service agencies may paint a rather bleak picture of the resources available to refugees, a closer examination of social resources in kinship and community networks may provide another perspective from which to assess problems and possibilities.

CHANGING ROLES, CHANGING FAMILIES

Traditional Roles, Changing Expectations

For many traditional societies, the family rather than the individual is the basic unit of society (Hayes, 1984). While there is a wide range of customs and cultures among the peoples of Southeast Asia, certain themes repeatedly arise. With the prevalence of patrilineal kinship among most Southeast Asian peoples, roles of family members were quite well defined, providing support, security and a sense of meaning to members (Lum, 1983). Filial piety, including the expectation of respect, duty and reverence for elders (particularly older men) was reinforced by principles of ancestor worship found both in Confucianism and Buddhism (Bengtson and Kuypers, 1971). Men and women had clearly defined roles in the divided labor of managing both rural and urban households. Children, particularly in the countryside, began contributing in gender-appropriate ways to subsistence activities as soon as they were old enough.

Among elder Asians, life satisfaction seems to revolve around the degree to which they can continue to occupy positions of respect and power within their families (Gelfand, 1982). Often they cling to traditional values, role structures and exchange patterns in an attempt to maintain some semblance of psychological continuity. This is consistent with Bultena's (1969) "continuity theory" which suggests that persons in later life seek to continue occupying the roles they held earlier, particularly those of high status. Roles older people traditionally held in their families included providing assistance (financial, housekeeping, child care), maintaining cultural traditions and values, decision-making, and offering advice and emotional support.

For refugee families it is clear that a major discrepancy exists between the traditional roles elders held in their homeland and those that are available to them in the United States. Although many elder refugees provide child care assistance to their families, they are no longer able to offer financial support, land or other material goods. Instead, they are increasingly dependent on their children and grandchildren for assistance. Their lack of understanding of American culture, as well as their inability to speak or read English, limits their credibility when advising their families on important decisions. Younger family members become the mediators with institutions such as schools and the welfare system, and are increasingly displacing elders in some of their leadership roles. Though elders try to maintain their role as transmitters of traditional values and customs, their grandchildren often reject that cultural heritage in an effort to assimilate into American society. As this "role emptying" takes place, the elderly, having little to offer family and community, are put in an unfavorable exchange position (Gozdziak, 1988).

Early studies have shown that while elders anticipate respect from their adult children, they cannot achieve the same level of authority which was obtained in the original culture (Ex, 1966; Wu, 1975). Studies of Chinese and Japanese immigrants in America indicate a continuing belief in maintaining the elder at home, but the level of family assistance is documented as declining. Filial piety is being increasingly challenged by younger assimilated Asian Americans (Ishizuka, 1978; Wu, 1975). In more recent studies of refugees, elders report spending most of their time "just sitting in a chair" (Gozdziak, 1988). Unable to use household appliances, many Hmong elders watch hours of television, understanding nothing of what they hear (Hayes, 1984). As a 67 year-old farmer explained through an interpreter to Hayes, "Where is my dignity if I cannot do anything for myself? Farming is everything I know" (Hayes, 1984, p. 67).

While the greatest discrepancies exist between traditional role expectations and role realization for elders, members of the other generations are equally stressed by changes that are required to adapt to the new environment. Adult children are caught in the middle, as they face life in a society in which "the emphasis on individualism, nuclear family autonomy in an urban-industrial milieu, and economic-racial discrimination against minorities creates pressures on the children of Asian elderly" (Lum, 1983). These pressures are echoed by Fujii (1976) and Kalish and Yuen (1971) who point to the dissolution of customary values and practices in light of economic stresses, geographic mobility, increasing reliance on public responsibility, extended life span, and lack of role models in the United States for care of the elderly.

Even in cases where adult children are anxious to assume their traditional roles in supporting their aging parents, the task is not an easy one. One Hmong woman reports:

> My parents were farmers in Laos. They cannot drive, read or speak English. My husband and I try to make them happy, but we cannot. They always talk of those relatives who are not with us. As children, we must be supportive to our old people, but we don't know how to help them. I try to change their thoughts by asking them about old customs, sickness remedies and making food, but this doesn't help. (Hayes, 1984, p. 95)

Refugees in the middle generation are faced not only with caring for their aging parents, but coping with shifts in power relationships with their own children. As an example, a Cambodian man spoke of how his son had been expelled from school. The boy left the house each morning at 8 a.m., and returned at 4 p.m. each day. Because the father depended on his son to decipher documents sent from the school, he was unaware of any problem until a neighbor spoke with him six months after the expulsion (personal communication with G. Weinstein-Shr).

Unable to help their children with school work, many Asian parents worry that they are losing their children's respect (Heinbach, 1983). In Hayes' 1984 study, parents reported concerns that schools were teaching their children "the American way," that is, not to obey or respect their parents. They reported that being corrected or criticized by their more English proficient children, no matter how respectfully or gently, was a source of embarrassment and sadness (Hayes, 1984, p. 93). Several Lao, Hmong and Cambodian adults in Philadelphia have expressed their concern about what will happen to them as they grow old in a country where their children's values are undergoing such radical change (personal communication with G. Weinstein-Shr).

When parents are under stress, children are not left untouched. The struggle to reconcile two sets of values is poignantly illustrated by a Vietnamese teen who wrote the following "letter to Ann Landers" as an English assignment:

> Dear Ann Landers, There is an American boy in my class who wants to take me out. I like him very much, and I think he respects and likes me. My parents say I can't see him at all because he's a foreigner. My American heart says I should be independent and do what I think is right, but my Vietnamese heart says I should obey my parents. What should I do? (Weinstein, 1980)

The dilemmas for younger children are no easier. The role of translator, interpreter and problem-solver is not a comfortable role when children take care of parents and grandparents. Unrealistic expectations of teachers concerning parent involvement are often sources of embarrassment to children. School personnel who call on children to translate for their parents, or who ask for parental support that parents are not equipped to give, may unwittingly contribute to the forces that segregate generations and that keep them from interacting in mutually supportive ways.

Clearly, within a family, the difficulties of any one generation has consequences for all of the others. The stresses on the family as a system are exacerbated by the different pace at which generations tend to acculturate. Elders usually have few opportunities to interact with Americans. They tend to stay home to provide child care or meet with one another at community gathering places. Conversation is usually about the past or about the wish to return to the homeland to resume life as it once was. With concerns about death and the afterlife of the spirit, many elders speak of returning to their homelands to die. Gozdziak (1988) documents a case of a woman who arranged to do just that.

Children and young adults, on the other hand, interact continually with Americans and American institutions in school and on the job. Those who have been born in America or those who were very young in flight have no memory or direct connection with the country of origin. It is not surprising that in contrast with their seniors, young people tend to be much more future-oriented, seeing that future in the American context. It has been suggested that the more rapidly children acculturate, the more likely it is that family conflict will occur (Alley, 1980). As English becomes the language of choice for young people, linguistic barriers add a serious obstacle to the bonding between generations that is already strained by growing gaps in experience, in values and world views.

PROSPECTS FOR THE FUTURE: SUMMARY AND CONCLUSION

In this article, we have made some preliminary observations about intergenerational relationships in Southeast Asian refugee families. As Sue and Morishima (1982) point out, while there are many studies of Chinese and Japanese Americans in the literature, few have focused on other Asian communities. We have drawn on related literature as well as on our experiences to highlight some of the difficulties and resources brought by refugees to the task of adjusting to life in a new country. It is clear that the move to America has had far-reaching impact on the structure of families and on the relations between the generations in those families. The nature of the impact and its consequences is yet to be examined systematically.

Whether refugee families can remain viable sources of strength and support for their members is yet to be determined. The stresses are enormous and the potential for conflict is great. In most communities, services have been developed to help refugees adjust to their new environment. However, these services are fragmented and tend to target specific age groups. Schools are only now beginning to recognize the importance of reaching out to parents to effectively serve the children in their care. Governmental efforts and resettlement agencies tend to concentrate exclusively on developing jobs programs for employable youth. Elderly refugees are generally ignored altogether.

To adequately address the complex needs of these newcomers, resettlement agencies and social service organizations must develop a more coordinated approach to service delivery that focuses on *the family* as a unit for adaptation. It is also essential that mainstream educational and human service networks work collaboratively with ethnic leaders to develop programs that are culturally appropriate and speak to the condition of each generation. This requires a deeper understanding of the communities themselves, and of the ways in which families do and/or can operate as supports for their members.

It is our conviction that the study of social process in refugee families holds promise for illuminating issues of concern to all who are interested in human relations and human services. As technology roars ahead and as America becomes increasingly culturally heterogeneous, rapid change and ethnic diversity will be the rule rather than the exception. By studying adaptation processes among people for whom change and culture contact are pivotal, we can gain understanding of processes that will become increasingly universal. Our growing insights can be used to inform policy that strengthens rather than divides families, nurturing in them a haven for members to cope with a world of uncertainty and change.

NOTE

1. Through Project LEIF, Learning English through Intergenerational Friendship, we have worked with more than 300 Lao, Hmong, Khmer, Chinese, Vietnamese and Latin refugees in Philadelphia. In this model project, American college youth are trained to teach English as a Second Language to refugee elders. For more on LEIF, see Weinstein 1988, 1989.

REFERENCES

Ascher, C. (1985). The social and psychological adjustment of Southeast Asian refugees. In *The Urban Review 17(2)* 147-152.

Alley, J. (1980). Better understanding of the Indochinese student. *Education 101*, 111-114.

Barney, G.L. (1981). The Hmong of Northern Laos. In *Glimpses of Hmong history and culture*. Washington, D.C. Center for Applied Linguistics.

Bengtson, V.L. and J.A. Kuypers. (1971). Generational differences and the developmental stake. *Aging and Human Development, 2*, 249-259.

Bultena, G. (1969). Life continuity and morale in old age. *The Gerontologist 9*, 251-253.

DeVos, G. (1978). Selective permeability and reference group sanctioning: Psychological continuities in role degradation. Paper presented as seminar on comparative studies in ethnicity and nationality, University of Washington-Seattle.

Downing, B. and S. Dwyer. (1981). Hmong refugees in an American city: A case study in language contact. M.S. University of Minnesota.

Downing, B. and D.P. Olney. (1982). *The Hmong in the West*. Minneapolis: Southeast Asian Refugees Studies Project.

Dunnigan, T. (1982). The importance of kinship in Hmong community development. University of Minnesota, M.S.

Ex, J. (1966). *Adjustment after migration*. The Hague.

Fujii, S.M. (1976). Older Asian American victims of double jeopardy. *Civil Rights Digest Fall*, 24-25.

Gans, H. (1962). *The urban villagers*. New York. The Free Press of Glencoe.

Gelfand, D. (1982). *Aging: The ethnic factor*. Boston: Little and Brown.

Goldstein, B. (1985). *Schooling for cultural transitions: Hmong girls and boys in American high schools*. University of Wisconsin-Madison. Unpublished doctoral dissertation.

Gozdziak, E. (1988). *Older refugees in the United States: From dignity to despair*. Washington, D.C.: Refugee Policy Group.

Haines, D., D. Rutherford, and P. Thomas. (1981). Family and community among Vietnamese refugees. *International Migration Review 15*, 312-32.

Hayes, C. (1984). *A study of older Hmong refugees in the United States*. Unpublished dissertation.

Heinbach, E. (1983). *Interview notes.* Cited in Hayes 1984.

Hullet, S. (1989). Where a ride to the doctor cost $20. *Aging*, 359.

Ishizuka, K. (1978). *The elder Japanese*. San Diego, CA: San Diego State University, Center on Aging.

Kalish, R.and S.Yuen. (1971). Americans of East Asian ancestry: Aging and the aged. *Gerontologist 11(1)*, 36-47.

Kunz, E. (1973). The refugee in flight: Kinetic models and form of displacement. *International Migration Review*.

Liebow, E. (1967). *Tally's Corner*. Boston. Little, Brown and Company.

Lum, D. (1983). Asian-Americans and their aged. In R. McNeeley and J. Colen (Eds.), *Aging in Minority Groups*. Beverly Hills: Sage Publications.

Moore, J. (1971). Mexican Americans and cities: A study in migration and the use of formal resources. *American Sociological Review*, Vol. 5.

Office of Refugee Resettlement. (1986). Report to congress: refugee resettlement. Washington, D.C.: Department of Health and Human Services.

Reder, S. (1982). A Hmong community's acquisition of English. In B. Downing & D. Olney (Eds), *The Hmong in the West*, Center for Urban Regional Affairs Minnesota.

Reder, S. (1985). *The Hmong resettlement study*. Volume 1 Final Report. Prepared by Literacy and Language Program, Northwest Regional Laboratory, for Office of Refugee Resettlement. Oregon.

Stack, C. B. (1974). *All our kin*. Harper and Row, N.Y.

Sue, S. and J. Morishima. (1982). The mental health of Asian Americans. San Francisco: Jossey-Bass.

Sussman, M.B. (1953). The help pattern in the middle-class family. *American Sociological Review, 18*, 22-28.

Sussman, M.B. (1959). The isolated family: Fact or fiction. *Social Problems, 6*, 333-340.

Torgoff, S. (1983). Immigrant women, the family, and work: 1850-1950. In *Ethnic immigration groups: The United States, Canada and England*. New York: Haworth Press.

Troll, L., Miller, S., Atchley, R. (1979). *Families in later life*. Belmont, CA: Wadsworth Publishing Company.

Weinstein, G. (1980). Teaching Reading to Refugees at Community College. Unpublished Manuscript.

Weinstein, G. (1982). Some social consequences of literacy. In D. Smith, P.I., *Using literacy outside of school: An ethno-graphic investigation*. Final report to NIE.

Weinstein, G. (1984). Literacy and second language acquisition: Issues and perspectives. *TESOL Quarterly, 18*, 3.

Weinstein-Shr, G. (1986). *From mountaintops to city streets: An ethnographic investigation of literacy and social process among the Hmong of Philadelphia*. Ph.D. dissertation, University of Pennsylvania.

Weinstein-Shr, G. (1988). Project LEIF, Learning English through Intergenerational Friendship: A manual for building community across generations and across cultures.

Weinstein-Shr, G. (1989). Breaking the linguistic and social isolation of refugee elders. *TESOL News, XIII*, October.

Wu, F. (1975). Mandarin-speaking aged Chinese in the Los Angeles area. *Gerontologist, 15*, 217-275.

The Impact of Grandparents
on Children's Outcomes in China

Toni Falbo

Grandparents have played a significant role in the rearing of children in the People's Republic of China. In many respects, this is due to the fact that many grandparents live with or close to their grandchildren. During the 80s, it was estimated that around 24% of urban households contained three generations, with the parents and children living in the grandparents' home (Tien and Lee, 1988). The percentage in rural China was higher, estimated to be around 40% (Tien and Lee, 1988). Even if the grandparents and children do not live in the same household, they frequently visit each other if they live in the same city or town or village.

Admittedly, part of the reason for the prevalence of three-generation households is that the young parents have nowhere else to live. Housing shortages are commonplace in the cities. When the opportunity arises, many Chinese parents and children move into their own households, leaving behind the grandparents. This modernday popularity of nuclear households in China can also be found in rural China; as soon as a family becomes rich enough, they begin building new houses for each nuclear family unit.

Despite the prevalence of three-generational households in China, little research has been done to examine the impact of grandparents on children's development. There has been speculation that with solely one child per household that the only child would be spoiled by the attention of four grandparents and two parents (popularly referred to as the 4-2-1 problem). Due to the government's one-child policy, about 90% of urban children born after 1979 have no

---

Toni Falbo may be contacted at the Population Research Center, University of Texas at Austin, Austin, TX 78712.

siblings; in rural China, as many as 40% of the children born after 1979 have no siblings (Kristof, 1990). The single study bearing on this subject (Jiao, Ji, and Jing, 1986) found that the schoolchildren with the most peer prestige were those who had siblings and lived in a three-generational household. The schoolchildren with the lowest prestige were only children who lived in nuclear households. The authors explained this finding in terms of the parents in a nuclear family spoiling their only child. This finding is somewhat inconsistent with the 4-2-1 problem in that the Jiao et al. results suggested the *absence* of grandparents and siblings led to less desirable outcomes.

With the help of Dudley Poston, Jr. and colleagues at Jilin University, I was able to conduct a survey of 1460 schoolchildren in Jilin Province, in northeastern China. The survey included items about the household structure, the preschool caretaker, and characteristics of the grandparents, such as their educational attainment and the frequency of their contact with their grandchildren.

HYPOTHESES

The first hypothesis examines the interaction between living with grandparents and siblings on children's academic and personality outcomes. If the 4-2-1 theory is correct, then only children living in a three-generational household will have lower outcomes than other children. However, if the Jiao et al. (1986) finding is reliable, then only children living in a nuclear household will have lower outcomes than other children.

The second hypothesis focuses on the relationship between the quality of contact with grandparents and children's outcomes. If Chinese grandparents have a positive impact, one would expect greater contact to be associated with more positive outcomes. Specifically, more contact with better educated grandparents would have a positive impact on children's outcomes, particularly their academic outcomes.

The third hypothesis concerns the impact of the children's preschool experience on their outcomes. Traditionally, grandparents have played a significant role in caring for preschool-aged children. Are children better off in preschool than under the supervision of their grandparents or parents? Given the relatively low level of educational attainment among the grandparents' and parents' generation, it is expected that children who attended preschool will outscore children who were cared for by grandparents.

METHOD

A survey of 1460 schoolchildren from the first and fifth grades was conducted in the summer of 1987. Information about the children was collected from one parent (usually the mother) and the child's teacher. The teachers reported the child's most recent language and math test score (these tests are taken each semester) and rated the child's personality using The 31 Attributes Checklist (Falbo, Poston, Ji, Jiao, Jing, Wang, Gu, Yin, and Liu, 1989). The parents completed a background questionnaire and The 31 Attributes Checklist about the target child.

Eight schools participated in the survey. Five were in the city of Changchun, the provincial capital, and three in rural areas adjacent to the capital. We selected first and fifth graders for our sample in order to include two types of children: those born before and after the one-child policy.

The children's outcomes were categorized into two types: personality and academic. The personality measure used here is the virtue score, which combines the checklist ratings of parents and teachers. As described in Falbo et al. (1989), factor analyses of the parents' and teachers' checklist evaluations were conducted separately and the results were similar for both parents and teachers. The primary factor which emerged had strong loadings from 15 of the items: gentleness, concern about being liked, selflessness, care about others' feelings, kindness, helpfulness, lack of willfulness, respect for property, lack of aggressiveness, respect for elders, modesty, honesty, obedience to class discipline, doing one's own homework, and sharing. These attributes are highly desired by adults in school-aged children in China. In fact, the Chinese think of these attributes in moral terms; to have them is moral, to not have them is immoral. Therefore, a scale was created that combined the parents' and teachers' evaluations on these 15 attributes and it was called the Virtue Scale. The scale scores ranged from 4 to 30, with a median of 25. The alpha coefficient was .81.

The academic achievement scores were divided into two types: language and mathematics. Each semester, the same tests are given to all children within grade in Jilin Province. The language scores ranged from 0 to 100 with a mean of 88.2. The math scores ranged from 0 to 100 with a mean of 86.6.

There were four basic grandparent variables: (1) whether the child lived in a three-generational or nuclear household, (2) the frequency of contact between the grandparent and child, (3) the educational attainment of the grandparents, and (4) the preschool caretaker of the child. All of these variables were based on information provided by the parents' response to a questionnaire. The contact variable ranged from 1 to 3, from rarely to often together. The educational attainment variable ranged from 1 to 7, i.e., illiterate to graduate degree.

RESULTS

The first hypotheses aimed to test the popular Chinese notion that only children suffer from the excessive attention of grandparents. This idea was tested in a variety of ways. First, a two-way multivariate analysis of variance was conducted with household type (nuclear vs. three-generational) and only child status (only vs. nononly) as the independent variables and the children's virtue and academic achievement scores as the dependent variables. If living with grandparents caused special problems for only children, then we would expect to find a significant interaction between the two independent variables.

The analysis did not yield a significant interaction. Indeed, the main effect of living in a nuclear or three-generational household was not significant. The only child status variable did yield a significant multivariate $F(3, 1333) = 38.13$, $p < .0001$. Subsequent univariate analyses indicated that only children outscored siblinged children in academic scores but not virtue scores. For virtue, the difference was nonsignificant.

The second hypothesis examined the quality of the contact between grandparents and the children's outcomes. A variable was created which reflected the interaction between frequency of contact and the grandparents' educational attainment. The contact quality variables were correlated with the children's outcomes and the results are presented in Table 1.

All of the correlations between the grandparent quality contact variables and the children's academic outcomes were positive and significant, indicating that more contact with better educated grandparents was associated with better school performance. For virtue, more contact with better educated grandfathers was associated with more positive personality attributes.

The third hypothesis concerns the relationship between preschool caretaker and children's outcomes. A multivariate analysis of variance was conducted with Caretaker (three levels: preschool, par-

Table 1

Correlations between Quality Contact and Children's Outcomes

Grandparents		Children's Outcomes	
	Language	Mathematics	Virtue
Maternal			
Grandfather	.17*	.15*	.05[b]
Grandmother	.11*	.11*	-.01
Paternal			
Grandfather	.22*	.23*	.10*
Grandmother	.20*	.20*	.04

Note: Varying numbers of grandparents were alive at the time of the survey so the sample sizes vary from 661 to 796.

* $p < .005$; [b] =borderline

ents, or grandparents) and the independent variable and the children's three outcome variables and the dependent variables. The analysis yielded a significant $F(6, 2620) = 18.16, p < .0001$. Subsequent univariate analyses indicated that the Caretaker variable produced a significant effect for the Language, $F(2, 1311) = 47.14, p < .0001$, and Math, $F(2, 1311) = 27.45, p < 0001$ scores. The means are presented in Table 2 and indicate that children performed better in school if they had attended preschool. Interestingly, the relative disadvantage of not attending preschool was less if the child was cared for by grandparents than by parents.

To understand this finding better, we compared the educational attainments of caretaking grandparents with those of caretaking parents and found that caretaking grandparents had greater educational attainments.

DISCUSSION

The results of this study suggest that Chinese grandparents have an impact on their grandchildren that extends beyond simply living with them. Contrary to the popular concern in modern China that grandparents overindulge their grandchildren, their cohabitation with children has no negative effects on either their personality or academic outcomes. This was found to be true regardless of whether the grandchild had siblings.

Specifically, more contact with better educated grandparents was positively and significantly associated with academic outcomes. Similarly, more contact with better educated grandfathers was positively and significantly associated with the child possessing a more desirable personality, as judged by both mothers and teachers. It is unclear why this relationship was found for quality contact with grandfathers and not grandmothers.

Having been cared for by grandparents before elementary school was associated with good academic performance, but not quite as good as having attended preschool. Given the better education of these grandparents relative to their parents, the child's time with grandparents probably prepared them better for school than time with their lesser educated parents. The parents in this sample consisted of those referred to in China as the "lost generation" because

Table 2

Children's Outcomes by Caretaker before Elementary School

| | | Children's Outcomes | |
Caretaker	Language	Mathematics	Virtue
Preschool (N=868)	90.3	88.6	23.8
Parent (N=242)	80.8	81.3	23.5
Grandparent (N=186)	89.4	84.9	24.0

Note: The Language and Mathematics means for Grandparent and Preschool are both significantly higher than that for Parent. Virtue did not vary with Caretaker.

they grew up during the Cultural Revolution, when schools were closed and many families were fragmented.

Rather than having a negative impact on only children as popular thinking claims, this study suggests that grandparents can have positive effects on their grandchildren, even on those without siblings. In urban environments, where most children have no siblings, it has become common for grandparents to gather up their grandchildren from their various schools and care for them until the parents come home from work. These grandchildren are cousins, but they use sibling terms when referring to each other. This sibling-like relationship is fostered by the grandparents who treat them as though they were siblings. Thus, when the extended family gets together on holidays and special events, the grandchildren play together like siblings. This transformation of cousins into siblings is fostered by grandparents and will probably facilitate the children's development of relationship skills.

To date, the evidence regarding the social skills and adjustment of only children in China is mixed, with the preponderance of larger scale studies indicating no differences between only children and others on personality characteristics (Feng, 1990). This may be due to the tendency of cousins to be treated like siblings, mentioned above. It is also worth noting that no consistent association between being an only child and personality characteristics has been found in the Western literature (Polit and Falbo, 1987).

REFERENCES

Falbo, T., Poston, D.L., Jr., Ji, G., Jiao, S., Jing, Q., Wang, S., Gu, Q., Yin, H. & Liu, Y. (1989). Physical, achievement and personality characteristics of Chinese children. *Journal of Biosocial Science, 21*, 483-495.

Feng, X. (1990). The present status and critique of the only child studies in China. *Jianghai Xuekan, No. 1.*

Jiao, S., Ji, G. & Jing, Q. (1986). Comparative study of behavioral qualities of only children and sibling children. *Child Development, 57*, 357-361.

Kristof, N. D. (1990). More in China willingly rear one child. *The New York Times, 139*, May 9.

Polit, D.F. & Falbo, T. (1987). Only children and personality development: A quantitative review. *Journal of Marriage and the Family, 49*, 309-325.

Tien, H.Y. & Lee, C.F. (1988). New demographics and old designs: The Chinese family and induced population transition. *Social Science Quarterly, 69*, 605-628.

Developing Informal Networks
of Caring
Through Intergenerational Connections
in School Settings

Carol H. Tice

The need to strengthen the American Family and to promote education with a strong emphasis on the work ethic bombards us. Newspaper stories, magazines, and TV commentators report daily updates on the war on drugs that has implications for the lives of every citizen, especially the young. The impact of the widespread sale and use of illegal drugs questions American values. Decisions must be made concerning the welfare of all family members. Sometimes alternative or foster families must serve as the only safe option for youths struggling to sustain healthy lives.

Increasing numbers of youths entering their early teens *must* make a conscious decision to "just say no" lest they find themselves caught in a spiral of greed with the lure of easy crack sales. In addition they confront a deadening of the mind and spirit as the experimental use of drugs turns to habit and addiction.

These dangers plague our schools, and cast shadows on families at every socioeconomic level. For the poor, the challenge of illegal drugs hangs as an oppressive cloud, preventing opportunity from rising beyond a minimal common denominator. The fallout will be felt for years to come by all our children, and by their children yet unborn. In order to cope with the drug problem there is a mandate for restoration of caring and commitment in families, schools, and

Carol H. Tice is Program Associate, Institute for the Study of Children and Families, Eastern Michigan University, Ypsilanti, MI 48197.

communities. Intergenerational programs can provide a means of promoting these fragile but important connections.

Since the early 1970s, programs that encourage the interaction of older adults with children and youths have become a common phenomenon. They are based in a variety of settings: elementary and secondary schools, community centers, libraries, churches, and social service agencies. They are developed and funded with the support of city, state, and federal governing, local school districts, community groups, or private foundations. Most programs are designed to benefit both age groups. Young people gain a sense of community and of the significance of the lifespan. Elders find themselves useful and have a heightened sense of belonging to the mainstream of society.

Anthropologists and historians of the family are probably more sensitive than most to the various dimensions of the relations among the generations. Margaret Mead noted that, in the post World War II industrialized world, "elders must also learn from the experience of children," because the culture has changed so drastically since they themselves were young. Furthermore, if children are to have access to the past, one means is "the presence of older people within their immediate community, if not their own grandparents, then someone else's grandparents" (Mead, 1976).

THE NEED: WHO IS ENTITLED TO A SENSE OF WELL-BEING?

The need for new and sustained efforts to link the age groups comes from social stresses on both the growing older population and the younger people who will eventually need to take care of aging parents and other family members. Life expectancy will be lengthened and the numbers of older people will increase. Within the next decade, approximately one out of every six persons in the nation will be over 65. The fastest growing segment of the population is in the over-80 age group.

Dwindling resources have sharpened the division between age groups, particularly at the level of national policy. The young have a claim on the national resources, as do the increasing numbers of older people. Both groups rely heavily on the community and government for needed social services and support. Citizens over 65 years of age, people with voter registration in hand and feel that they have "paid their dues" will outnumber those under 14 years of age by the year 2000. The social, political and economic consequences of that population shift will demand the attention of social institutions, policy-makers, and legislative bodies. Meeting the needs of older people with respect to housing, health care, and social activity that lends meaning and purpose to the latter years have educational dimensions for the elderly and society at large.

Some needs of the youths are similar. They include the needs for housing, health care, and the development of appropriate activities and meaningful relationships. However, with most of life ahead of them, youth's need for education remains unique and central to finding a productive place in today's world. Changes in society have created pressing challenges with respect to education excellence for job success in the marketplace. This imperative lies in juxtaposition with issues of equity in education opportunity. Who is entitled to a sense of well-being throughout the lifespan? Whose responsibility is it that prosperity takes place? Does well-being belong only to those whose families have already made their way in the world and have resources and influence to pass on to their children? The question of the use of resources becomes more complex as one looks at the relationships between new immigrants and minority populations, the latter having lived in this country for generations but without full entitlement. Public education continues to serve a key function in unlocking the answers to questions of equity and excellence, but the solutions are not as easily at hand.

EDUCATION:
CHALLENGES THAT INVOLVE FAMILIES

Students of all ages come to school from a context of their family's situation with respect to health, economic stability, language experience, expertise in interpersonal relationships, and values. For many youth, public schooling is a major entry-way to economic stability through awareness of career opportunities, job skill training, and an educational experience that has meaning with respect to productive employment. Radical job market changes have shifted work opportunities from a large number of hard laborers to high-tech functions, requiring training for complex thinking and expertise.

With the setting of higher education standards for performance and graduation, and the need for more highly trained workers in the world of work, an alarming school dropout rate becomes all the more serious. While statistics vary, unacceptable numbers of youths entering the 8th grade will drop out before completing high school. In large cities, the number of dropouts is even higher. Dropout rates for Native American, Hispanic, and Black youth are at the top of the scale. Widening the gap between citizens with economic opportunity through college or advanced education and those who remain "barely educated" has implications for the economic foundation of marriage and families. It has further impact on the society at large. American citizens use vast resources each year in unemployment, welfare, and other costs for dropouts and their families. The need to stay in school through graduation and beyond becomes the society's economic imperative.

In spite of the fact that consequences of schooling are great, some students continue to do poorly. This may not always be a matter of conscious choice. Living in families that are at or below the poverty line, with one or more parents who is an alcoholic or drug addict, or trying to cope with physical and/or sexual abuse all impact on how a young person is able to attend school and focus on the challenges of lessons to be learned.

In its final report, Youth and America's Future: The William T. Grant Foundation's Commission on Work, Family, and Citizenship (1988, p. 3) states: "Young people's experiences at home, at school, in the community, and at work are strongly interconnected, and our response to problems that arise in any of these domains must be equally well integrated."

Intergenerational programs can help address the need for integrated response to encompassing learning challenges. In order for programs to go beyond the activity stage and move to addressing some of the deeper needs of children and youth—as well as older adults, one needs to explore how things have been done in the past with respect to the family and the schools.

THE FAMILY AS EDUCATOR

The family, as the oldest and most deeply rooted human institution, has been the primary context through which children have learned who they are, how they fit into society, and where they acquire a vision of what they might become. Connections between generations in the family have provided the "cement" which bonded families, giving information and identity with the past, which created depth and meaning to the present. This sense of where the family has come from, and where it is now in relationship to characteristics and values that define that particular family, provide and important resource for charting and securing the future. This is true for the older members with respect to health status, to life expectancy, and to developing a sense of contentment. The need for intergenerational connections is even greater among today's children and youth. They have more choices to make than their parents had when they were young. Those decisions are thrust upon them at earlier and earlier ages, and have serious and long-lasting consequences.

There was a time when grandparents, who had either lived in the household or nearby, played a vital role in the care giving and upbringing of the child. Integrated with the process of nurturing, stories of days gone by were told, giving children some understanding of the reality of the world before they, and even their parents, were born. Learning to picture things as they were long ago gave children and youths the capabilities to dream about and try to imagine what it could be like in the future. Because the contact with older people was frequent, ongoing, and sustained, the young had time and freedom to explore choices and consequences in a safe and limited manner. What a relief it was to discover that grandpa had played pranks in his youth, or that grandma had "chosen" grandpa long before he even noticed her—such an "unladylike" thing to do! Insights like these protected youths against the feelings of being "strange" and unworthy of belonging as they experienced adolescence with its myriad of challenges, including urges for risk-taking actions.

In return for investing in the nurture of the young, the older generation's sense of belonging was secure and affirmed. For the most part, they felt useful, needed, and loved. As age brought greater infirmity to the elders, the young were present to provide care and support to those who had played an important part in their own development. The whole of the life cycle was experienced—what it meant to grow up, have children, to complete life's major tasks and to grow old. "Through a grandmother's voice and hands the end of life is known at the beginning" (Mead, 1977).

For hundreds of years the family was viewed as an economic unit and as an important place for learning about work and its relationship to well-being. Every member had tasks to perform in order for the group as a whole to function as a working ecology. Members of the family worked together and played together. Leisure time was often spent in activities that included everyone in some way. Work and leisure merged in activities such as barn raisings or celebrations after the neighbors had labored together to bring in the harvest. Even holiday festivities had a work/play equation. Getting ready for the feast and traditional celebrations was largely carried out in the home with everyone helping. Preparing food together gave ample opportunity to pass on traditions, customs, and anecdotes that strengthened family identity while the peeling, slicing, and dicing was carried out by the women. The men had their own clearly defined tasks where similar conversations took place.

Children and youth learned their work skills and habits within caring relationships. Mothers taught their daughters to do women's things, and men taught their sons to do men's things. There was a relatively small range of work options open when a youth was ready to make the decisions that would lead him or her into the world of work. While work opportunities were not limited by what the family had done to make a living, they were largely determined by the experiences the youth had received while being a member of the family. Professionals tended to rear children who became professionals. College and university graduates anticipated having children who would follow in their footsteps. Similarly, if the family had experienced dysfunction and problems, the cycle often continued into the next generation.

Not everything was predetermined by family background and experience. History books are full of individuals who stepped out of poverty—particularly out of the immigration experience—to make the American Dream come true. Even though the self-made individual often set out alone to achieve in extraordinary ways, the notion of the family as an economic unit and as educator for future work was intact with most people. Youths who worked outside the family structure were apprenticed to people often known to them. There was vivid expectation that industriousness and hard work could produce results in becoming what a youth set out to become. A strong sense of responsibility to one's family and to the neighborhood and community was the expectation.

Within the extended family, children and youths learned what was necessary to keep the larger community strong and steady through natural disasters such as floods, tornadoes, and a summer's draught. Memorabilia, photographs, and stories passed on survival strategies during wars—whether small and localized, or worldwide. Social traditions, practiced and carried on primarily through the family structure, provided a framework for life to go on in spite of disaster. The oldest people could remember what had been done in years past when there was no harvest, or how the orphans had been divided up after parents had been killed in some common disaster or in an epidemic. The transition of this survival knowledge was carried out informally from generation to generation.

The rural or urban neighborhood served as a framework of checks and balances beyond the family walls for children and youths growing up. Older people such as maiden aunts and grandparents provided a watchful eye from porch swings or upstairs windows while children and youths explored their own world, testing the limits of their increasing freedom. If a boundary of safety or morality was pushed too far, the influence of family and neighbors served as a reminder to use restraint for safety sake, or to come back "into line" with the rest of the community's values.

SCHOOLS AS INTERGENERATIONAL INSTITUTIONS

Schools, from their earliest existence, have served as places where unifying values could be celebrated by the community and reinforced with the young. The role and function of families as compared to schools were clearly defined and quite different. It was the family's responsibility, along with the church and religious institutions, to instruct and guide for moral character and personal values. The school was designed to teach basic academic skills. Sometimes there was an overlap when reading and writing exercises were integrated with phrases obviously designed to guide the youth down an industrious and righteous path. Examples from an 1879 *McGuffey Reader* illustrate: "Pride, not nature, craves much," "Folly is never pleased with itself," "What cannot be cured must be endured" (1879, p. 14).

With intact families and stable communities, the separation of practical skills such as coping in times of disaster, or developing work experience, and the more academic pursuits such as the study of English or of French Literature could exist separately. It is understood that both forms of knowledge could continue to exist because the survival skills were passed on informally from generation to generation. The rules for survival were clear, and each new change in the world seemed to come in sequence at a pace that the people living in stable surroundings could deal with in time, and most importantly together.

Public education, with its emphasis on literacy in areas of literature, languages, mathematics, and sciences, is a connection between the generations. The assumption is made that insights and information from the past are worthy and perhaps even essential for those who will be responsible for the future. The intergenerational connections here are implicit, but nonetheless based in reality. Books, papers, orator, debate are all a part of the vehicle of transmission.

More explicit expressions of the compact are found in programs that bring the old and young together. In early America, the school, along with churches and neighborhood institutions like granges in rural areas and settlement houses in urban settings, have served as major places where families could meet together around a common social interest. Throughout our country's history, gatherings in schools have brought the generations together in recognition of educational goals and achievement such as speech and music programs, drama presentations, and graduation exercises. To be in school, or in some way associated with schools was a mark of status and personal success in the eyes of the community. In more recent times, sports competitions and class reunion events have provided people of all ages ways of belonging to and identifying with an alma mater, as well as staying close to youthful energy throughout the lifespan.

While the use of schools as a socially organizing institution across the generations through special events is clearly evident, the role of public schooling in a democratic society continues to be the subject of debate. Some argue that schools should be primarily an instrument of social reform, while others promote the notion that schools should leave hands off social issues which lie outside the realm of instruction in the three R's. The relationships between schools and families continually raise questions of who is responsible for the many and complex facets of a child's development.

By the turn of the century, parent groups, usually women as a major force, worked to promote school/home relationships that sought the well-being of children (primarily in urban settings) through advocacy for feeding the poor, cleaning up the streets, and assisting immigrant children in adjusting to American values and customs (Kagan, 1989).

The Community School Movement in the 50s expanded the concept of the use of schools to include the entire community. A vision of lifelong education and productive use of leisure within school environments was set forth. School buildings were open for use by different age groups long after the regular students had gone home for the day. These activities continued and were expanded during the summer months. In addition to recreational opportunities, among the many classes for adults were Literacy Training, English as a Second Language, and Home Arts.

In the 60s, school volunteer programs brought parents involvement into the school building during the regular K-12 program. Mothers, and sometimes fathers, could be found assisting in media centers, school offices, and in some classrooms. This new involvement greatly expanded participation of parents beyond the traditional role of home room mothers providing cookies for school events.

School volunteer programs set the stage for including older adults in school settings. First attempts at this larger concept of the Parents as Volunteers Movements used the talents of older volunteers as tutors. These efforts continue to be popular throughout the country. It soon became evident that the use of senior citizens' help with students had far more potential than simply helping the young person complete an assignment given by the teacher. Since many children and youth were living apart from their own grandparents, there were benefits from just being present together.

Intergenerational relationships are restorative. They bring together what technology, mobility and age grouping have pulled apart. At their best, they can incubate a sense of caring between individuals and between generations by replacing isolation and fragmentation with reciprocity and coherence. The interchange between the generations contributes to the understanding of the world by children and youth, to a sense of purpose for the aging, and to social wholeness.

Reports attempting to assess the state of the art in intergenerational programming indicate a steady increase from the early 70s. "The loss or eroding of the transfer of knowledge, practices, beliefs, and values within families from older generations to the young requires and alternative structure. Although modern conditions of life have not dramatically altered the need for generational bonding, the ways and means such needs are fulfilled have changed" (Sussman and Pfeifer, 1982, p. 3).

The States Speak (Romani, 1985) indicates documented activity linking the generations in special ways in 45 states, with schools serving as the primary focus for local programs. Tutorial initiatives, cultural exchanges, and efforts to promote health and human services are among the types of efforts being made to bring the old and young together. Review of the state responses to the survey conducted by New Age, Inc. "clearly indicates that provision of this missing ingredient (nurturing of children) in family life is a principal reason underlying the initiation of many of the current intergenerational programs" (Romani, 1985, p. 6). This emphasis brings into focus not only the uses of schools, but also the role of schools in efforts to create productive and caring citizens.

An in-depth study, *Children and Youth with Older Adults: Descriptions of Meaningful and Creative Activities and Relationships*, (Sussman and Pfeifer, 1982), discusses the role of government in fostering intergeneration programming. The 1981 White House Conference on Aging with mini-conferences held for the purpose of identifying and promoting programs fostering intergenerational exchange and cooperation was identified as providing impetus to programs utilizing exchanges of activities involving several generations.

ACTION has been working intergenerationally since the establishment of the Peace Corps over 20 years ago. These values of the public and private sectors working together across the generations in the spirit of volunteerism has increased over the years with the establishment of the Retired Senior Volunteer Program (RSVP) which assists older people in volunteering, in many places in their communities. Intergenerational programs in schools is one example of this type of activity.

The Foster Grandparent program was started in 1965 by ACTION to create opportunities for low-income seniors over 60 to work with children who are mentally and physically handicapped, who suffer sight or hearing disorders, language impairment, or a specific learning disability. They also serve children who have been abused or neglected, juvenile offenders, and those in need of foster care. The Foster Grandparent is paid a small, non-taxable stipend.

Thousands of local independent intergenerational programs have been established over the past two decades. These initiatives involve very young children in preschool programs, and continue through the age spectrum to include university opportunities for older learners, as well as service-learning programs. The Elvirita Lewis Foundation of Palm Springs, California, started the first Intergenerational Child Care Center in 1976. Many similar centers are now supported with funds from the California State Legislature. This serves as an example of how a local initiative has spurred intergenerational activity at the statewide level. Many states have Intergenerational Child Care Centers and/or preschool programs. A notable example is the Preschool Program at Messiah Village — a retirement community in Mechanicsburg, Pennsylvania. Interviews conducted with 14 key administrative and professional staff of Messiah Village indicated "Almost universal favorable reaction to the intergenerational program" (Sussman and Pfeifer, 1982, p. 3).

Elementary, Junior High, and High School programs often have a tutorial focus, using retirees to complement and supplement educational resources in schools. Teaching-Learning Communities (T-LC) programs, started in Ann Arbor, Michigan in 1971, emphasize the potential for lifelong development and learning. Neighborhood schools become centers where people of all ages can both teach and learn. An emphasis on mentoring focuses on personal and social development as a necessary component in a youth's educational development. The caring relationship often becomes reciprocal, so that the youths have experience in caring for others as well as receiving encouragement and support from the older volunteers. In a recent report, *Partner in Growth: Elder Mentors and At-Risk Youth*, the case is made for increasing the opportunity for older adults to work as mentors with adolescents so that they can better "navigate the treacherous course to adulthood." "An accumulation of longitudinal research suggests that adult relationships—provided not only by parents, but by grandparents, neighbors, and other interested adults—are a common factor among resilient children who achieve success despite growing up in disadvantaged and stressful circumstances" (Freedman, 1988, p. i).

With increasing numbers of schools and community groups involving older adults, children, and youth in exchanges that have educational, social, and personal benefits, the need for program assistance and training has emerged. "Our best hope for the future is to embark on an affirmative action program to bring the generations together. The old have myriad skills and experiences that, in the right context, can be of great value to young people. The old are the carriers of cultural values. They provide a sense of continuity in an uncertain and often frightening world. Bringing the generations together is a delicate process. We must ensure that intergenerational contact is developed under the best possible conditions, without competition and with a sense of shared purpose" (Roybal, 1985, pp. 7-8).

Many groups across the country have stepped forth to fill the need for training in developing intergenerational programs "with a sense of shared purpose." A coalition of national leaderships was established in 1986 as Generations United, including over 111 national agencies serving youth or older people. Co-sponsored by the Child Welfare League of America and the National Council on the Aging, the group stimulates and strengthens intergenerational policy and program. Issues may deal with children and youth or the elderly, but the emphasis is on how the needs and challenges of both groups interrelate and impact on each other. Needs such as housing, food, medical care, and employment directly touch the lives of people in all age categories. Policies and service programs working across the generations can address these needs more effectively and *economically* than a more segregated approach. In the final analysis, however, each service area must rely on educational efforts to realize long-term benefits for clients and communities. National groups can promote education, but it is in local communities, schools, and families where the direct teaching and learning must take place. The role of both family and school can be strengthened by activities shared by young and old alike. Through this process, traditional culture and values are restored, enhanced, and once more made relevant to daily life. Informal networks of support and concern often result. These, in turn create a constellation of caring that promotes healthly choices and productive lifestyles throughout the lifespan.

REFERENCES

Freedman, M. (1988). *Partners in growth: Elder mentors and at-risk youth*. Philadelphia: Public/Private Ventures.

Kagan, S. (1989, January 18). Family Support Programs and the Schools. *Education Week*.

McGuffey's Fifth Eclectic Reader. (1879). Revised edition. Cincinnati & New York: Van Antwerp-Brogg & Co.

Mead, M. (1976, November 3). Unpublished interview at Teaching-Learning Communities, Ann Arbor Public Schools. Ann Arbor.

Mead, M. (1977, February 8). Unpublished interview at Museum of Natural History. New York.

Mead, M. (1978, March 3). Unpublished interview at Museum of Natural History. New York.

Romani, J. (1985). *The States speak*, Ann Arbor: New Age, Inc.

Roybal, E. (1985). Commentaries. In K. Struntz & S. Reville (Eds.), *Growing together: An intergenerational sourcebook*, 1, (pp. 7-8). Washington, DC: American Association of Retired Persons and The Elvirita Lewis Foundation.

Sussman, M. & Pfeifer, S. (1982). *Children and Youth Connecting With Older Adults: Description of Meaningful and Creative Activities and Relationships*. Report funded by The William T. Grant Foundation. Newark, DE: Department of Individual and Family Studies, The University of Delaware.

Youth and America's Future: William T. Grant Commission on Work, Family, and Citizenship. (1988). *The forgotten half: Pathways to success for America's youth and young families*. Washington, DC: Author.